T0275991

Current Clinical Practice

Series editor
Neil S. Skolnik

More information about this series at http://www.springer.com/series/7633

Joel J. Heidelbaugh

Editor

Men's Health
in Primary Care

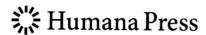 Humana Press

Editor
Joel J. Heidelbaugh, MD, FAAFP, FACG
Departments of Family Medicine and Urology
University of Michigan Medical School
Ann Arbor, NY, USA

Current Clinical Practice
ISBN 978-3-319-26089-1   ISBN 978-3-319-26091-4   (eBook)
DOI 10.1007/978-3-319-26091-4

Library of Congress Control Number: 2015960810

Springer Cham Heidelberg New York Dordrecht London

Printed on acid-free paper

Humana Press is a brand of Springer
Springer International Publishing AG Switzerland is part of Springer Science+Business Media
(www.springer.com)

Acknowledgments

For my patients, my students and residents, my mentors, and my colleagues

For the advancement of men's health worldwide

With deepest gratitude to my coauthors for their inspiration and contributions

And to my family for their love and support

Preface

What is men's health? "Guy problems. You know, prostate and genital problems. They die of heart attacks and strokes mostly. Working out at the gym. Oh yeah, some cancers too. And stupid, risky behaviors. Guys like to take chances, and don't always think about what might happen to them. We should know better. Yeah, that should just about cover it…" [1].

While the above answer is quite superficial in its scope, it should be widely acknowledged that men on the worldwide arena share the common factor that they are at a higher risk of premature death from the majority of adverse health conditions that we would expect to affect men and women equally. Ultimately, men's health as a subgenre of medicine needs to progress beyond a discussion simply reflecting morbidity and mortality statistics, urology, and sexual function concerns, to focus on the circumstances that influence men to either seek or not seek preventive and holistic medical care.

In the past decade, the field of men's health has begun to evolve and gain some modest traction, not simply as an answer to "women's health," but more formally to recognize, research, and address medical and social issues predicated upon inherent disparities affecting the male gender. However, creating a distinct field of "men's health" is still an admirable goal, one that should be multidisciplinary and should focus on the unique biopsychosocial factors that impact the health of men across the life cycle.

In reviewing the currently available primary care and specialty-oriented men's health-affiliated journals and textbooks, I continue to see a growing need for primary care clinicians to have a multidisciplinary and evidence-based reference guide to the diseases and disorders that affect male patients of all ages, with a comparative epidemiologic focus. Although the majority of references for this target audience on general pediatric and adult medical problems are considered to be comprehensive and up to date, few are specifically targeted at those diseases and disorders that unequally affect male patients. Hopefully, future provisions of men's health will be supported through such legislature as the Affordable Care Act, which should help to improve many parameters of healthcare outcomes in men.

The collection of authors assembled for this textbook represents a cohort of nationally and recognized scholars, clinicians, and researchers, many of whom are the leading experts on their respective topics. They have provided current evidence-based reviews and practice recommendations on best practice strategies to approach common clinical concerns and disorders in men's health.

I would like to sincerely thank all of the authors who donated their extremely valuable time and energy to believe and participate in this textbook project. A very special thanks is given to Patrick Carr and his excellent staff at Springer for their assistance in the production and timely publication of this textbook.

It is my hope that this textbook spawns a broader interest in recognizing and addressing disparities in men's health and provides a practical reference for learners and clinicians who care for common disorders in male patients across the globe.

Best wishes

Reference

1. Random male patient interview conducted by editor, when soliciting advice on what to include in a textbook on men's health, Ypsilanti Health Center, Ypsilanti, Michigan, June 11, 2004. Appears in Heidelbaugh JJ (ed.) *Clinical Men's Health: Evidence in Practice*. Philadelphia, PA: Saunders/Elsevier, 2008

Ypsilanti, MI   Joel J. Heidelbaugh
Ann Arbor, MI

Series Editor Introduction

As a practicing primary care physician, I take care of many men who suffer from chronic diseases including hypertension, high cholesterol, diabetes, heart disease, COPD, and BPH. I also have noticed that many men first present to the doctor at the insistence of their spouses, an observation that is not mine alone. While I knew that men have a shorter life expectancy than women, I had not given much thought to the fact that from their first year of life onward, despite many occupational and social advantages when compared to women, men are more likely to die at any given age than their female counterparts. I had not thought a lot about the possibility that this increase in mortality may be partly attributable to behavioral choices and the consequent chronic diseases that men suffer from. Like a boy who grows up in the forest and never gives much thought that the trees may simultaneously form and obscure the landscape, I had never thought much about social determinant of men's health. I had never given direct attention to the distinct interaction between male expectations, stresses, the behavioral choices that are often a by-product of these stresses and expectations, as well as their relation to chronic disease and mortality.

It is seldom, after 30 years in the practice of medicine, to be provoked to think anew about a common problem that influences the health of the patients that I take care of each and every day. This book provokes such thought and provides data and the commentary which sheds new light on this common issue. For this, the authors deserve our thanks and attention.

Neil Skolnik, MD
Professor of Family and Community Medicine
Temple University School of Medicine

Associate Director
Family Medicine Residency Program
Abington Memorial Hospital

Contents

1 Men's Health in 2010s: What Is the Global Challenge?.................... 1
   Roland J. Thorpe, Jr. Derek M. Griffith, Keon L. Gilbert,
   Keith Elder, and Marino A. Bruce

2 Masculinity in Men's Health: Barrier or Portal
   to Healthcare? 19
   Derek M. Griffith, Keon L. Gilbert, Marino A. Bruce,
   and Roland J. Thorpe Jr.

3 Health-Seeking Behavior and Meeting the Needs
   of the Most Vulnerable Men... 33
   Keon L. Gilbert, Keith Elder, and Roland J. Thorpe Jr.

4 Providing Preventive Services to Men:
   A Substantial Challenge? 45
   Masahito Jimbo

5 The Evidence-Based Physical Examination
   of the Child and Adolescent Male....................................... 57
   David A. Levine and Makia E. Powers

6 Caring for the Adolescent Male... 89
   Cullen N. Conway, Samuel Cohen-Tanugi, Dennis J. Barbour,
   and David L. Bell

7 The Evidence-Based Well Male Examination in Adult Men 103
   Mark J. Flynn

8 Promoting Cardiovascular Health in Men 125
   Michael Mendoza and Colleen Loo-Gross

9 Male Sexual Health 145
   Harland Holman and Mark Armstrong

10 **Sexually Transmitted Infections in Men** 165
    Charles Kodner

11 **Benign Prostatic Hyperplasia and Lower Urinary
    Tract Symptoms** 197
    Abdul Waheed

12 **Testicular, Scrotal, and Penile Disorders** 225
    Michael A. Malone and Ahad Shiraz

13 **Hypogonadism: The Relationship to Cardiometabolic
    Syndrome and the Controversy Behind Testosterone
    Replacement Therapy** 249
    Joel J. Heidelbaugh, Anthony Grech, and Martin M. Miner

14 **Prostate Cancer: A Primary Care Perspective** 269
    Robert Langan

15 **Caring for Men Who Have Sex with Men** 283
    Jim Medder

Index 301

Contributors

Mark Armstrong, DO Department of Family Medicine, Spectrum Health, Grand Rapids, MI, USA

Dennis J. Barbour, Esq Partnership for Male Youth, Washington, DC, USA

David L. Bell, MD, MPH Columbia University Medical Center, New York, NY, USA

Marino A. Bruce, PhD, MSRC, MDiv, CRC Department of Criminal Justice and Sociology, Jackson State University, Jackson, MS, USA

Center for Health of Minority Males (C-HMM), Myrlie Evers-Williams Institute for the Elimination of Health Disparities, University of Mississippi Medical Center, Jackson, MS, USA

Samuel Cohen-Tanugi Columbia University Medical Center, New York, NY, USA

Cullen N. Conway, MPH Columbia University Medical Center, New York, NY, USA

Keith Elder, PhD, MPH, MPA Department of Health Management and Policy, College for Public Health and Social Justice, Saint Louis University, St. Louis, MO, USA

Mark J. Flynn Family Medicine Residency, Naval Hospital Camp Pendleton, Camp Pendleton, CA, USA

Keon L. Gilbert, DrPH, MA, MPA Department of Behavioral Sciences and Health Education, Salus Center, College for Public Health and Social Justice, St. Louis, MO, USA

Anthony Grech, MD Departments of Family Medicine and Internal Medicine, University of Michigan Medical School, Ann Arbor, MI, USA

Derek M. Griffith, PhD Institute for Research on Men's Health, Center for Medicine, Health and Society, Vanderbilt University, Nashville, TN, USA

Joel J. Heidelbaugh, MD Departments of Family Medicine and Urology, University of Michigan Medical School, Ann Arbor, MI, USA

Harland Holman, MD Spectrum Family Medicine, Family Medicine Residency Clinic, Grand Rapids, MI, USA

Masahito Jimbo, MD, PhD, MPH Department of Family Medicine and Urology, University of Michigan, Ann Arbor, MI, USA

Charles Kodner, MD Department of Family and Geriatric Medicine, University of Louisville School of Medicine, Louisville, KY, USA

Robert Langan, MD Department of Family Medicine, St. Luke's University Hospital, Bethlehem, PA, USA

David A. Levine, MD Department of Pediatrics, Morehouse School of Medicine, Atlanta, GA, USA

Colleen Loo-Gross, MD, MPH Department of Family Medicine, University of Rochester—Highland Hospital, Rochester, NY, USA

Michael A. Malone, MD Department of Family and Community Medicine, Penn State College of Medicine, Hershey, PA, USA

Jim Medder, MD, MPH Department of Family Medicine, University of Nebraska Medical Center, Omaha, NE, USA

Michael Mendoza, MD, MPH, MS Department of Family Medicine, University of Rochester—Highland Hospital, Rochester, NY, USA

Department Public Health Sciences, University of Rochester—Highland Hospital, Rochester, NY, USA

Martin M. Miner, MD Department of Family Medicine and Urology, Warren Alpert School of Medicine, Brown University, Providence, RI, USA

Men's Health Center, The Miriam Hospital, Providence, RI, USA

Makia E. Powers, MD, MPH Department of Pediatrics, Morehouse School of Medicine, Atlanta, GA, USA

Ahad Shiraz, MD Department of Family and Community Medicine, Penn State College of Medicine, Hershey, PA, USA

Roland J. Thorpe Jr., PhD Department of Health, Behavior and Society, Program for Research on Men's Health, Hopkins Center for Health Disparities Solutions, Johns Hopkins Bloomberg School for Public Health, Baltimore, MD, USA

Abdul Waheed, MD Department of Family and Community Medicine, Penn State University College of Medicine, Milton S. Hershey Medical Center, Hershey, PA, USA

Chapter 1
Men's Health in 2010s: What Is the Global Challenge?

Roland J. Thorpe Jr., Derek M. Griffith, Keon L. Gilbert, Keith Elder, and Marino A. Bruce

In recent decades, there has been a dramatic increase in attention toward men's health internationally in the popular press and scientific literature [1–3]. A number of factors have contributed to this heightened awareness of men's health. These include the recognition that there are different body image and health-related issues for men: the increase in the use of reproductive/sexual health medications (e.g., phosphodiesterase type 5 inhibitors), weight loss/maintenance programs for men (e.g., Weight Watchers

R.J. Thorpe Jr., PhD (✉)
Department of Health, Behavior and Society, Program for Research on Men's Health,
Hopkins Center for Health Disparities Solutions, Johns Hopkins Bloomberg School of Public
Health, 624 N. Broadway, Suite 708, Baltimore, MD 21205, USA
e-mail: rthorpe@jhsph.edu

D.M. Griffith, PhD
Institute for Research on Men's Health, Center for Medicine, Health and Society,
Vanderbilt University, PMB #351665, 2301 Vanderbilt Place, Nashville, TN 37235-1665, USA
e-mail: derek.griffith@vanderbilt.edu

K.L. Gilbert, DrPH, MA, MPA
Department of Behavioral Sciences and Health Education, Salus Center, College for Public
Health and Social Justice, 3545 Lafayette Ave, St. Louis, MO 63104, USA
e-mail: kgilber9@slu.edu

K. Elder, PhD, MPH, MPA
Department of Health Management and Policy, College for Public Health and Social Justice,
Saint Louis University, 3545 Lafayette Ave., Room 369, St. Louis, MO 63104, USA
e-mail: kelder2@slu.edu

M.A. Bruce, PhD, MSRC, MDiv, CRC
Department of Criminal Justice and Sociology, Jackson State University,
18830, 360 Dollye M.E. Robinson Building, Jackson, MS 39217, USA

Center for Health of Minority Males (C-HMM), Myrlie Evers-Williams Institute for the
Elimination of Health Disparities, University of Mississippi Medical Center,
2500 North State Street, Jackson, MS 39212, USA
e-mail: mbruce@umc.edu

© Springer International Publishing Switzerland 2016
J.J. Heidelbaugh (ed.), *Men's Health in Primary Care*, Current Clinical Practice,
DOI 10.1007/978-3-319-26091-4_1

Online for Men, Nutrisystem® For Men), and the emergence of reports documenting men's poor health outcomes in Europe, Asia, and other parts of the world [2–5]. However, there continues to be a substantial paucity of research, practice, and advocacy focused on improving the lives of men worldwide and within the USA.

Around the world, men experience premature mortality compared to women [2, 3, 6]. This is somewhat paradoxical given that men have historically had social and economic advantages that are often associated with being male that do not appear to be associated with better health outcomes [7, 8]. Although there is mounting evidence that premature mortality is largely due to men tending to engage in high-risk-taking behaviors [9], premature mortality is likely a result of a more broad and complex set of social, behavioral, physiological, and psychosocial factors that are commonly unaddressed in most men's health research [6, 8, 10–16]. Failure to understand relationships between these factors will continue to impede the progress of the nascent field of men's health.

The objectives of this chapter are to (1) define men's health, (2) describe the health profile of men, (3) discuss the challenges of providing adequate men's health, (4) discuss the impact of the Affordable Care Act (ACA) on preventive healthcare for men, and (5) provide future directions for improving men's health worldwide.

What Is Men's Health?

Men's health has been categorized into four general areas: (a) conditions that are unique to men (e.g., prostate cancer and erectile dysfunction), (b) diseases or illnesses that are more prevalent in men (e.g., cardiovascular disease, stroke), (c) health problems for which risk factors are different in men (e.g., obesity), and (d) health issues for which different interventions to achieve improvements in health and well-being at the individual or the population level are required for men (e.g., access to care) [17, 18]. Most men's health dispositions are considered to be modifiable because the primary causes are social and behavioral—rather than biological [19]. Moreover, behaviors that affect health outcomes may account for up to 40 % of mortality irrespective of gender [20]. Because men are more likely than women to engage in over 30 hazardous behaviors that have been known to increase their risk of injury, morbidity, and mortality, health behaviors help to explain gender differences in health outcomes [9]. This notion underscores the importance of adequately defining and studying men's health.

Are We Improving the Lives of Men?

Life Expectancy

In most countries throughout the world, males are more likely than females to die sooner at every age across the life course, and the gap has not improved in the last decades [2, 3, 6]. For example, when comparing the life expectancy at birth of males in the USA to that of males in 21 other highly developed countries (e.g., Australia,

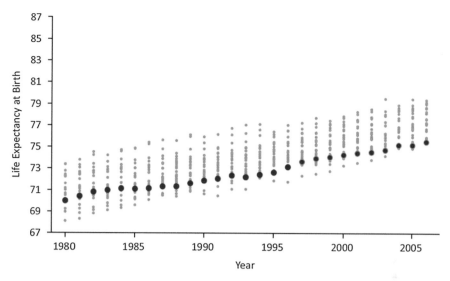

Fig. 1.1 US male life expectancy at birth relative to 21 other high-income countries, 1980–2006. *Notes: Red circles* depict newborn life expectancy in the USA. *Grey circles* depict life expectancy values for Australia, Austria, Belgium, Canada, Denmark, Finland, France, Iceland, Ireland, Italy, Japan, Luxembourg, the Netherlands, New Zealand, Norway, Portugal, Spain, Sweden, Switzerland, the UK, and West Germany. *Source:* National Research Council (2011, Figs. 1–3)

Canada, Japan, Sweden, the UK), the life expectancy of males in the USA has consistently remained in the bottom tertile since the 1980s [21] (Fig. 1.1). Furthermore, males in the USA have the lowest life expectancy when compared to men in other highly developed countries [21].

The medical and technological advances in the USA over the last century have extended the length in which people live by approximately 30 years (Fig. 1.2). However, the gender difference in life expectancy in the USA has widened across the majority of the twentieth century and into the first decade of the twenty-first century. By comparing males in the USA to other males around the world and to females in the USA, this emphasizes the myriad of factors on several levels that impact men's health outcomes and provides additional opportunities to improve men's health in the USA.

Across racial and ethnic groups, men on average live shorter lives than women throughout the twentieth century and into the twenty-first century (Fig. 1.3). In addition to the differences in life expectancy between men and women, racial disparities in health among men are substantial with black men in the USA exhibiting the shortest life expectancy of any racial/ethnic group of men and Asian and Latino men having the longest life expectancy compared to white men [10, 22, 23]. Indeed there is some evidence to suggest that racial disparities are decreasing [24, 25], yet, for the majority of health indicators, racial and ethnic disparities in health among men persist [14, 15, 26]. These data make health disparities among groups of men a keen focus at local, state, and federal public health agendas [27, 28].

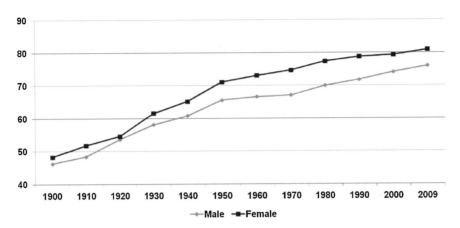

Fig. 1.2 Life expectancy by sex, 1900–2009. *Source:* 1990–1940 National Vital Statistics Report, Vol. 50, No. 6, March 21, 2002, Table 12; 1995–1990 US National Center for Health Statistics, "Health, United States, 2003," Table 27; 2000–2009: US National Center for Health Statistics, "Health, United States, 2011," Table 22

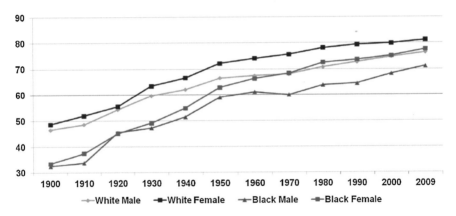

Fig. 1.3 Life expectancy by race and sex, 1900–2009. *Source:* 1990–1940 National Vital Statistics Report, Vol. 50, No. 6, March 21, 2002, Table 12; 1995–1990 US National Center for Health Statistics, "Health, United States, 2003," Table 27; 2000–2009: US National Center for Health Statistics, "Health, United States, 2011," Table 22

Mortality, Morbidity, and Leading Causes of Death

The US age-adjusted mortality rates for the total population and by gender are presented in Fig. 1.4. Although there has been a continuous decline in the age-adjusted mortality rates for the past seven decades for women and men, the age-adjusted mortality rates are higher for men when compared to women and when compared to the US population. Furthermore, regarding the men's health literature in the USA, research on men of color (e.g., African Americans, Hispanics, Asians, American Indian or Alaskan Native, Pacific Islanders) is scant [8, 26]. Yet, men of color account

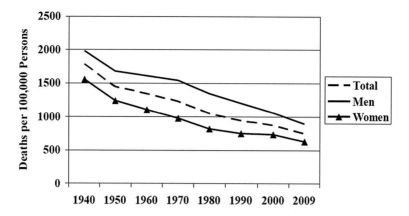

Fig. 1.4 Age-adjusted mortality rates by sex, 1940–2009. *Source*: US National Center for Health Statistics, "National Vital Statistics Reports," Vol. 60, No. 3, December 29, 2011, Table 1

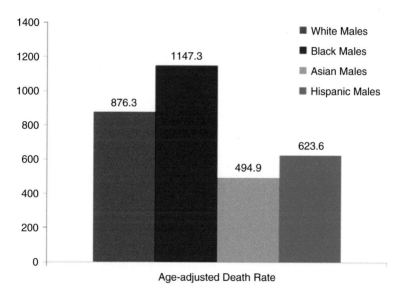

Fig. 1.5 Age-adjusted mortality rates by race/ethnicity among males, 2009. *Source*: US National Center for Health Statistics, "National Vital Statistics Reports," Vol. 60, No. 3, December 29, 2011, Tables 1 and 2. [1]Data for Hispanics is based on estimates

for a considerable amount of the reported gender difference in mortality [9, 29]. African American men have the highest rates of age-adjusted mortality, and Asian men have the lowest, with White men and Hispanic/Latino men falling between these two groups (Fig. 1.5). These data support the need for additional research in the USA focusing on the health of racial/ethnic men, particularly African American men.

Chronic medical conditions encompass the majority of the leading causes of mortality for males in the USA, with heart disease and cancer being the top two leading causes of death for men (Table 1.1). Over one-third of adult men have some form of

Table 1.1 Leading causes of death in men by race/ethnicity, 2009

Rank	White males	African American males	American Indian/Alaska native males	Asian/Pacific Islander males	Hispanic males
1	Heart disease	Heart disease	Heart disease	Cancer	Heart disease
2	Cancer	Cancer	Cancer	Heart disease	Cancer
3	Unintentional injury	Unintentional injury	Unintentional injury	Stroke	Unintentional injury
4	Respiratory disease	Stroke	Diabetes mellitus	Unintentional injury	Stroke
5	Stroke	Homicide	Liver disease and cirrhosis	Diabetes mellitus	Diabetes mellitus
6	Diabetes mellitus	Diabetes mellitus	Suicide	Respiratory disease	Liver disease and cirrhosis
7	Suicide	Respiratory disease	Respiratory disease	Influenza/pneumonia	Homicide
8	Alzheimer's	Nephritis	Stroke	Suicide	Suicide
9	Influenza/pneumonia	HIV disease	Influenza/pneumonia	Nephritis	Respiratory disease
10	Nephritis	Septicemia	Homicide	Alzheimer's	Influenza/pneumonia

Source: National Center for Health Statistics: National Vital Statistics Reports, Deaths: Leading Causes for 2009, Vol. 61, No. 7, October 26, 2012, Tables 1 and 2 "Deaths, percentage of total deaths, and death rates for the 10 leading causes of death in selected age groups, by race, ethnicity, and sex, US 2009"

heart disease [30], and nearly one in two men will develop cancer at some point in their lifetime [31]. It is important to note that only three of the leading causes of death for men are not considered to be directly related to chronic diseases: unintentional injuries (including drug overdose), suicide, and influenza/pneumonia. These statistics are noteworthy because there are significant opportunities to consider behaviors that might impede the progress or delay the onset of chronic conditions.

Race and ethnicity can be useful proxies for a man's exposure to health-harming environments and substances, social disadvantage, and health-promoting resources [32]. Understanding the poor status of men's health and premature death includes considering how racialized and gendered social determinants of health shape men's lives and experiences, particularly through economic and environmental factors [13, 14, 27]. The differences among males by race and ethnicity are highlighted in Table 1.1. Heart disease is the leading cause of death for all racial and ethnic groups of males except Asian/Pacific Islanders, for whom cancer is the leading cause of death; these leading causes of death have remained the same for decades. Hence, only modest progress has been achieved in advancing men's health and addressing disparities in mortality in men's health in the USA. Improving the quality of lives of men in the USA could lead to improved life expectancy and a higher ranking when compared to males from other international countries.

Why Is Creating/Providing Adequate Men's Health Such a Challenge?

It has been established that the bulk of factors associated with the leading causes of death among men can be linked to the social determinants. Gender is one of the most important social determinants of health and health-related behavior, particularly for men, but the study of men's health and well-being have not always conceptualized men as gendered beings [33–35]. A gendered analysis of male behavior can further our understanding of the larger contextual influences upon men's lives, social roles, and other factors that influence men's health [36–38].

Gender is one of the most commonly collected but least understood variables in research [39]. Despite the volume of research that has examined the role that masculinity plays in men's health outcomes, we still know relatively little about specific social–biological pathways through which gendered arrangements become embodied as differences in health among men or between males and females [39]. Gendered processes—social relations and practices associated with biological sex—are the complex array of social relations and practices attached to gender that are rooted in biology and shaped by environment and experience [33, 39]. Thus, most health outcomes for men are the result of factors associated with both sex and gender, but researchers often fail to consider both. Furthermore, gender is both a structural characteristic that helps to define systems of social inequality and an individual level experience. It is critical to explore how it is understood, experienced, and practiced daily at both levels [40–42]. The theories that have been used to explain men's health rarely examine the unique mechanisms and pathways that explain differences between men and women or among men [7].

Health scientists and practitioners should also consider the impact of psychosocial stress on men's lives and men's health. Stress is a socially patterned and contextual phenomenon affected by cultural, economic, and social factors and structures [43–44] that shape the social gradient in health [45–47]. Much of the literature on stress and coping in men builds on an interactional model of stress that highlights the social and cultural context of stress and coping [48] and argues that *perceptions of stressors* are the primary determinants of behavior and health status [49].

Stress directly and indirectly contributes to high rates of unhealthy behaviors, chronic disease, and premature mortality among men [6]. Psychological research on men's health and masculinity often presents stress as an acontextual, psychological construct with universal mechanisms and pathways [49], yet characteristics (e.g., race, ethnicity, life stage) that are socially meaningful in their societal context [50, 51] shape what aspects of life are deemed stressful. Research has highlighted the importance of examining how social and cultural expectations of men and women shape their behavioral strategies for coping with stress; these patterns may help explain not only racial disparities in health outcomes but how these patterns vary by gender as well [46, 48, 52]. What remains unclear, however, is how men's conceptions of various aspects of masculinity may shape men's physiological or behavioral response to stress [6, 48, 53, 54].

Across disciplines theories of masculinity have historically presumed that there is one, universally accepted definition of masculinity [29, 55]. However, what masculinity means to men and the salience of different aspects of masculinity that change over the adult life span [56] may vary by race, ethnicity, socioeconomic status (SES), and geographic location [57]. Each phase of the life cycle can be distinguished in part by a man's efforts to fulfill role performance goals [36, 53]: educational and professional preparation in the preadult and early adult years, being a provider for himself and his family in the middle adult years, and dignified aging as men move into and through older adulthood [53, 58]. These goals represent social and cultural pressures that change as men age, and these strains are rooted in efforts to perform certain masculinities and fulfill social roles and responsibilities [50].

According to Pyke [59], this focus on the primacy of the success of the male career legitimizes hegemonic notions of masculinity and gender inequality. Men who are unable to attain the masculine hegemonic ideals of white, heterosexual middle- and upper-class men may make use of other constructs of masculinity and personal assets to conceptualize and enact what they deem the most important aspects of masculinity [59]. This is an important distinction to make because it highlights how manhood is inherently racialized and class bound [60], which has direct implications on provisions of healthcare for the man, his family, and his community.

Is the ACA Appropriately Poised to Improve the Preventive Healthcare of Men?

The Patient Protection and Affordable Care Act (ACA) of 2010 is a piece of US legislation that was written to provide access to healthcare for all American citizens. A key element of the approach to provide universal healthcare coverage was to expand Medicaid coverage for low-income wage earners. As a result, the ACA would have the potential to have a greatly positive impact on men's health in the USA because men who did not qualify for state-sponsored health insurance prior to ACA could now have access to some form of coverage. In many cases, the financial barriers to healthcare services have been reduced considerably by ACA.

There are also other provisions in ACA that could improve health outcomes among underserved men and reduce and eliminate existing racial/ethnic disparities. These include free coverage of preventive care services, investments in the development of health teams and medical homes to manage chronic conditions in minority communities, and greater emphasis on methods to improve language services and community outreach in underserved communities. The extension of affordable insurance coverage through the new health insurance marketplace in 2014 was designed to ensure that individuals have a choice for quality, affordable health insurance. Subsidies were also to be provided so that all Americans who desired health insurance could afford it. Lastly, the ACA increased funding for community health centers, which provide comprehensive medical care for everyone regardless of their ability to pay. These provisions would allow health centers to double the number of patients that they see over the next several years. This is particularly salient for underserved communities as the majority of the 20 million patients receiving healthcare at community health centers are low income, uninsured, or are members of racial/ethnic minority groups [61].

While these policy-level solutions target all Americans, low-income minority men have perhaps the greatest potential to benefit given the social and economic constraints that impair their ability to seek timely and appropriate medical care. It is also important to note that the benefits of ACA are not limited to men of color born in the USA. Males make up the majority of undocumented immigrants, with a large segment of this group being classified as Hispanic or Latino. Undocumented immigrants are not penalized or required to purchase health insurance; however, immigrant men may qualify for state and local health programs such as community health and migrant clinics under the ACA [62]. This access to healthcare could have implications for millions of minority immigrant men whose primary access to healthcare prior to ACA was the emergency room [63].

The ACA is a pathway that can enhance the health of men overall; however, the future remains unclear about the manner and degree to which this law improves men's health. A caveat is that each state in the USA can select its level of ACA coverage. As such the states with the greatest need for Medicaid expansion have only adopted portions of the ACA. States with the highest level of unemployment, poverty, and poor health outcomes for men (e.g., Alabama, South Carolina, Louisiana,

Mississippi, and Texas) have refused to expand Medicaid in the manner outlined in the ACA. Millions of minority native and immigrant men will continue to have restricted access to healthcare because of the financial and legal barriers to health insurance that provide opportunities for preventative rather than acute care [64].

Men's health will move forward as the national healthcare narrative changes, yet there must be a national commitment to men's health over the life span. This must involve a greater commitment of resources via the federal government to fund research and provide specified training of researchers and clinicians who will focus on men's health. As important, the narrative must change concerning where healthcare is generated for men. The doctor's office is absolutely integral to healthcare delivery, yet public health, healthcare organizations, and schools must improve the awareness, particularly for young boys and men, that health and health maintenance is produced outside of the doctor's office [65]. Aggressive investment in all facets of men's health research, practice, and promotion will position the USA to make significant advancements in the health of males from infancy to advanced age across the globe.

Future Directions for Improving Men's Health

Advancing our knowledge of men's health and health disparities is critical to improving the lives of men worldwide. This involves a sustainable public health and medical infrastructure that is conducive and appropriate for men. Below are some recommendations that should be considered by researchers, policymakers, and practitioners. First, understanding men's health and men's health disparities requires an interdisciplinary approach. Currently much of the work is viewed through individual disciplinary perspectives, which limit our ability to critically think about men and their lives with a wider and perhaps more comprehensive conceptual framework [29]. The contexts in which men live are comprised of social, economic, and political structures that intersect to shape life chances in ways that influence behaviors that can have implications for men's health indicators and outcomes. Such an initiative requires health scientists and practitioners to consider the health of men as a function of both individual and environmental factors. A focus on comprehensive men's health must be more than a pursuit to understand biological mechanisms associated with gender-specific diseases such as prostate cancer and erectile dysfunction. There is considerable room to explore the environments and ways in which men live that elevate their risks for disability, disease, and premature death. Such exploration extends beyond disciplinary boundaries and calls for investigator teams comprised of individuals from the health sciences, social sciences, and the humanities. Interdisciplinary teams are well poised to address some of the complex issues associated with men's health, thereby increasing the likelihood that health indicators and outcomes would markedly improve.

Second, the effort to understand and improve men's health requires a consideration of the existing theoretical frameworks. Sound theories afford scholars the opportunity to provide evidence-based information that can lead to health-promoting strategies and policy-relevant solutions targeted toward explicating disparities among and improving the lives of men. Three theoretical frameworks that are fundamental to advancing men's health and men's health disparities, intersectionality, life course, and environmental affordances, will be discussed briefly.

The bulk of research in the scientific literature tends to examine the independent determinants of health behaviors and health outcomes. Many of the socially defined and socially meaningful characteristics influencing men's health are inextricably intertwined and cannot be fully appreciated as factors that operate independently or additively [40, 50, 66]. Health and social scientists have established that race, ethnicity, sexual identity and orientation, disability status, and geography are critical determinants of men's health; however, they are rarely integrated into efforts to explain men's physical health and health behaviors [8, 26, 67]. Intersectionality provides a framework where scholars can understand how the nexus critical determinants of men's health operate together to impact health outcomes. Furthermore, this framework provides an opportunity to understand the sources of stress in men's lives; it is critical to recognize how gender, race, socioeconomic class, life stage, and other factors form new and dynamic social and cultural expectations that provide an important context for men's daily lives and health [50].

The life course perspective is another lens that can be very useful in understanding men's health because it tenders three important features: (1) the opportunity to identify how social and economic circumstances (e.g., education, family formation, work history) interrelate across the life course, shaping or being shaped by physical and mental health; (2) the insight to understanding both the cumulative effect of gendered norms, beliefs, and roles over the life course and shifts in expressions of masculinity as one ages [8, 68]; and (3) the timing of significant experiences in life that might contribute to patterns of health [69–71]. Two well-studied frameworks that have a life course perspective are cumulative disadvantage theory (CDA) [72, 73] and the weathering hypothesis [74, 75]. Cumulative disadvantage theory posits that early advantage or disadvantage can lead to increasing differentiation in opportunities and experiences over the life course, which results in heterogeneity in adult health status [76, 77]. This is a useful framework for examining differences in health between men and women, as well as the variability in health and functioning among men. The weathering hypothesis articulates focuses on explaining how health declines in Blacks begin prematurely in early adulthood and as a consequence of long-term and compound exposure to unfavorable social–environmental, psychosocial, and economic conditions [74]. Both frameworks articulate the process by which social disadvantages and stressors accumulate over the life course [70]. However, there is a paucity of work that uses either one of these frameworks on the health and well-being of men.

The third framework—the environmental affordances framework—can provide insight into behavioral responses of men to the stressors of the social context in which they dwell. Jackson and Knight [48] argue that stressful social and economic living conditions combined with restricted access to a range of potential resources to manage those conditions may contribute to behavioral responses to stress that may adversely affect health outcomes; their testable, theory-driven model is also designed to explain the fact that African Americans tend to have lower rates of mood/anxiety disorders and other psychiatric diagnoses than Caucasians, but African Americans tend to have higher rates of chronic physical health conditions than Caucasians [52, 78]. Taken altogether, Jackson and colleagues argue that psychological stress can lead to coping strategies that are shaped by what is accessible in people's environment and behaviors that are considered gender-appropriate coping strategies. For men, these typically include tobacco use, physical inactivity, and alcohol and illicit substance abuse [48]. These social and economic conditions contribute to chronic stress, increase risk for poor health outcomes, and reduce chances for social or economic success over time [79, 80]. Thus, advances in understanding how stress and stressors impact disparities in men's health at different points in the life course are essential toward improving the lives of racial/ethnic minority men. In addition, there is a focus on explicating how biological, behavioral, and social processes operate across the life course to create divergent health trajectories [71, 81, 82].

A third recommendation for men's health professionals to consider involves the integration of the social determinants of health into future studies and interventions. Factors such as poverty, education, geography, family, race and ethnicity, incarceration, unemployment, and underemployment have been identified as important social determinants of health and healthcare for men [42, 83–86]. Moreover these factors have implications for disease manifestation, treatment adherence, physical functioning, and premature death [87]. However, the manner through which social determinants have implications for men's health has been largely ignored in the effort to understand and address poor outcomes among vulnerable and underserved men [71, 86, 88].

The last recommendation, which is a huge challenge in the USA, is to heighten the awareness and increase the allocation of resources committed to understanding the leading causes of men's health and the determinants of men's health behaviors. *Healthy People 2020* set forth 10-year national objectives for promoting health and preventing disease among US residents, with a focus on achieving increased quality and years of healthy life and the reduction and elimination of health disparities. Indeed it is a progress to have explicit goals for men's health for the first time; however, *Healthy People 2020* only includes goals for men's sexual and reproductive health, prostate cancer screening and mortality, and incidence and prevalence of AIDS cases and hepatitis B transmission [89]. The selection of these topics reflects more about our cultural beliefs that men's health is synonymous with men's sexual functioning, sexual risk behavior, and virility, rather than the leading causes of mortality for men or their high-risk health behaviors. Thus, the difficulty in obtaining a more comprehensive view of men's health in the USA remains elusive. The creation of a national men's health report akin to the European and Asian reports is a desperately needed and viable solution. This report would allow researchers, policymakers, and advocacy persons to determine potential areas that are amenable to interventions, to formulate and implement such interventions, and to improve healthcare outcomes.

Conclusion

Over the past two decades, the world has become smaller and more connected. Recent events like the Ebola outbreak demonstrate how health incidents in one corner of the globe can have implications for another. Improving the health of men and boys, regardless of their country of origin or social station in life, can have far-reaching ripple effects. Healthy men can be present and available to make positive contributions to their families and communities. Reducing the considerable social and economic costs associated with disease, disability, and premature death should be a global priority. As such, men's health and community organizations are encouraged to partner with universities, national institutes, and international agencies to leverage their resources and create a network of researchers, practitioners, clinicians, and policymakers to improve the lives of all men. Funding agencies should be encouraged to support research and programs that focus on men's health disparities and include addressing the social determinants of health [85, 88, 90]. Research on men's health and related disparities are often overlooked or seen as competing with women's and children's health [6, 91]. In spite of these alleged distinctions, it is important to understand that men's health and the disparities that exist among them are directly related to the health of women, families, and their communities worldwide. We can no longer afford to allow health scientists and practitioners to ignore the health of minority men in particular, men in general, and the factors impacting them. A focus on men's health is critical for the health of families, communities, and society around the globe.

References

1. Watkins DC, Griffith DM. Practical solutions to addressing men's health disparities: guest editorial. Int J Men's Health. 2013;12(3):187–94.
2. European Commission. The state of men's health in Europe-report. Directorate General for Health & Consumers; 2011.
3. Tong SF, Low WY, Ng CJ. Profile of men's health in Malaysia: problems and challenges. Asian J Androl. 2011;13(4):526–33.
4. Courtenay WH. Dying to be men. New York: Routledge; 2011.
5. White AK. Report on the scoping study of men's health. London: The Department of Health; 2001.
6. Williams DR. The health of men: structured inequalities and opportunities. Am J Public Health. 2003;93(5):724–31.
7. Robertson S. Understanding men and health: masculinities, identity, and well-being. Maidenhead: Open University Press; 2007.
8. Griffith DM, Thorpe Jr RJ. Men's physical health and health behaviors. In: Wong YJ, Wester SR, editors. APA handbook of the psychology of men and masculinities, APA handbooks in psychology series. Washington, DC: American Psychological Association; 2016. p. 709–30.
9. Courtenay WH. Constructions of masculinity and their influence on men's well-being: a theory of gender and health. Soc Sci Med. 2000;50(10):1385–401.
10. Thorpe Jr R, Wilson-Frederick S, Bowie J, Coa K, Clay O, Laveist T, Whitfield K. Health behaviors and all-cause mortality in African American Men. Am J Men's Health. 2013;7(Suppl):8S–18S.

11. Courtenay WH. Key determinants of the health and well-being of men and boys. Int J Men's Health. 2003;2(1):1.
12. Warner DF, Hayward MD. Early-life origins of the race gap in men's mortality. J Health Soc Behav. 2006;47(3):209–26.
13. Young AMW. Poverty and men's health: global implications for policy and practice. J Men's Health. 2009;6(3):272.
14. Treadwell H, Braithwaite K. Men's health: a myth or a possibility? J Mens Health Gend. 2005;2(3):382–6.
15. Treadwell HM, Ro M. Poverty, race, and the invisible men. Am J Public Health. 2003;93:705–7.
16. Young AMW, Meryn S, Treadwell HM. Poverty and men's health. J Mens Health. 2008;5(3):184–8.
17. Meryn S, Young AMW. Making the global case for men's health. J Men's Health. 2010;7(1):2–4.
18. Sabo D, Gordon G, editors. Men's health and illness: gender, power and the body. London: Sage; 1995.
19. Featherstone B, Rivett M, Scourfield J. Working with men in health and social care. Thousand Oaks, CA: Sage; 2007.
20. McGinnis MJ, Williams-Russo P, Knickman JR. The case for more active policy attention to health promotion. To succeed, we need leadership that informs and motivates, economic incentives that encourage change, and science that moves the frontiers. Health Aff (Millwood). 2002;21(2):78–93.
21. National, R. C. U., Woolf S, Aron L. US health in international perspective: shorter lives, poorer health. Washington, DC: National Academies Press; 2013.
22. Dressler WW, Oths KS, Gravlee CC. Race and ethnicity in public health research: models to explain health disparities. Ann Rev Anthropol. 2005;34:231–52.
23. Braboy Jackson P, Williams DR. The intersection of race, gender and SES: health paradoxes. In: Schulz AJ, Mullings L, editors. Gender, race, class & health: intersectional approaches. San Francisco, CA: Jossey-Bass; 2006. p. 131–62.
24. Harper S, Lynch J, Davey Smith G. Trends in black-white life expectancy gap in the United States, 1983–2003. JAMA. 2007;297(11):1224–32.
25. Hambleton IR, Jeyaseelan S, Howitt C, Sobers-Grannum N, Hennis AJ, Wilks RJ, Harris EN, MacLeish M, Sullivan LW, US Caribbean Alliance for Health Disparities Research Group. Cause of death disparities in the African diaspora: exploring differences among shared-heritage populations. Am J Public Health. 2015;105 Suppl 3:S491–8.
26. Griffith DM, Metzl JM, Gunter K. Considering intersections of race and gender in interventions that address U.S. men's health disparities. Public Health. 2011;125(7):417–23. doi:10.1016/j.puhe.2011.04.014.
27. Pease B. Racialised masculinities and the health of immigrant and refugee men. In: Broom A, Tovey P, editors. Men's health: body, identity and context. Chichester: Wiley; 2009. p. 182–201.
28. Williams S, Giorgianni S. Survey of state public health department resources for men and boys: identification of an inadvertent and remediatable service and health disparity. Am J Mens Health. 2010;4(4):344–52.
29. Courtenay W. A global perspective on the field of men's health: an editorial. Int J Mens Health. 2002;1(1):1.
30. Go AS, Mozaffarian D, Roger VL, Benjamin EJ, Berry JD, Borden WB, Bravata DM, Dai S, Ford ES, Fox CS, Franco S, Fullerton HJ, Gillespie C, Hailpern SM, Heit JA, Howard VJ, Huffman MD, Kissela BM, Kittner SJ, Lackland DT, Lichtman JH, Lisabeth LD, Magid D, Marcus GM, Marelli A, Matchar DB, McGuire DK, Mohler ER, Moy CS, Mussolino ME, Nichol G, Paynter NP, Schreiner PJ, Sorlie PD, Stein J, Turan TN, Virani SS, Wong ND, Woo D, Turner MB. Heart disease and stroke statistics—2013 update: a report from the American Heart Association. Circulation. 2013;127(1):e6–e245. doi:10.1161/CIR.0b013e31828124ad.

31. American Cancer Society. Cancer facts & figures 2013. Atlanta, GA: American Cancer Society; 2013.
32. LaVeist TA. On the study of race, racism, and health: a shift from description to explanation. Int J Health Serv. 2000;30(1):217–9.
33. Evans J, Frank B, Oliffe JL, Gregory D. Health, Illness, Men and Masculinities (HIMM): a theoretical framework for understanding men and their health. J Men's Health. 2011;8(1): 7–15.
34. Kimmel MS. The gendered society. New York: Oxford University Press; 2000.
35. Kimmel MS, Hearn J, Connell R. Handbook of studies on men and masculinities. Thousand Oaks, CA: Sage; 2005.
36. Griffith DM, Gunter K, Allen JO. Male gender role strain as a barrier to African American men'sphysicalactivity.HealthEducBehav.2011;38(5):482–91.doi:10.1177/1090198110383660.
37. Mankowski E, Maton K. A community psychology of men and masculinity: historical and conceptual review. Am J Community Psychol. 2010;45(1):73–86. doi:10.1007/s10464-009-9288-y.
38. Watts R. Advancing a community psychology of men. Am J Community Psychol. 2010;45(1):201–11. doi:10.1007/s10464-009-9281-5.
39. Springer KW, Mager Stellman J, Jordan-Young RM. Beyond a catalogue of differences: a theoretical frame and good practice guidelines for researching sex/gender in human health. Soc Sci Med. 2012;74(11):1817–24.
40. Coles T. Negotiating the field of masculinity. Men Masculinities. 2009;12(1):30–44. doi:10.1 177/1097184x07309502.
41. Weber L, Parra-Medina D. Intersectionality and women's health: charting a path to eliminating health disparities. In: Demos V, Segal MT, editors. Advances in gender research: gender perspectives on health and medicine. Amsterdam: Elsevier; 2003. p. 181–230.
42. Bruce MA, Roscigno VJ, McCall PL. Structure, context, and agency in the reproduction of black-on-black violence. Theor Criminol. 1998;2:29–55.
43. Aldwin CM. Stress, coping and development: an integrative perspective. New York: Guilford; 2007.
44. Meyer IH, Schwartz S, Frost DM. Social patterning of stress and coping: does disadvantaged social statuses confer more stress and fewer coping resources? Soc Sci Med. 2008;67(3): 368–79.
45. Orpana HM, Lemyre L, Kelly S. Do Stressors explain the association between income and declines in self-rated health? A longitudinal analysis of the national Population Health Survey. Int J Behav Med. 2007;14(1):40–7.
46. Bruce M, Griffith DM, Thorpe Jr RJ. Stress and kidney disease. Advances in Chronic Kidney Disease. 2015;22(1):46–54.
47. Turner RJ, Avison WR. Status variations in stress exposure: implications for the interpretation of research on race, socioeconomic status, and gender. J Health Soc Behav. 2003;44:488–505.
48. Jackson JS, Knight KM. Race and self-regulatory health behaviors: the role of the stress response and the HPA axis. In: Schaie KW, Carstensen LL, editors. Social structure, aging and self-regulation in the elderly. New York: Springer; 2006. p. 189–240.
49. Skinner EA, Edge K, Altman J, Sherwood H. Searching for the structure of coping: a review and critique of category systems for classifying ways of coping. Psychol Bull. 2003;129:216–69.
50. Griffith DM. An intersectional approach to men's health. J Men's Health. 2012;9(2):106–12. doi:10.1016/j.jomh.2012.03.003.
51. Snow RC. Sex, gender, and vulnerability. Global Public Health. 2008;3(Suppl):58–74.
52. Jackson JS, Knight KM, Rafferty JA. Race and unhealthy behaviors: chronic stress, the HPA axis, and physical and mental health disparities over the life course. Am J Public Health. 2010;100(5):933–9. doi:10.2105/ajph.2008.143446.
53. Bowman PJ. Research perspectives on Black men: role strain and adaptation across the adult life cycle. In: Jones RL, editor. Black adult development and aging. Berkeley, CA: Cobb & Henry Publishers; 1989. p. 117–50.

54. Bowman PJ. Role strain and adaptation issues in the strength-based model: diversity, multi-level, and life-span considerations. Couns Psychol. 2006;34(1):118–33.
55. Creighton G, Oliffe JL. Theorising masculinities and men's health: a brief history with a view to practice [Report]. Health Sociol Rev. 2010;19(4):409–18.
56. Griffith DM, Gunter K, Watkins DC. Measuring masculinity in research on men of color: findings and future directions. Am J Public Health. 2012;102 Suppl 2:S187–94.
57. Hammond WP, Mattis JS. Being a man about it: manhood meaning among African American men. Psychol Men Masculinity. 2005;6(2):114–26. doi:10.1037/1524-9220.6.2.114.
58. Erickson EH. Identity and the life cycle. New York: Norton; 1980.
59. Pyke KD. Class-based masculinities the interdependence of gender, class, and interpersonal power. Gender Soc. 1996;10:527–49.
60. Summers MA. Manliness and its discontents: the Black Middle-class and the transformation of masculinity, 1900–1930. Chapel Hill, NC: University of North Carolina Press; 2004.
61. Bureau of Primary Health Care. Uniform data system. In help wanted the state of unmet need for primary health care in America. Bethesda, MD: National Association of Community Health Centers; 2012.
62. Passel J, Capps R, Fix M. Undocumented immigrants: facts and figures. Washington, DC: Urban Institute; 2004.
63. Cox C, Levitt L. The individual mandate: how sweeping? The Henry J. Kaiser Family Foundation: Health Reform Source; 2012. http://healthreform.kff.org/notes-on-health-insurance-and-reform/2012/march/the-individual-mandate-how-sweeping.asp.
64. The Henry J. Kaiser Foundation. Status of state action on medicaid expansion decision; 2015. http://kff.org/health-reform/state-indicator/state-activity-around-expanding-medicaid-under-the-affordable-care-act/.
65. Elder K, Wiltshire J, McRoy L, Campbell D, Gary L, Safford M. Men and differences by racial/ethnic group in self-advocacy during the medical encounter. J Men's Health. 2010;7(2):133–44.
66. Warner DF, Brown TH. Understanding how race/ethnicity and gender define age-trajectories of disability: an intersectionality approach. Soc Sci Med. 2011;72(8):1236–48.
67. Bowleg L, Teti M, Massie JS, Patel A, Malebranche DJ, Tschann JM. 'What does it take to be a man? What is a real man?': ideologies of masculinity and HIV sexual risk among Black heterosexual men. Cult Health Sex. 2011;13(5):545–59.
68. Watkins DC. Depression over the adult life course for African American Men: toward a framework for research and practice. Am J Mens Health. 2012;6(3):194–210.
69. George LK. What life-course perspectives offer the study of aging and health. In: Settersten RAJ, editor. Invitation to the life course: toward new understandings of later life. Amityville, NY: Baywood; 2002. p. 161–88.
70. Thorpe Jr RJ, Kelley-Moore J. Life course theories of race disparities: a comparison of cumulative dis/advantage perspective and the weathering hypothesis. In: LaVeist TAI, editor. Race, ethnicity, and health. 2nd ed. San Francisco, CA: Jossey-Bass; 2013. p. 355–75.
71. Thorpe Jr RJ, Duru OK, Hill CV. Advancing racial/ethnic minority men's health using a life course approach. Ethn Dis. 2015;25(3):241–4.
72. Merton RK. The Matthew effect in science: the reward and communication system of science. Science. 1968;159(3810):55–63.
73. Dannefer D. Cumulative advantage/disadvantage and the life course: cross-fertilizing age and social science theory. J Gerontol Soc Sci. 2003;58B(6):S327–37.
74. Geronimus AT. The weathering hypothesis and the health of African-American women and infants: evidence and speculations. Ethn Dis. 1992;2(3):207–21.
75. Geronimus AT. Understanding and eliminating racial inequalities in women's health in the United States: The role of the weathering conceptual framework. J Am Med Women's Assoc (1972). 2001;56(4):133–6. 149–50.
76. Kelley-Moore J, Lin J. Widening the view: capturing 'unobserved' heterogeneity in studies of age and the life course. In: Settersten R, Angel J, editors. Handbook of sociology of aging. New York: Springer; 2011. p. 51–70.

77. Dannefer D, Kelley-Moore JA, Huang W. Opening the social: sociological imagination in life course studies. In: Shanahan MJ, Mortimer JT, Johnson MK, editors. Handbook of life course. 2nd ed. New York: Springer; 2015. p. 87–110.
78. Mezuk B, Rafferty JA, Kershaw KN, Hudson D, Abdou CM, Lee H, Eaton WW, Jackson JS. Reconsidering the role of social disadvantage in physical and mental health: stressful life events, health behaviors, race, and depression. Am J Epidemiol. 2010;172(11):1238–49. doi:10.1093/aje/kwq283.
79. Massey DS. Segregation and stratification: a biopsychosocial perspective. DuBois Rev Soc Sci Res Race. 2004;1(1):7–25.
80. Massey DS, Denton NA. American Apartheid: segregation and the making of the underclass. Cambridge, MA: Harvard University Press; 1988.
81. Ben-Shlomo Y, Kuh D. A life course approach to chronic disease epidemiology: conceptual models, empirical challenges and interdisciplinary perspectives. Int J Epidemiol. 2002;31(2):285–93.
82. Kuh D, Shlomo YB. A life course approach to chronic disease epidemiology, 2. Oxford: Oxford University Press; 2004.
83. Marmot M. Action on health disparities in the United States: commission on social determinants of health. JAMA. 2009;301(11):1169–71.
84. Marmot M, Allen JJ. Social determinants of health equity. Am J Public Health. 2014;104(S4):S517–9.
85. Xanthos C, Treadwell HM, Holden KB. Social determinants of health among African American men. J Mens Health. 2010;7(1):11–9.
86. Treadwell HM, Young AMW, Rosenberg MT. Want of a place to stand: social determinants and men's health. J Men's Health. 2012;9(2):104–5.
87. Bruce MA, Griffith DM, Thorpe Jr RJ. Social determinants of men's health disparities. Fam Community Health. 2015;38(4):281–3.
88. Thorpe R, Richard P, Bowie J, Laveist T, Gaskin D. Economic burden of men's health disparities in the United States. Int J Men's Health. 2013;12(3):195–212.
89. Porsche DJ. Healthy Men 2020. Am J Men's Health. 2010;4(1):5–6. doi:10.1177/1557988309361158.
90. Gadson SL. The third world health status of Black American Males. J Natl Med Assoc. 2006;98:488–91.
91. Bonhomme J, Young A. The health status of black men. In: Braithwaite RL, Taylor SE, Treadwell HM, editors. Health issues in the black community. 3rd ed. San Francisco, CA: Jossey-Bass; 2007. p. 73–95.

Chapter 2
Masculinity in Men's Health: Barrier or Portal to Healthcare?

Derek M. Griffith, Keon L. Gilbert, Marino A. Bruce, and Roland J. Thorpe Jr.

In the United States and most countries in the world, males are more likely than females to die in their first year of life and at every age across the remainder of the life course [1]. Strong and consistent evidence suggests that health behaviors play a key role in the etiology of most of the leading causes of death among men [2–6]. Men often use health behaviors in daily interactions to help them negotiate social power and social status, and these health practices can either undermine or promote health [5]. Men are more likely than women to engage in over 30 behaviors that have been known to increase their risk of injury, morbidity, and mortality. How men

D.M. Griffith, PhD (✉)
Institute for Research on Men's Health, Center for Medicine,
Health and Society, Vanderbilt University, PMB #351665, 2301 Vanderbilt Place,
Nashville, TN 37235-1665, USA
e-mail: derek.griffith@vanderbilt.edu

K.L. Gilbert, Dr.PH, MA, MPA
Department of Behavioral Sciences and Health Education, College for Public Health and
Social Justice, Saint Louis University, Salus Center, 3545 Lafayette Avenue,
St. Louis, MO 63104, USA
e-mail: kgilber9@slu.edu

M.A. Bruce, PhD, MSRC, MDiv, CRC
Department of Criminal Justice and Sociology, Jackson State University,
18830, 360 Dollye M.E. Robinson Building, Jackson, MS 39217, USA

Center for Health of Minority Males (C-HMM), Myrlie Evers-Williams Institute for the
Elimination of Health Disparities, University of Mississippi Medical Center,
2500 North State Street, Jackson, MS 39216, USA
e-mail: mbruce@umc.edu

R.J. Thorpe Jr., PhD
Department of Health, Behavior and Society, Program for Research on Men's Health,
Hopkins Center for Health Disparities Solutions, Johns Hopkins Bloomberg School of Public
Health, 624 N. Broadway, Suite 708, Baltimore, MD 21205, USA
e-mail: rthorpe@jhsph.edu

© Springer International Publishing Switzerland 2016
J.J. Heidelbaugh (ed.), *Men's Health in Primary Care*, Current Clinical Practice,
DOI 10.1007/978-3-319-26091-4_2

think about and project an image of themselves as men and respond to gendered social norms and pressures is often implicated in explanations of men's premature death due to stress and unhealthy behaviors (e.g., reckless driving, alcohol and drug abuse, risky sexual behavior, high-risk sports, and leisure activities) [7, 8]. Thus, there is a need for health research and practice that is gender sensitive in relation to men's lives and to understand masculinities in relation to health and illness [9], which may come through understanding the relationship between masculinity and diverse aspects of men's health.

Masculinity has primarily been operationalized and studied as a static factor that resides solely in each man's individual psychology [10], but masculinity is often signified by beliefs and behaviors that change over time and that are practiced in everyday social and cultural patterns, practices, and relations [10–12]. Across the life span, the stressors associated with beliefs and expectations about men's behavior, economic opportunities, and social marginalization can directly and indirectly contribute to men having poor health behaviors and high rates of morbidity from preventable diseases [1]. Increasingly, masculinity is being conceptualized and framed to be best understood in the context of social and cultural factors [4, 13, 14]. While masculinity is considered to be an important determinant of men's health, the study of men's health and well-being has not always conceptualized men as gendered beings [9, 15, 16]. Surprisingly, little research has empirically examined the relationship between masculinity and men's health [9].

In this chapter, we will discuss masculinity and how it may affect men's health and health-related behavior. We will begin by discussing how masculinity is conceptualized and measured, how masculinity and manhood shape men's health behaviors, and then how men define health. We will conclude with a brief discussion of environmental factors that shape how men engage in health-related behaviors that not only influence their health outcomes but are used to demonstrate their identities as men.

Masculinity in Men's Health

Since the 1970s, US-based studies on men have focused primarily on identifying the main elements of masculinity, assuming them to be equally relevant for all men, and then quantifying the extent to which these elements are present in individual men [11]. Hegemonic masculinity is the idealized cultural standard of masculinity that exists in a specific time, place, and culture; it sets the ideal of how to be a man and sets the standard by which all men are judged [17–19]. Early work examining the relationship between masculinity and health was dominated by the assumption that biological sex played a primary role in determining health behaviors, but recently, scholars have paid increasing attention to the health implications of gendered expectations and normative gender roles on men's health [20, 21]. Men will often prefer to risk their physical health and well-being rather than be associated with traits they or others may perceive as feminine [9, 14, 22]. Though public health campaigns such as "Real Men Get Checked," "Real Men Wear Gowns," and "Real Men, Real Depression" convey the important message that masculinity and men's health are not inherently at odds, health-promoting behaviors often are associated with femininity and health-harming behaviors are linked with masculinity, and men's adherence to masculine ideals is thought to help explain the disparity between men's and women's health outcomes [5, 18, 21, 23, 24].

While men often recognize that there may be a hegemonic, cultural ideal of masculinity, individual men frequently define and experience their masculinities by drawing on facets of hegemonic masculinity which they have the capacity to perform [17]. Men piece together aspects of hegemonic masculinity to establish their own standards and meanings of masculinity. As they seek to establish and regularly reinforce that their masculine identities are valid in the context of their everyday lives [17], men may respond to masculine ideals by reformulating them, shaping them along the lines of their own abilities, perceptions, and strengths, and then defining their masculine identity along these new lines.

In research on men's health, there is a need to examine three key factors associated with masculinity: *how different conceptions of masculinity are related to health*; *how notions of masculinity are constructed and embedded in social, economic, and political contexts and institutions*; and *how culture and subcultures influence how men develop their gender identities and how they respond to health issues* [25, 26]. Some researchers are beginning to explore the centrality of masculinity versus racial identity and cultural beliefs in men's identities and health [27–30]. Research on African American, Asian American, and Latin American men is finding that there are forms of manhood that diverge from hegemonic masculine norms [31–34] and that experiences of discrimination and racism may highlight stigmatized identities (e.g., race, ethnicity, sexual minority status) in their daily experience more than masculinity [35, 36]. African American, Asian American, and Latin American men often seek ways to integrate hegemonic masculine norms with their racial and ethnic identities in ways that create new standards of masculinity that are racial and ethnic specific [34, 36].

In addition, one of the key areas that is emerging in both the quantitative and qualitative men's health research is how sexual orientation, sexual identity, and traditional conceptualizations of masculinity intersect to affect the health behaviors and health outcomes of men [37–41]. The minority stress model posits that the vigilance that "men who have sex with men" may have in expecting to experience discrimination based on their sexual identity may lead them to internalize negative social attitudes and conceal their sexual orientation, increasing stress-related mental and physical health concerns [42]. Gay men also have consistently higher rates of steroid use associated with body image issues and different standards of what the ideal masculine body should look like [40].

Conceptualizing and Measuring Masculinity

Within any society, there can exist a hierarchy of masculinities that are compared to a dominant or hegemonic ideal [18]. In the United States, the normative form of hegemonic masculinity is defined by race (white), sexual orientation (heterosexual),

SES (middle class), and possessing certain traits: assertiveness, dominance, control, physical strength, and emotional restraint [5, 9, 11]. Though it is useful to determine if men adhere to hegemonic ideals of masculinity, hegemonic masculinity does not have uniform meanings and negative influence within and across men's lives [4, 11]. Masculinity is defined in diverse ways that vary by race, ethnicity, class, sexual identity, disability status, and other factors, but are organized around a common membership in the category of "man" [36].

Masculinity is often defined in relational terms as that which is not feminine [9, 43]. Measures of masculinity serve as the operational definitions of masculinity in empirical studies [11, 44]. How we operationally define masculinity in men's health helps to determine how well we have captured gendered constructs that are relevant to health. We will briefly describe selected groups of measures of masculinity. Space does not permit an exhaustive review, but see reviews by Loue [45], Smiler [11], and Thompson [46] for a more thorough discussion of measures of masculinity.

The Male Role Norms Inventory [47] and its subscales measure men's adherence to hegemonic male norms. The Conceptions of Masculinity Scale [39], one of the few measures of masculinity designed specifically with and for gay men, assesses perceptions that masculinity is defined by men's sexual behavior, social behavior, and physical appearance. The Meaning of Masculinity Scale [39] measures a specific, traditional form of gay men's masculinity. Factors associated with male norms such as the salience of norms, subjective norms, and conformity to norms (e.g., Conformity to Masculine Norms Inventory [48], Male Gender Norms scales, Salience of Traditional Masculine Norms [49]) have been used in research to highlight different aspects of psychological stressors that affect men's health and health practices. Measures of male norms assess the degree to which men indicate their level of agreement or disagreement to an array of dominant cultural norms of masculinity in the United States [47, 48, 50, 51]. Measures of attitudes and feelings about the hegemonic gender roles males often perform (e.g., Gender Role Conflict Scale, Male Gender Role Stress Scale [52], Male Subjective Norms [53]) highlight key psychological stressors in the lives of males that result from discrepancies between how men perceive their personal characteristics and how they perceive men are expected to behave. Measures of masculine conceptions or ideologies examine the degree to which men feel that they are able to fulfill a single form of stereotypically masculine roles [46]. Conformity to Masculine Gender Norms describes men's perceptions of their ability to adhere to traditional masculine norms. Measures of gender role conflict or stress assess ideologies and beliefs about the meaning of being male and the extent to which one endorses or internalizes cultural norms and values of masculinity and the male gender role [54].

While there is considerable research utilizing these scales, there remains surprisingly little empirical research examining how measures of masculinity are associated with, or predictive of, health behaviors or health outcomes [44]. The studies that have included measures of masculinity and health outcomes have had inconsistent findings. Some studies found positive relationships between masculinity and health, while others reported more negative associations [55]. For example, Levant and colleagues (2013) found that masculine risk-taking and self-reliance were negatively related to health behavior measures but that emotional control, primacy of work, and winning were positively related [55, 56]. This complexity is echoed in the work of Gordon and colleagues who found that toughness was related to both more exercise and increased junk food consumption [57]. Engaging in positive health behaviors and being rational and decisive and making autonomous decisions also may draw on hegemonic ideals of masculinity, highlighting that masculinity may not only be associated with risky behavior [4]. The work on masculinity and health is particularly limited to men who are not college students at 4-year colleges and universities, a very selective and non-generalizable group to males in the United States. There also is a paucity of work focusing on masculinity and health across the globe [58]. One area where there is particularly little is in studying how these measures of masculinity are associated with the health of middle-aged and older men, across racial and ethnic groups.

While Kimmel asserts that homophobia is a core characteristic of hegemonic masculinity, studies of Latin and African American men are finding that these men's definitions of manhood may not include homophobia, violence, physical domination, or emotional isolation [32, 36, 59]. Machismo is measured as a combination of traditional machismo (i.e., hypermasculine traits such as dominance) and caballerismo (i.e., nurturing qualities, family centeredness, social responsibility, and emotional connectedness) [60]. The values espoused in caballerismo and black manhood are most congruent with feminist masculinities that include being an ethical human being, having emotionally healthy relationships with others, being involved with activism in the community, and rejecting aspects of hegemonic masculinity (e.g., objectification of women, physical and sexual domination of women, and homophobia) [32, 33, 36, 59]. The work on Asian American men and masculinity highlights how this group of men has historically been viewed as hypermasculine and effeminate simultaneously [34]. The notion that there is a singular masculinity that represents the hegemonic ideals of a particular racial or ethnic group is a misnomer; the concept of Asian American masculinity, for example, is one that was not defined by that specific population [34]. Thus, masculinity is complex, can be related to desirable as well as undesirable behaviors, and resides both within the psychology of men and their interactions with their social environment [11].

Stress, Masculinity, and Men's Health Behavior

Stress directly and indirectly contributes to high rates of unhealthy behaviors, chronic disease diagnoses, and premature mortality among men [1]. Smoking, alcohol and substance abuse, unhealthy eating, sedentary behavior, and poor sleep all are behaviors that are adversely affected by stress [61]. In the context of medicine and public health, men's self-representation and internalization of notions of masculinity and masculine social norms and pressures are often implicated in explanations of men's premature death due to stress and unhealthy behaviors (e.g., interpersonal violence, reckless driving, alcohol and drug abuse, risky sexual behavior, high-risk sports, and leisure activities) [7–9, 14, 22]. These behaviors often are culturally sanctioned ways of distinguishing among males and between males and females and may help explain the association between masculinity and men's risky and unhealthy behaviors [5, 9].

These behaviors also may be affected by men's experiences of psychosocial stress. For example, Whitehead's (1997) Big Man Little Man Complex argues that men are trying to achieve a level of respectability through economic success, educational attainment, and social class status while simultaneously demonstrating prowess along the social and cultural dimensions of traditional masculinity: virility, sexual prowess, risk-taking, physical strength, hardiness, etc. [62]. These factors highlight that masculinity may lead to stress and coping that results from trying to achieve success in areas of respectability and risky behaviors that may represent traditional aspects of masculinity (e.g., eating large portions, alcohol abuse, substance use, speeding while driving, risky types of physical activity, high numbers of sexual partners, inconsistent safe sexual practices). The aspects of masculinity that men find stressful and use to define themselves and that they try to portray to others appear to change over time.

Masculinity Changes over Time

Because the fundamental meaning of masculinity and the salience of different aspects of masculinity change over the life course, it is critical to consider how both the notions of masculinity change over time and the importance of key health behaviors changes over time [4, 9]. Each phase of life can be distinguished, in part, by men's efforts to fulfill salient role performance goals [7, 63]: educational and professional preparation in the preadult and early adult years, being a provider for himself and his family in the middle-adult years, and dignified aging as men move through older adulthood [63, 64]. While these goals may not be universal, it remains critical to recognize that there are social and cultural pressures that men experience and that these pressures and strains, which may be rooted in efforts to fulfill salient roles, change as men age [25]. Some of the masculinities men try to perform when they are younger tend to demonstrate their physical strength, sexual prowess, and risk tolerance, but as men age, they tend to also want to demonstrate more positive aspects of masculinity: being a responsible father, provider, and husband/partner [14, 32, 63]. These changes in notions of masculinity highlight the positive aspects of masculinity that can be the foundation for interventions to promote healthy behaviors, lifestyles, and outcomes [53, 65–68]. In sum, age-related dimensions of gendered behaviors also demonstrate how masculinities are related to leading causes of death among men at different ages.

From ages 15 to 44 years, the leading cause of death among men is unintentional injury, including accidental drug overdose, which remains a leading cause of death through age 64 years. Often in younger ages, these injuries and accidents are presumed to be the result of reckless and risky social behaviors, while in middle and older ages, it is presumed that these patterns are the result of work-related injuries.

Homicide is a leading cause of death for men only from ages 15 through age 44 years, while suicide remains a top 4 leading cause of death from ages 15 to 54 years (and drops to 8th in the 55–64-year age range). Heart disease and cancer are the leading causes of death for men age 45 years and older. For example, the risk of being diagnosed with and dying from cancer, diabetes, and heart disease increases with age [69, 70]. While men are diagnosed with hypertension at a higher rate than women until age 45 years, from ages 45 to 64 years, the percentages of men and women with hypertension are similar. After 65 years of age, women are diagnosed with hypertension at a higher rate than men [70]. These data emphasize the importance of incorporating a life course perspective in our explanations of men's health and men's health disparities [71–73].

Social Determinants of Masculinity and Men's Health

Understanding the poor health status of men includes considering how masculinities and gendered social determinants of health (e.g., social norms and expectations of biological males of a certain age) shape men's lives and experiences, particularly through economic and environmental factors [33, 74–76]. There is a tendency to blame men for their poor health behavior and not to consider the wider social and economic determinants of men's health or men's health behavior that we have included in research on racial disparities, SES inequalities, and women's health [77]. All men do not benefit equally from the social, economic, and political benefits of being a man; many men are marginalized by race, ethnicity, sexual orientation, and class and unable to achieve aspects of hegemonic masculinity that may be achieved by their peers of other socially defined groups [76]. Racism, segregation, economic discrimination, and other structural forces have limited the ways some men can define themselves in relation to hegemonic masculine norms (e.g., fulfilling the role of economic provider, moving their families into desirable housing and neighborhood conditions, and accumulating wealth to pass on to their children and grandchildren) [14, 32, 35, 44, 63, 78, 79].

Disproportionate poverty, likelihood of working in low-paying and dangerous occupations, residence in proximity to polluted environments, exposure to toxic substances, experiences of threats and realities of crime, as well as consistently worrying about meeting basic needs all differentially affect socially defined groups of men [24, 26]. Understanding the basis of poor status of men's health as well as premature death includes looking at multiple social determinants of health including poverty, poor educational opportunities, underemployment and unemployment, incarceration, and social and racial discrimination—all challenging and influencing poor men, African American men and Latin American men, and their capacity to achieve gendered goals and maintain good health [75].

The health and masculinities of African American, Asian American, and Latin American men are understudied [26, 75, 80], despite these men often accounting for much of the reported difference in mortality globally between men and women [5, 10]. The health and healthcare of African American men and Latin American men and other marginalized groups of men are overlooked, not prioritized, and not considered an area of focus in many countries [75]. While the health of these men is important, it is equally vital to focus on the unique challenges and needs of African American, Asian American, and Latin American men. Furthermore, despite the differences in masculinities and social determinants of health, it is noteworthy that all poor health behaviors are not worse in racial and ethnic minority groups of men when they are compared with white men [81].

How Do Men Conceptualize Health?

How men conceptualize masculinity is an important determinant of men's health-related decisions and is the strongest predictor of men's health behaviors [9, 82]. Men are often stereotyped as being unwilling to ask for help, support, and health-related services. While to some degree this may be true, this notion also is an over-simplification. It is not that men do not value their health or recognize the importance of health, but men often do not think about their health until poor health impairs some aspect of their lives (e.g., sexual relationships, employment, physical activity) or roles (e.g., provider, father, significant other) that is considered a higher priority because it is associated with notions of manhood and the way men are defined by their families, friends, and communities [63, 83, 84]. Some men may define health based on diagnoses of illnesses or biological and physiological processes; however, Robertson (2006) found that men's definitions of health may be influenced by their perceptions of what it means to be a man. In his study of how men negotiate hegemonic masculinity and health, Robertson (2006) found that men related their perceptions of health to their general lifestyle and well-being (e.g., drinking and eating in moderation), engagement in healthy behavior (e.g., regular physical activity, adequate sleep), and ability to fulfill socially important roles (e.g., provider, partner, father). Additionally, Ravenell and colleagues (2006) found that some men may define health broadly and in relation to other aspects of their lives that may have little to do directly with their own individual health. Some men have conceptualized being "healthy" as being able to fulfill social roles, such as holding a job, providing for family, protecting and teaching their children, and belonging to a social network [85]. Prioritizing success in fulfilling key social roles at the expense of one's health is consistent with various theories that link gender and health [13, 21, 35, 44, 84, 86].

Conclusion

Snow (2008) argues that it is the phenotype of sex, or whether a person is judged to look male or female by others, that triggers a variety of gendered social expectations, responsibilities, and obstacles whose importance and impact are shaped both by global and local forces; this gendered experience incurs health risks unrelated to chromosomal sex, genetics, or genomics. Masculinity has been linked to less social support, lower rates of medical help seeking, less frequent condom use, less social connection with other men, and more homophobia, alcohol/drug use, sexual partners, and cardiovascular stressors [21]. There is conflicting evidence regarding whether higher scores on masculinity confer health advantages or disadvantages, and more work is needed to tease out these factors [4].

Much in the same way that the sex genotype does not cause health outcomes linked to males [87], phenotypic (e.g., race, ethnicity), social (e.g., sexual orientation, social class, economic position), and cultural (e.g., religion, racial identity, ethnic identity, values) characteristics beyond sex are a necessary precondition for understanding men's health [25, 26]. The gendered expectations that are imposed on members of each sex are shaped by race, ethnicity, and other key social characteristics and identities. If we are to understand the sex and gender vulnerabilities of males, it is critical to consider how sex and gender intersect with other key factors to shape men's health outcomes [25, 26].

Health promotion interventions have remained focused on the aspects of identity that are most congruent with the disease epidemiology (i.e., we should focus on ethnic identity because people's health outcomes vary significantly by ethnicity), rather than considering personal characteristics that also may influence the behavior of interest (e.g., gender, age, religion) [88]. Research in health behavior has recognized that masculinity and other factors influence health behavior, but they have yet to be incorporated effectively to understand the multilevel factors that influence how and where we intervene to improve health behavior [26]. Masculinity is not something that simply resides in the minds of individual men; masculinity is learned, shaped, and reproduced through interpersonal relationships with other men and women and within various contexts such as neighborhoods, schools, and faith-based organizations [4]. Men's health behaviors are the product of their own thoughts about what it means to be a male and a man and how their social network, social norms, and larger cultural context consider these issues [4].

It is important to consider that health-promoting behavior can be a strategy men use to demonstrate their masculine identity that may increase their health risk and unhealthy behavior or health-promoting behaviors, particularly, as men age, may be a strategy men use to demonstrate age-appropriate masculinities [25]. It is critical for healthcare providers to ask men how they define their health and what their priorities and life goals are now and connect the medical information shared with them to these definitions and goals.

References

1. Williams DR. The health of men: structured inequalities and opportunities. Am J Public Health. 2003;93(5):724–31.
2. Thorpe Jr R, Wilson-Frederick S, Bowie J, Coa K, Clay O, Laveist T, et al. Health behaviors and all-cause mortality in African American men. Am J Mens Health. 2013;7(4 Suppl):8S–18S.

3. Robertson S. Theories of masculinities and health-seeking practices. "Nowhere Man" Men's Health Seminar. Belfast, Ireland: Nowhere Man Press; 2008.
4. Creighton G, Oliffe JL. Theorising masculinities and men's health: a brief history with a view to practice. Health Sociol Rev. 2010;19(4):409–18.
5. Courtenay WH. Constructions of masculinity and their influence on men's well-being: a theory of gender and health. Soc Sci Med. 2000;50(10):1385–401.
6. Courtenay WH. Key determinants of the health and well-being of men and boys. Int J Men's Health. 2003;2(1):1.
7. Griffith DM, Gunter K, Allen JO. Male gender role strain as a barrier to African American men's physical activity. Health Educ Behav. 2011;38(5):482–91.
8. Peterson A. Future research agenda in men's health. In: Tovey ABP, editor. Men's health: body, identity and social context. West Sussex: Wiley-Blackwell; 2009. p. 202–13.
9. Evans J, Frank B, Oliffe JL, Gregory D. Health, Illness, Men and Masculinities (HIMM): a theoretical framework for understanding men and their health. J Men's Health. 2011;8(1):7–15.
10. Courtenay W. A global perspective on the field of men's health: an editorial. Int J Mens Health. 2002;1(1):1.
11. Smiler A. Thirty years after the discovery of gender: psychological concepts and measures of masculinity. Sex Roles. 2004;50(1):15–26.
12. Moynihan C. Theories in health care and research: theories of masculinity. BMJ. 1998;317(7165):1072–5.
13. Robertson S. 'I've been like a coiled spring this last week': embodied masculinity and health. Sociol Health Illn. 2006;28(4):433–56.
14. Bruce MA, Roscigno VJ, McCall PL. Structure, context, and agency in the reproduction of black-on-black violence. Theor Criminol. 1998;2(1):29–55.
15. Kimmel MS, Hearn J, Connell R. Handbook of studies on men and masculinities. Thousand Oaks, CA: Sage; 2005.
16. Kimmel MS. The gendered society. New York, NY: Oxford University Press; 2000.
17. Coles T. Finding space in the field of masculinity. J Sociol. 2008;44(3):233–48.
18. Connell RW. Masculinities. Oxford: Polity; 1995.
19. Connell RW, Messerschmidt JW. Hegemonic masculinity: rethinking the concept. Gend Soc. 2005;19(6):829–59.
20. Broom A, Tovey P. Introduction: men's health in context. Men's health: body, identity, & social context. Chichester: Wiley-Blackwell; 2009. p. 1–5.
21. Robertson S. Understanding men and health: masculinities, identity, and well-being. Maidenhead: Open University Press; 2007.
22. Messerschmidt JW. Crime as structured action: doing masculinities, race, class, sexuality, and crime: Rowman & Littlefield; 2013.
23. Courtenay WH, Keeling RP. Men, gender, and health: toward an interdisciplinary approach. J Am Coll Health. 2000;48(6):243–6.
24. Sabo D. The study of masculinities and men's health: an overview. In: Kimmel M, Hearn J, Connell RW, editors. Handbook of studies on men and masculinities. Thousand Oaks, CA: Sage; 2005. p. 326–52.
25. Griffith DM. An intersectional approach to men's health. J Men's Health. 2012;9(2):106–12.
26. Griffith DM, Metzl JM, Gunter K. Considering intersections of race and gender in interventions that address U.S. men's health disparities. Public Health. 2011;125(7):417–23.
27. Carter R, Williams B, Juby H, Buckley T. Racial identity as mediator of the relationship between gender role conflict and severity of psychological symptoms in black, Latino, and Asian Men. Sex Roles. 2005;53(7):473–86.
28. Liu WM, Iwamoto DK. Asian American Men's Gender Role Conflict: The Role of Asian Values, Self-Esteem, and Psychological Distress. Psychol Men Masculinity. 2006;7(3):153–64.

29. Liu WM, Iwamoto DK. Conformity to masculine norms, Asian values, coping strategies, peer group influences and substance use among Asian American men. Psychol Men Masculinity. 2007;8(1):25–39.
30. Mahalik JR, Pierre MR, Wan SSC. Examining racial identity and masculinity as correlates of self-esteem and psychological distress in Black men. J Multicult Couns Dev. 2006;34(2):94–104.
31. Estrada F, Arciniega GM. Positive masculinity among Latino men and the direct and indirect effects on well-being. J Multicult Couns Dev. 2015;43(3):191–205.
32. Hammond WP, Mattis JS. Being a man about it: manhood meaning among African American men. Psychol Men Masculinity. 2005;6(2):114–26.
33. Griffith DM. I AM a Man: manhood, minority men's health and health equity. Ethn Dis. 2015;25(3):287–93.
34. Shek YL. Asian American masculinity: a review of the literature. J Men's Stud. 2007;14(3):379–91.
35. Griffith DM, Ellis KR, Allen JO. Intersectional approach to stress and coping among African American men: men's and women's perspectives. Am J Mens Health. 2013;7(4S):16–27.
36. Hurtado A, Sinha M. More than men: Latino feminist masculinities and intersectionality. Sex Roles. 2008;59(5-6):337–49.
37. Bowleg L, Teti M, Massie JS, Patel A, Malebranche DJ, Tschann JM. 'What does it take to be a man? What is a real man?': ideologies of masculinity and HIV sexual risk among Black heterosexual men. Cult Health Sex. 2011;13(5):545–59.
38. Crawford I, Allison K, Zamboni B, Soto T. The influence of dual-identity development on the psychosocial functioning of African-American gay and bisexual men. J Sex Res. 2002;39(3):179.
39. Halkitis P, Green K, Wilton L. Masculinity, body image, and sexual behavior in HIV-seropositive gay men: a two-phase formative behavioral investigation using the Internet. Int J Men's Health. 2004;3(1):27.
40. Halkitis PN, Moeller RW, DeRaleau LB. Steroid use in gay, bisexual, and nonidentified men-who-have-sex-with-men: relations to masculinity, physical, and mental health. Psychol Men Masculinity. 2008;9(2):106.
41. Vogel DL, Heimerdinger-Edwards SR, Hammer JH, Hubbard A. "Boys don't cry": examination of the links between endorsement of masculine norms, self-stigma, and help-seeking attitudes for men from diverse backgrounds. J Couns Psychol. 2011;58(3):368–82.
42. Meyer IH. Prejudice, social stress, and mental health in lesbian, gay, and bisexual populations: conceptual issues and research evidence. Psychol Bull. 2003;129(5):674.
43. Malebranche DJ, Fields EL, Bryant LO, Harper SR. Masculine socialization and sexual risk behaviors among black men who have sex with men. Men Masculinities. 2009;12(1):90–112.
44. Griffith DM, Gunter K, Watkins DC. Measuring masculinity in research on men of color: findings and future directions. Am J Public Health. 2012;102 Suppl 2:S187–94.
45. Loue S. Measures of sex, gender, gender role, and sexual orientation. Assessing race, ethnicity and gender in health. New York, NY: Springer; 2006. p. 136–51.
46. Thompson E, Pleck J, Ferrera D. Men and masculinities: scales for masculinity ideology and masculinity-related constructs. Sex Roles. 1992;27(11):573–607.
47. Levant RF. The male role: an investigation of contemporary norms. J Ment Health Couns. 1992;14(3):325.
48. Mahalik JR, Locke BD, Ludlow LH, Diemer MA, Scott RPJ, Gottfried M, et al. Development of the conformity to masculine norms inventory. Psychol Men Masculinity. 2003;4(1):3–25.
49. Hammond WP, Matthews D, Mohottige D, Agyemang A, Corbie-Smith G. Masculinity, medical mistrust, and preventive health services delays among community-dwelling African-American men. J Gen Intern Med. 2010;25(12):1300–8.
50. Levant R, Richmond K. A review of research on masculinity ideologies using the Male Role Norms Inventory. J Men's Stud. 2007;15(2):130.

51. Levant RF, Pollack WS, editors. A new psychology of men. New York, NY: Basic Books; 2003.
52. Eisler RM, Skidmore JR. Masculine gender role stress: scale development and component factors in the appraisal of stressful situations. Behav Mod. 1987;11:123–36.
53. Hammond WP, Matthews D, Corbie-Smith G. Psychosocial factors associated with routine health examination scheduling and receipt among African American men. J Natl Med Assoc. 2010;102(4):276.
54. O'Neil J, Helms B, Gable R, David L, Wrightsman L. Gender-role conflict scale: college men's fear of femininity. Sex Roles. 1986;14(5):335–50.
55. Levant RF, Wimer DJ. Masculinity constructs as protective buffers and risk factors for men's health. Am J Men's Health. 2014;8(2):110–20. doi:10.1177/1557988313494408.
56. Levant RF, Wimer DJ, Williams CM. An evaluation of the Health Behavior Inventory-20 (HBI-20) and its relationships to masculinity and attitudes towards seeking psychological help among college men. Psychol Men Masculinity. 2011;12(1):26.
57. Gordon DM, Hawes SW, Reid AE, Callands TA, Magriples U, Divney A, et al. The many faces of manhood examining masculine norms and health behaviors of young fathers across race. Am J Men's Health. 2013;7(5):394–401. doi:10.1177/1557988313476540.
58. Jones D. A WEIRD view of human nature skews psychologists' studies. Science. 2010;328(5986):1627.
59. Estrada F, Rigali-Oiler M, Arciniega GM, Tracey TJG. Machismo and Mexican American men: an empirical understanding using a gay sample. J Couns Psychol. 2011;58(3):358–67.
60. Arciniega GM, Anderson TC, Tovar-Blank ZG, Tracey TJG. Toward a fuller conception of machismo: development of a traditional machismo and caballerismo scale. J Couns Psychol. 2008;55(1):19.
61. Bruce MA, Griffith DM, Thorpe Jr RJ. Stress and the kidney. Adv Chronic Kidney Dis. 2015;22(1):46–53.
62. Whitehead TL. Urban low-income African American men, HIV/AIDS, and gender identity. Med Anthropol Q. 1997;11(4):411–47.
63. Bowman PJ. Research perspectives on Black men: role strain and adaptation across the adult life cycle. In: Jones RL, editor. Black Adult Development and Aging. Berkeley, CA: Cobb & Henry Publishers; 1989. p. 117–50.
64. Erickson EH. Identity and the life cycle. New York, NY: Norton; 1980.
65. Addis ME, Mahalik JR. Men, masculinity, and the contexts of help seeking. Am Psychol. 2003;58(1):5–14.
66. Galdas PM, Cheater F, Marshall P. Men and health help-seeking behaviour: literature review. J Adv Nurs. 2005;49(6):616–23.
67. Griffith DM, Allen JO, Gunter K. Social and cultural factors that influence African American men's medical help-seeking. Res Soc Work Pract. 2011;21(3):337–47.
68. Neighbors HW, Jackson JS. The use of informal and formal help: four patterns of illness behavior in the black community. Am J Community Psychol. 1984;12(6):629–44.
69. Society AC. Cancer Facts and Figures 2013. Atlanta: American Cancer Society, 2013.
70. Go AS, Mozaffarian D, Roger VL, Benjamin EJ, Berry JD, Borden WB, et al. Heart Disease and Stroke Statistics—2013 update: a report from the American Heart Association. Circulation. 2013;127(1):e6–e245.
71. Thorpe Jr RJ, Kelley-Moore J. Life course theories of race disparities: a comparison of cumulative dis/advantage perspective and the Weathering Hypothesis. In: LaVeist TA, Isaac LA, editors. Race, ethnicity, and health. 2nd ed. San Francisco, CA: Jossey-Bass; 2013. p. 355–74.
72. Thorpe RJ, Richard P, Bowie J, Laveist T, Gaskin D. Economic burden of men's health disparities in the United States. Int J Men's Health. 2013;12(3):195–212.
73. Thorpe Jr RJ, Duru K, Hill C. Advancing racial/ethnic minority men's health using a life course approach. Ethn Dis. 2015;25(3):241–4.
74. Young AMW. Poverty and men's health: global implications for policy and practice. J Men's Health. 2009;6(3):272.

75. Treadwell H, Braithwaite K. Men's health: a myth or a possibility? J Mens Health Gend. 2005;2(3):382–6.
76. Pease B. Racialised masculinities and the health of immigrant and refugee men. In: Broom A, Toveye P, editors. Men's health: body, identity and context. Chichester: Wiley; 2009. p. 182–201.
77. Crawshaw P. Critical perspectives on the health of men: lessons from medical sociology. Crit Public Health. 2009;19(3):279–85.
78. Griffith DM, Johnson JL. Implications of racism for African American men's cancer risk, morbidity and mortality. In: Treadwell HM, Xanthos C, Holden KB, Braithwaite RL, editors. Social determinants of health among African American men. New York, NY: Jossey-Bass; 2013. p. 21–38.
79. Summers MA. Manliness and its discontents: the black middle-class and the transformation of masculinity, 1900–1930. Chapel Hill, NC: University of North Carolina Press; 2004.
80. Treadwell HM, Ro M. Poverty, race, and the invisible men. Am J Public Health. 2003;93:705–7.
81. Warner DF, Hayward MD. Early-life origins of the race gap in men's mortality. J Health Soc Behav. 2006;47(3):209–26.
82. Garfield CF, Isacco A, Rogers TE. A review of men's health and masculinity. Am J Lifestyle Med. 2008;2(6):474–87.
83. Bowman PJ. Role strain and adaptation issues in the strength-based model: diversity, multi-level, and life-span considerations. Couns Psychol. 2006;34(1):118–33.
84. Bird CE, Rieker PP. Gender and health the effects of constrained choices and social policies Cambridge. New York, NY: Cambridge University Press; 2008. Available from: http://search.ebscohost.com/login.aspx?direct=true&scope=site&db=nlebk&db=nlabk&AN=221290.
85. Ravenell JE, Johnson WE, Whitaker EE. African American men's perceptions of health: a focus group study. J Natl Med Assoc. 2006;98:544–50.
86. James SA, Hartnett SA, Kalsbeek WD. John Henryism and blood pressure differences among black men. J Behav Med. 1983;6(3):259–78.
87. Snow RC. Sex, gender, and vulnerability. Glob Public Health. 2008;3 Suppl 1:58–74.
88. Griffith DM, Thorpe Jr RJ. Men's physical health and health behaviors. In: Wester SR, Joel Wong Y, editors. APA handbook on the psychology of men and masculinities. Washington, DC: American Psychological Association; 2015:709–730.

Chapter 3
Health-Seeking Behavior and Meeting the Needs of the Most Vulnerable Men

Keon L. Gilbert, Keith Elder, and Roland J. Thorpe Jr.

Introduction

Men seek and ask for help in many different ways compared to women when it comes to their health. It has been well documented that men are less likely to have a usual source of healthcare and are less likely to utilize healthcare services, even when they have access to these services. For minority men (African American, Hispanic, and Latino), these healthcare-seeking behaviors are worse and are often structured by socioeconomic factors, which increases their risk for morbidity and mortality from preventable diseases. Men who are missing from healthcare settings may avoid these settings because they do not acknowledge their risk for chronic diseases, may experience challenges with navigating through healthcare settings (e.g., making appointments, transportation issues), or have difficulties with establishing trusting relationships with their providers. For minority men, their engagement with healthcare settings may be further diminished as a result of

K.L. Gilbert, Dr. PH, MA, MPA (✉)
Department of Behavioral Sciences and Health Education, Salus Center, College
for Public Health and Social Justice, 3545 Lafayette Avenue, St. Louis, MO 63104, USA
e-mail: kgilber9@slu.edu

K. Elder, PhD, MPH, MPA
Department of Health Management and Policy, College for Public Health and Social Justice,
Saint Louis University, 3545 Lafayette Avenue, Room 369, St. Louis, MO 63104, USA
e-mail: kelder2@slu.edu

R.J. Thorpe Jr., PhD
Department of Health, Behavior and Society, Program for Research on Men's Health,
Hopkins Center for Health Disparities Solutions, Johns Hopkins Bloomberg School
of Public Health, 624 N. Broadway, Suite 708, Baltimore, MD 21205, USA
e-mail: rthorpe@jhsph.edu

© Springer International Publishing Switzerland 2016
J.J. Heidelbaugh (ed.), *Men's Health in Primary Care*, Current Clinical Practice,
DOI 10.1007/978-3-319-26091-4_3

experiences of discrimination within these settings. Men who are engaged, have trusting relationships, and feel confident about managing their health are more likely to be adherent to treatment plans and exhibit positive health behaviors and health outcomes. To improve men's healthcare-seeking behaviors, researchers, practitioners, and clinicians will need to consider individual, economic, and social determinants of men's healthcare-seeking behaviors and relevant barriers toward improvement.

Men's health remains a relatively recent area of study compared to women's health in the United States (USA) and internationally [1–3]. Men's health has gathered momentum around the world since the late 1980s and early 1990s due to gaps in health status and health-seeking behavior between men and women. Men are more disconnected from healthcare compared to women. The W.K. Kellogg Foundation noted in the early 1990s "a growing concern, and now with alarm, the absence of men of all ages in the waiting rooms of clinics and other healthcare providers" [4]. From 1997 to 1998, doctor visits for annual examinations and preventive services were 100 % higher for women than for men [5]. This problem with men accessing healthcare has persisted decades later as men are 24 % less likely than women to have visited a doctor within the past year, but are 32 % more likely to be hospitalized [6]. However, minority men are least likely to access healthcare and their health outcomes are even more dire than their Caucasian counterparts [7]. African American (AA) men's health is considerably worse than other race-gender groups, with AA men disproportionately suffering from preventable diseases, being disproportionately disabled by them, and suffering disproportionately higher mortality, relative to European American (EA) men [1].

Research suggests that male gender socialization teaches men that they are invulnerable to illness or that asking for help, such as for medical problems, is a sign of weakness and continues to persist, particularly in AA men [8–10]. Avoidance of healthcare providers by men has been offered as a partial explanation for the increased mortality rates from several chronic diseases and the persistent disparities that have been observed in hypertension, heart disease, diabetes, and lung, colorectal, and prostate cancers when compared to Caucasian men [10–13]. Disparities in healthcare and health outcomes have been identified across race/ethnicity with minority men faring the worst on many health outcomes [14–16]. Overall, minorities are less likely to participate during the medical encounter and AA and Hispanic men are less likely to self-advocate during the medical encounter [17, 18]. Furthermore, AA and Hispanic men are less likely than Caucasian men to effectively manage their chronic condition [19–21]. AA men also have a shorter life span than any other group in the USA [11]. The Affordable Care Act (ACA) lays the foundation for a partnership with patients as health outcomes are linked to physician payment [22]. In particular, the ACA encourages shared decision which is associated with better health outcomes [23–26]. The literature shows that overall the health of AA, Hispanic, and Latino men lags behind that of Caucasian men and AA men's health is at a crisis point due to the disparate burden of the diseases.

Root Causes of Disparities in Healthcare

The collective experiences of AA men appear to be distinctive from Caucasian men and AA women—this is partly attributable to race- and gender-based differences in economic and social life, health burden, and experiences of inequity in the healthcare system—which could impact AA men's healthcare utilization and perceptions of healthcare [27–30]. In addition, studies have shown various barriers to improving men's health behaviors [31]. Men often express fear of diagnosis, stress and role strain, lack of awareness and access to good information (from self and peers), medical mistrust, and relationships with healthcare providers [32]. One factor that promotes use of preventative health services is having a usual source of care, which can improve routine screening and care. As a result of many men in the USA lacking insurance, they are less likely than women to have a usual provider and usual source of care.

An Institute of Medicine (IOM) report described how the social hierarchy that exists in the USA plays an important role in explaining differences in the quality of care provided to minorities [33]. These differences occur in the context of historical and contemporary social inequities; are impacted by a variety of sources, including conscious or unconscious stereotyping; and are not explained by racial and ethnic differences in treatment refusal rates [33]. How people of different racial, ethnic, cultural, and gender groups are perceived remains part of a growing body of literature focusing on racism and bias within public health and healthcare [34–36]. That is, healthcare organizations are beholden to societal institutions and forces through funding streams, government mandates, and the practices of individual staff members [37–39]. For example, public health departments are constrained by government bodies that confer legal authorization to function and that provide their funding. Funders of health can structure the values and operating principles by which staff are evaluated and promoted which may influence the quality of care delivered and the resulting health outcomes of patients in those facilities. At the same time, as the conduits to resources and providers of critical services, health departments can have the capacity to control AA communities' power, agency, and ability to access resources and services [39–41]. Hence, an essential starting point for appreciating the complexity of institutional racism in today's healthcare system is to recognize the existence of inequities in the delivery and quality of healthcare [42].

Navigating Healthcare Systems

Racial disparities in quality of healthcare may involve one or more of several factors. Possible explanations include organizational factors within facilities and health plans or systems, including complex appointment or referral systems or long waiting times, simple lack of providers within any reasonable traveling distance or time, and poor understanding of how best to mobilize local community organizations that principally serve African American residents. Other matters, such as the racial and ethnic concordance (or lack thereof) between patients and clinicians, may have effects on patient care-seeking behaviors or satisfaction with care (101–104). Moreover, cognitive and decision-making processes may differ by culture and ethnic group, meaning that choices and preferences may not be mutually understood or acted upon [43]. Research has also demonstrated that poor health literacy may be a key intermediate variable, since poor health literacy is differentially distributed among racial and ethnic groups and is associated with difficulty obtaining appropriate care [33, 44].

Health-Seeking Behaviors and Barriers

When men do not seek help, or healthcare, they can burden the healthcare system [45]. There are many factors that contribute to men's health-seeking behaviors that are shaped by male socialization and the lack of socializing males to and within the healthcare system. Many men exhibit treatment fears and help-seeking stigma that are fueled by psychological factors such as restricted emotional expression and not expressing negative emotions [45–47]. There are four central areas related to men and healthcare-seeking behaviors: access, awareness of their health needs, inability to express their emotions, and lack of social networks [45]. Our focus is largely on health behaviors here. Health behavior is a function of health status [48]; hence, it is important to understand the health beliefs and behaviors of men across race and ethnicity in order to improve their health outcomes.

For example, abuse of alcohol and illegal drugs is more common among men than women, and research has demonstrated that alcohol use among various populations is associated with the presence of masculine attitudes [13, 49]. Substance abuse may occur as a response to stress, physiological addiction, difficult life circumstances, and other environmental factors [50]. These life challenges may be further magnified by the fact that men are socialized to value economic independence. Low-income men may be at increased risk for substance abuse because of the daily stresses they face and the socially sanctioned nature of substance use as a coping strategy for men. Men with limited educational and employment opportunities may turn to alcohol and other drugs as an escape from their inability to live up to one of the major tenets of male gender socialization in our society [51].

AA men in their middle-adult years often evaluate their sense of manhood against their ability to fulfill their roles as provider, husband, father, employee, and community member [46, 52, 53], and often to maintain this sense of manhood, many men engage in unhealthy behaviors. Avoidance of healthcare providers by men has been offered as a partial explanation for the increased mortality rates from heart disease among men [10, 12, 13]. However, what further complicates this story is socioeconomic position. Men in lower socioeconomic positions also may conform more to traditional male role norms, which allows them to diminish their vulnerabilities [54]. As noteworthy, trust appears to benefit men's health-seeking behavior and adherence to their treatment plans [55].

Mistrust of the healthcare system remains an important issue with men, particularly AA men in the southern US states, due to the history of unethical mistreatment and racial discrimination which at times were highly prevalent (e.g., Tuskegee syphilis experiment) [56]. Racial and ethnic minorities are more prone than Caucasians to distrust the healthcare establishment, and historically minority men have had less access to culturally competent providers [57–59]. Southern US AAs are more likely than Caucasians to report perceived racial barriers to care [60] and AA men are more likely than AA women to report perceived discrimination [61–65]. Perceived discrimination and mistreatment are associated with poorer medical adherence and delays in seeking healthcare [66–69]. In addition, higher levels of trust in the healthcare system are associated with better adherence to recommended care, greater patient satisfaction, and better outcomes [70–73].

Self-Management and Self-Advocacy

Self-management positively influences health outcomes by increasing persons' involvement in the control of their health conditions [74]. Negative emotional states, social factors, and chronic life stressors have been found to hinder men's ability to manage their health [75]. Additionally, there are significant racial/ethnic differences in perceived difficulty with self-care behaviors [76–78], which, for men, is significantly influenced by self-confidence [79]. Self-confidence refers to the belief that one is capable of performing those behaviors required to attain a certain outcome and could be applied specifically to beliefs about self-care behaviors [80]. Research has also found that men with high levels of self-confidence were able to engage in more health-promoting and health-monitoring behaviors. Confidence in self-management is influenced by patient empowerment [81]. Higher levels of self-confidence in men as measured by self-efficacy were associated with being more likely to report better medication adherence and hypertension control. Higher self-efficacy has been closely linked to active participation in cardiovascular disease risk-reduction strategies in minority populations [82], positive behavior change [83], patient empowerment [84], and chronic disease management. Men as patients can become empowered as they gain new knowledge about their health. This knowledge may come as a result of better relationships and communication with their providers and their own search for information. As men gain new knowledge, they may also acquire new skills and capacities to manage their chronic conditions which will make them co-participants in the healthcare encounter. As providers improve communication, build rapport, engage patients, and develop accountability systems to monitor patient outcomes, patients and providers will improve their relationships.

Another important factor to better manage and increase men's confidence to manage their health is involvement. The positive benefits of patient involvement extend beyond the medical encounter [23, 24, 26, 85–88]. Patients who are well informed are more capable of monitoring their health, coping with their illness, and adhering to treatment [89]. Self-advocacy extends beyond patient involvement; it encompasses gathering and using information to advance health [90]. Health information seeking has increased in the USA, and it is associated with patient empowerment, positive health management, patient follow-up, and patient treatment decision making [91, 92]. Rooks and colleagues found health information seeking was associated with changing approach to managing health and better understanding of how to treat illness [93]. However, studies have found racial and ethnic minority men are less likely to use the health information sought during the medical encounter [18, 94].

Health information is an important factor contributing to the poor health status of the most vulnerable men; however, access to culturally appropriate information is important as well (NCI 2006). Possible explanations for poor access to culturally appropriate health information include organizational factors within facilities and health plans or systems, including complex appointment or referral systems or long waiting times, simple lack of providers within any reasonable traveling distance or time, and poor understanding of how best to mobilize local community organizations that principally serve African Americans. Other matters, such as the racial and ethnic concordance (or lack thereof) between patients and clinicians, may have effects on patient care-seeking behaviors or satisfaction with care [95–98].

Literacy levels of men remain a significant predictor in determining how appropriate health information is for AA men and other high-risk men to improve patient awareness of diseases and treatments [99]. AA men obtain health information using the Internet, television, and print media such as magazines, pamphlets, and books [100] and prefer to receive health messages from effective speakers who embody characteristics they can model such as clergies, community leaders, active community members, and health professionals [101]. As a result, studies have found that identifying and developing culturally appropriate health promotion messages for AA men would be beneficial toward improving the health outcomes of African American men [99–102].

Next Steps to Improve Health-Seeking Behavior

Improving the health-seeking behavior of the most vulnerable men will require a comprehensive approach. Traditionally, patients with multiple comorbidities are identified as complex patients [103–114]; however, this definition might be too restrictive [115]. Safford and colleagues [115] contend that complexity extends beyond having multiple comorbidities, proposing that it includes socioeconomic, behavioral, cultural, and environmental factors [115]. Safford and colleagues propose that patient complexity is a function of "the interactions between biological, cultural, environmental, socioeconomic, and behavioral forces" (Vector Model of Complexity). The health-seeking behavior of men is complex, and if healthcare providers address only one facet, as we have seen, the result is likely to be less than optimal for men [116]. Thus, to improve health-seeking behavior of men and the most vulnerable men (minority), one must address all the vectors that impact health-seeking behavior in men and how men interface with the healthcare system. The aforementioned remains somewhat difficult because men's health remains under-studied and systematically underfunded. However, the Patient Protection and Affordable Care Act (ACA) is a step in the right direction in addressing men's health. The ACA emphasizes preventive care and population health partnered with primary health. This type of partnership is absolutely necessary to improve health-seeking behavior in men as it addresses matters outside of the medical encounter that challenge health-seeking behavior for men. Lastly, one of the critical inclusions in the ACA is the role of accountability for physicians. With increased accountability and monitoring of patient outcomes, we will expect that we will see an increase in men's use of preventive healthcare services, as well as their engagement in the healthcare system in meaningful ways that will reduce their burden of disease and minimize costs to the healthcare system.

References

1. Rich J, Ro M. A poor man's plight: uncovering the disparity in men's health. Battle Creek, MI: Kellogg Foundation; 2002.
2. Sabo D. Understanding men's health: a relational and gender sensitive approach. Cambridge, MA: Harvard Center for Populations and Development Studies; 1999.
3. Yamey G. Health minister announces initiatives on men's health. BMJ. 2000;320(7240):961.
4. W.K. Kellogg Foundation. What about men? Exploring the inequities in minority men's health. Battle Creek, MI: W.K. Kellogg Foundation; 2002.
5. National Center for Health Statistics. Utilization of Ambulatory Medical Care by Women: United States, 1997–98. Hyattsville, MD; 2001.
6. Agency for Healthcare Research and Policy. Health Men. www.ahrq.gov/patients-consumers/patientinvolvement/health-men/index.html. Accessed November 1, 2015.
7. National Center for Health Statistics. Health, United States, 2013: With Special Feature on Prescription Drugs. Hyattsville, MD; 2014.
8. Griffith DM, Gunter K, Allen JO. Male gender role strain as a barrier to African American men's physical activity. Health Educ Behav. 2011. doi:10.1177/1090198110383660.
9. Ornelas IJ, Amell J, Tran AN, Royster M, Armstrong-Brown J, Eng E. Understanding African American men's perceptions of racism, male gender socialization, and social capital through photovoice. Qual Health Res. 2009;19(4):552–65. doi:10.1177/1049732309332104.
10. Nicholas DR. Men, masculinity, and cancer: risk-factor behaviors, early detection, and psychosocial adaptation. J Am Coll Health. 2000;49(1):27–33.
11. Harvey IS, Alston RJ. Understanding preventive behaviors among mid-Western African-American men: a pilot qualitative study of prostate screening. J Men's Health. 2011;8(2):140–51.
12. Staples R. Health among African American males. In: Sabo D, Gordon F, editors. Men's health and illness: gender, power and the body. Thousand Oaks, CA: Sage; 1995. p. 121–38.
13. Helgeson VS. Masculinity, men's roles, and coronary heart disease. In: Sabo D, Gordon F, editors. Men's health and illness: gender, power and the body. Thousand Oaks, CA: Sage; 1995. p. 68–104.

14. Adler NE, Rehkopf DH. US disparities in health: descriptions, causes, and mechanisms. Annu Rev Public Health. 2008;29:235–52.
15. Satcher D. Our commitment to eliminate racial and ethnic health disparities. Yale J Health Poliy Law Ethics. 2001;1:1.
16. Williams DR. Adult health status: patterns, paradoxes, and prospects. America becoming: racial trends and their consequences, vol. 2; 2001. p. 371.
17. Cooper-Patrick L, Gallo JJ, Gonzales JJ, Vu HT, Powe NR, Nelson C, Ford DE. Race, gender, and partnership in the patient-physician relationship. JAMA. 1999;282(6):583–9. doi:10.1001/jama.282.6.583.
18. Elder KT, Wiltshire JC, McRoy L, Campbell D, Gary LC, Safford M. Men and differences by racial/ethnic group in self advocacy during the medical encounter. J Mens Health. 2010;7(2):135–44.
19. Lorig KR, Ritter PL, Jacquez A. Outcomes of border health Spanish/English chronic disease self-management programs. Diabetes Educ. 2005;31(3):401–9.
20. Lorig KR, Ritter PL, Laurent DD, Plant K. Internet-based chronic disease self-management: a randomized trial. Med Care. 2006;44(11):964–71. doi:10.1097/01.mlr.0000233678.80203.c1.
21. Utz SW, Steeves RH, Wenzel J, Ivora Hinton P, Jones RA, Andrews D, Muphy A, Oliver MN. "Working hard with it": self-management of type 2 diabetes by rural African Americans. Fam Community Health. 2006;29(3):195–205.
22. Internal Revenue Service, Department of the Treasury, Employee Benefits Security Administration, Department of Labor, Centers for Medicare Medicaid Services, Department of Health. Coverage of certain preventive services under the Affordable Care Act. Final rules. Fed Regist 2013; 78(127): 39869–99.
23. Kaplan SH, Gandek B, Greenfield S, Rogers W, Ware JE. Patient and visit characteristics related to physicians' participatory decision-making style. Results from the Medical Outcomes Study. Med Care. 1995;33(12):1176–87.
24. Kaplan SH, Greenfield S, Ware Jr JE. Assessing the effects of physician-patient interactions on the outcomes of chronic disease. Med Care. 1989;27(3 Suppl):S110–127.
25. Oshima Lee E, Emanuel EJ. Shared decision making to improve care and reduce costs. N Engl J Med. 2013;368(1):6–8. doi:10.1056/NEJMp1209500.
26. Sherbourne CD, Hays RD, Ordway L, DiMatteo MR, Kravitz RL. Antecedents of adherence to medical recommendations: results from the Medical Outcomes Study. J Behav Med. 1992;15(5):447–68.
27. Carpenter WR, Godley PA, Clark JA, Talcott JA, Finnegan T, Mishel M, Bensen J, Rayford W, Su LJ, Fontham ETH. Racial differences in trust and regular source of patient care and the implications for prostate cancer screening use. Cancer. 2009;115(21):5048–59.
28. Musa D, Schulz R, Harris R, Silverman M, Thomas SB. Trust in the health care system and the use of preventive health services by older black and white adults. Am J Public Health. 2009;99(7):1293–9.
29. Williams DR. The health of men: structured inequalities and opportunities. Am J Public Health. 2003;93(5):724–31.
30. Williams DR, Mohammed SA. Discrimination and racial disparities in health: evidence and needed research. J Behav Med. 2009;32(1):20–47.
31. Cheatham C, Barksdale D, Rogers S. Barriers to health care and health seeking behaviors faced by Black men. J Am Acad Nurse Pract. 2008;20(11):555–63.
32. Griffith DM, Mason M, Yonas M, Eng E, Jeffries V, Plihcik S, Parks B. Dismantling institutional racism: theory and action. Am J Community Psychol. 2007;39(3):381–92.
33. Smedley BD, Stith AY, Nelson AR. Unequal treatment: confronting racial and ethnic disparities in healthcare. Washington, DC: National Academies Press; 2002.
34. Ford CL, Airhihenbuwa CO. The public health critical race methodology: Praxis for antiracism research. Soc Sci Med. 2010;71:1390–8. doi:10.1016/j.socscimed.2010.07.030.
35. Jones CP. Levels of racism: a theoretic framework and a Gardener's Tale. Am J Public Health. 2000;90(8):1212–5. doi:10.2105/AJPH.90.8.1212.

36. Jones CP, Truman BI, Elam-evans LD, Jones CA, Jones CY, Jiles R, Rumisha SF, Perry GS. Using "socially assigned race" to probe white advantages in health status. Ethn Dis. 2008;18:496–504.
37. Trubek LG, Das M. Achieving equality: healthcare governance in transition. Am J Law Med. 2003;29:395–421.
38. Byrd WM, Clayton LA. Race, medicine, and health care in the United States: a historical survey. J Natl Med Assoc. 2001;93(3 Suppl):11S–34S.
39. Dreachslin JL, Weech-Maldonado R, Dansky KH. Racial and ethnic diversity and organizational behavior: a focused research agenda for health services management. Soc Sci Med. 2004;59(5):961–71.
40. Morgan G. Images of organization. 2nd ed. Thousand Oaks, CA: Sage Publications; 1997.
41. Boyd NM, Angelique H. Rekindling the discourse: organizational studies in community psychology. J Community Psychol. 2002;30:325–48.
42. Sullivan LW. Missing persons: minorities in the health professions, a report of the Sullivan Commission on Diversity in the Healthcare Workforce. 2004.
43. Hiatt RA, Rimer BK. A new strategy for cancer control research. Cancer Epidemiol Biomarkers Prev. 1999;8:957–64.
44. Pignone M, DeWalt DA, Sheridan S, et al. Interventions to improve health outcomes for patients with low literacy. A systematic review. J Gen Intern Med. 2005;20(2):185–92.
45. White A, Banks I. Men and help seeking. In: Kirby RS, Carson CCI, White A, Kirby M, editors. Men's health. 3rd ed. New York, NY: Taylor & Francis Group; 2009. p. 505–14.
46. Hammond WP, Mattis JS. Being a man about it: manhood meaning among African American men. Psychol Men Masculinity. 2005;6(2):114–26. doi:10.1037/1524-9220.6.2.114.
47. White A. Men's health in the 21st century. Int J Men's Health. 2006. doi:10.3149/jmh.0501.1.
48. Brown LJ, Bond MJ. An examination of the influences on health-protective behaviours among Australian men. Int J Men's Health. 2008;7(3):274–87.
49. Lemle R, Mishkin ME. Alcohol and masculinity. J Subst Abuse Drugs. 1989;6(4):213–22.
50. Chaffin M, Kelleher K, Hollenberg J. Onset of physical abuse and neglect: psychiatric substance abuse and social risk factors from prospective community data. Child Abuse Neglect. 1996;20:191–203.
51. Batholomew LK, Parcel GS, Kok G, Gottlieb NH. Intervention mapping: designing theory and evidence based health promotion programs. Mountain View, CA: Mayfield Publishing; 2001.
52. Ray R. The professional allowance: how socioeconomic characteristics allow some men to fulfill family role expectations better than other men. Int J Sociol Fam (Spl Iss Intersectionality). 2008;34(2):327–51.
53. Bowman PJ. Research perspectives on Black men: role strain and adaptation across the Black adult male life cycle. In: Jones R, editor. Black adult development and aging. Verkeley, CA: Cobb and Henry; 1989. p. 117–50.
54. Powell-Hammond W, Siddiqi AA. Social determinants of medical mistrust among African American men. In: Treadwell HM, Xantos C, Holden KB, editors. Social determinants of health among African American men. San Francisco, CA: Jossey Bass; 2013. p. 135–60.
55. Elder K, Ramamonjiarivelo Z. Wiltshire J et al. Trust, medication adherence, and hypertension control in Southern African American men. 2012;102(12):2242–5.
56. Gamble VN. Under the shadow of Tuskegee: African Americans and Health Care. Am J Public Health. 1997;87:1773–8.
57. Boulware LE, Cooper LA, Ratner LE, LaVeist TA, Powe NR. Race and trust in the health care system. Public Health Rep. 2003;118(4):358–65.
58. Corbie-Smith G, Thomas SB, St George DM. Distrust, race, and research. Arch Intern Med. 2002;162(21):2458–63.
59. McGary H. Distrust, social justice, and health care. Mt Sinai J Med. 1999;66(4):236–40.
60. Fowler-Brown A, Ashkin E, Corbie-Smith G, Thaker S, Pathman DE. Perception of racial barriers to health care in the rural South. J Health Care Poor Underserved. 2006;17(1):86–100.

61. Banks KH, Kohn-Wood LP, Spencer M. An examination of the African American experience of everyday discrimination and symptoms of psychological distress. Community Ment Health J. 2006;42(6):555–70.
62. Dion KL. The social psychology of perceived prejudice and discrimination. Can Psychol. 2001;43:1–10.
63. Harrell JP, Merritt M, Kalu J. Racism and mental health. In: Jones RL, editor. Hampton, VA: Cobb and Henry; 1998. p. 247–80.
64. Krieger N. Embodying inequality: a review of concepts, measures, and methods for studying health consequences of discrimination. Int J Health Serv. 1999;29(2):295–352.
65. Williams DR, Williams-Morris R. Racism and mental health: the African American experience. Ethn Health. 2000;5(3–4):243–68.
66. Casagrande SS, Gary TL, LaVeist TA, Gaskin DJ, Cooper LA. Perceived discrimination and adherence to medical care in a racially integrated community. J Gen Intern Med. 2007; 22(3):389–95.
67. Corbie-Smith G, Thomas SB, Williams MV, Moody-Ayers S. Attitudes and beliefs of African Americans toward participation in medical research. J Gen Intern Med. 1999;14(9):537–46.
68. LaVeist TA, Nickerson KJ, Bowie JV. Attitudes about racism, medical mistrust, and satisfaction with care among African American and white cardiac patients. Med Care Res Rev. 2000;57 Suppl 1:146–61.
69. Nickerson KJ, Helms JE, Terrell F. Cultural mistrust, opinions about mental illness, and black students' attitudes toward seeking psychological help from white counselors. J Couns Psychol. 1994;41(3):378–85.
70. Mechanic D. Managed care, rationing, and trust in medical care. J Urban Health. 1998;75(1): 118–22.
71. Mechanic D, Schlesinger M. The impact of managed care on patients' trust in medical care and their physicians. JAMA. 1996;275(21):1693–7.
72. Safran DG, Taira DA, Rogers WH, Kosinski M, Ware JE, Tarlov AR. Linking primary care performance to outcomes of care. J Fam Pract. 1998;47(3):213–20.
73. Thom DH, Ribisl KM, Stewart AL, Luke DA. Further validation and reliability testing of the Trust in Physician Scale. The Stanford Trust Study Physicians. Med Care. 1999;37(5): 510–7.
74. Chen Y, Zhang X, Hu X, Deng Y, Chen J, Li S, Zhang C, Wang J, Liu Z, Hao Y. The potential role of a self-management intervention for benign prostate hyperplasia. Urology. 2012.
75. Brown CT, Emberton M. Self-management for men with lower urinary tract symptoms. Curr Prostate Rep. 2009;7(3):111–6.
76. Aguilar R. Men's health: managing type 2 diabetes in men. J Fam Pract. 2012;61(6):S16.
77. Liburd LC, Namageyo-Funa A, Jack Jr L. Understanding "masculinity" and the challenges of managing type-2 diabetes among African-American men. J Natl Med Assoc. 2007;99(5):550.
78. Misra R, Lager J. Ethnic and gender differences in psychosocial factors, glycemic control, and quality of life among adult type 2 diabetic patients. J Diabetes Complications. 2009;23(1):54–64.
79. Loeb SJ, Steffensmeier D, Kassab C. Predictors of self-efficacy and self-rated health for older male inmates. J Adv Nurs. 2011;67(4):811–20.
80. Joekes K, Van Elderen T, Schreurs K. Self-efficacy and overprotection are related to quality of life, psychological well-being and self-management in cardiac patients. J Health Psychol. 2007;12(1):4–16.
81. Williams K, Bond M. The roles of self-efficacy, outcome expectancies and social support in the self-care behaviours of diabetics. Psychol Health Med. 2002;7(2):127–41.
82. Olivarius NF, Beck-Nielsen H, Andreasen AH, Horder M, Pedersen PA. Randomised controlled trial of structured personal care of type 2 diabetes mellitus. Br Med J. 2001; 323(7319):970–5.
83. Cohen H, Britten N. Who decides about prostate cancer treatment? A qualitative study. Fam Pract. 2003;20(6):724–9.

84. Anderson RM, Funnell MM, Butler PM, Arnold MS, Fitzgerald JT, Feste CC. Patient empowerment. Results of a randomized controlled trial. Diabetes Care. 1995;18(7):943–9.
85. Barsky AJ, Kazis LE, Freiden RB, Goroll AH, Hatem CJ, Lawrence RS. Evaluating the interview in primary care medicine. Soc Sci Med Med Psychol Med Sociol. 1980;14A(6): 653–8.
86. Greenfield S, Kaplan S, Ware Jr JE. Expanding patient involvement in care. Effects on patient outcomes. Ann Intern Med. 1985;102(4):520–8.
87. Greenfield S, Kaplan SH, Ware Jr JE, Yano EM, Frank HJ. Patients' participation in medical care: effects on blood sugar control and quality of life in diabetes. J Gen Intern Med. 1988;3(5):448–57.
88. Stewart MA. Effective physician-patient communication and health outcomes: a review. CMAJ. 1995;152(9):1423–33.
89. Sanders Thompson VL, Talley M, Caito N, Kreuter M. African American men's perceptions of factors influencing health-information seeking. Am J Mens Health. 2009;3(1):6–15.
90. Vessey JA, Miola ES. Teaching adolescents self-advocacy skills. Pediatr Nurs. 1997; 23(1):53–6.
91. Bartlett YK, Coulson NS. An investigation into the empowerment effects of using online support groups and how this affects health professional/patient communication. Patient Educ Couns. 2011;83(1):113–9.
92. Tu HT, Cohen GR. Striking jump in consumers seeking health care information. Track Rep. 2008;20:1–8.
93. Rooks RN, Wiltshire JC, Elder K, BeLue R, Gary LC. Health information seeking and use outside of the medical encounter: is it associated with race and ethnicity? Soc Sci Med. 2012;74(2):176–84.
94. Wiltshire J, Cronin K, Sarto GE, Brown R. Self-advocacy during the medical encounter: use of health information and racial/ethnic differences. Med Care. 2006;44(2):100–9.
95. Mueller KJ, Ortega ST, Parker K, Askenazi PK. Health status and access to care among rural minorities. J Health Care Poor Underserved. 1999;10:230–49.
96. Eng E, Smith J. Natural helping functions of lay health advisors in breast cancer education. Breast Cancer Res Treat. 1995;35:23–9.
97. Earp JA, Eng E, O'Malley MS, Altpeter M, Rauscher G, Mayne L, Matthews HF, Lynch KS, Qaqish B. Increasing the use of mammography among older, rural African American women: results from a community trial. Am J Public Health. 2002;92(4):646–54.
98. Lopez E, Eng E, Robinson N, Wang C. Photovoice as a community based participatory research method. In: Israel B, Eng E, Schulz AJ, Parker D, editors. Methods in community based participatory research for health. San Francisco: Wiley; 2005. p. 326–48.
99. Bennett CL, Ferreira MR, Davis TC, Kaplan J, Weinberger M, Kuzel T, Seday MA, Sartor O. Relation between literacy, race, and state of presentation among low-income patients with prostate cancer. Journal of Clinical Oncology. 1998;16(9):3101–4.
100. Thompson Sanders V, Cavazos-Rehg P, Tate K, Gaier A. Health Education Research. Cancer information seeking among African Americans. J Cancer Educ. 2008;23:92–101.
101. Friedman DB, Thomas TL, Owens OL, Hebert JR. It takes two to talk about prostate cancer: a qualitative assessment of African American men's and women's cancer communication practices and recommendations. Am J Men's Health. 2012;6(6):472–84.
102. Griffith DM, Pichon LC, Campbell B, Allen JO. YOUR blessed health: a faith based CBPR approach to addressing HIV/AIDS among African Americans. AIDS Educ Prevent. 2010;22(3):203–17.
103. de Jonge P, Huyse FJ, Stiefel FC. Case and care complexity in the medically ill. Med Clin North Am. 2006;90(4):679–92.
104. Durso SC. Using clinical guidelines designed for older adults with diabetes mellitus and complex health status. JAMA. 2006;295(16):1935–40.
105. Elliott RA, Ross-Degnan D, Adams AS, Safran DG, Soumerai SB. Strategies for coping in a complex world: adherence behavior among older adults with chronic illness. J Gen Intern Med. 2007;22(6):805–10.

106. Francis CK. Hypertension, cardiac disease, and compliance in minority patients. Am J Med. 1991;91(1A):29S–36S.
107. Huyse FJ, Stiefel FC, de Jonge P. Identifiers, or "red flags," of complexity and need for integrated care. Med Clin North Am. 2006;90(4):703–12.
108. Kerr EA, Heisler M, Krein SL, Kabeto M, Langa KM, Weir D, Piette JD. Beyond comorbidity counts: how do comorbidity type and severity influence diabetes patients' treatment priorities and self-management? J Gen Intern Med. 2007;22(12):1635–40.
109. Lyketsos CG, Dunn G, Kaminsky MJ, Breakey WR. Medical comorbidity in psychiatric inpatients: relation to clinical outcomes and hospital length of stay. Psychosomatics. 2002;43(1):24–30.
110. Ofili E, Igho-Pemu P, Bransford T. The prevention of cardiovascular disease in blacks. Curr Opin Cardiol. 1999;14(2):169–75.
111. Shea S, Misra D, Ehrlich MH, Field L, Francis CK. Predisposing factors for severe, uncontrolled hypertension in an inner-city minority population. N Engl J Med. 1992;327(11): 776–81.
112. Textor SC. Managing renal arterial disease and hypertension. Curr Opin Cardiol. 2003;18(4):260–7.
113. Wolff JL, Starfield B, Anderson G. Prevalence, expenditures, and complications of multiple chronic conditions in the elderly. Arch Intern Med. 2002;162(20):2269–76.
114. Yates JW. Comorbidity considerations in geriatric oncology research. CA Cancer J Clin. 2001;51(6):329–36.
115. Safford MM, Allison JJ, Kiefe CI. Patient complexity: more than comorbidity. The vector model of complexity. J Gen Intern Med. 2007;22 Suppl 3:382–90.
116. Miller NH, Hill M, Kottke T, Ockene IS. The multilevel compliance challenge: recommendations for a call to action. A statement for healthcare professionals. Circulation. 1997;95(4): 1085–90.

Chapter 4
Providing Preventive Services to Men: A Substantial Challenge?

Masahito Jimbo

Introduction

When organizing preventive healthcare for men, primary care physicians face several challenges. First, many preventive care services are both time and labor intensive, adding stress and strain to the already sparse resources of physicians and their staff. Second, patients often bring multiple, competing agendas to the visit, adding even more time pressure to the provision of preventive services; it is in these visits that acute care often takes precedence over preventive care [1]. Third, many primary care practices do not possess an adequate system to ensure timely provision of preventive healthcare services and adequate follow-ups for abnormal and/or unexpected results to their patients. Lastly, general biopsychosocial characteristics of male patients may place them at a unique disadvantage compared to women and need to be considered.

This chapter seeks to address these various challenges in more detail. In particular, challenges unique to providing preventive healthcare to men will be highlighted. Subsequently, steps that should be taken in the ambulatory care setting to ensure that men are receiving the appropriate preventive care at the right intervals, and abnormal findings are followed up or referred expeditiously, will be discussed. Finally, methods in which practices may address the unique facilitators and barriers that male patients bring to their own healthcare will be proposed.

In this chapter, "men" are defined as adult males aged 18 years or older. The discussion of organizing preventive healthcare in men will be limited to within the ambulatory healthcare setting, including private physician offices and academic and community health centers. Community-targeted interventions requiring the

M. Jimbo, MD, PhD, MPH (✉)
Department of Family Medicine and Urology, University of Michigan,
1018 Fuller Street, Ann Arbor, MI 48104, USA
e-mail: mjimbo@med.umich.edu

© Springer International Publishing Switzerland 2016
J.J. Heidelbaugh (ed.), *Men's Health in Primary Care*, Current Clinical Practice,
DOI 10.1007/978-3-319-26091-4_4

participation of larger organizations, including commercial health plans and state and federal agencies, will be outside the scope of this chapter.

Challenges to Implementing Appropriate Preventive Healthcare

Substantial time and effort are required to provide adequate and appropriate preventive healthcare services. One study estimated that 7.4 h per work day would be required for physicians to implement all of the preventive services recommended by the United States Preventive Services Task Force (USPSTF) for their patients [2]. Obviously, this is a time allotment that primary care physicians simply do not have, especially with their responsibility to provide care for both acute and chronic illnesses, in addition to preventive care that includes behavioral and psychosocial counseling [1].

Most primary care offices lack systems to ensure timely implementation and follow-up of preventive healthcare for all patients. This is not surprising, since adequate provision of preventive healthcare requires multiple steps that include:

- Identifying specific preventive care measures recommended at the appropriate interval
- Notifying the patient of the recommended preventive care
- Scheduling the patient for the appropriate preventive care services, which may or may not require an office visit
- Ensuring that the patient followed up with the preventive care
- Obtaining the results from screening tests and determining their significance
- Notifying the patient of the results in a timely fashion

  - If normal, scheduling the patient for recommended preventive care at the next appropriate interval
  - If abnormal, arranging for appropriate follow-up and/or referral

- Ensuring that the patient followed through with the follow-up and/or referral
- Obtaining the results of the follow-up and/or referral
- Referring the patient for further testing and management if indicated

  This complex series of steps is further complicated by several factors including:

- Various recommended time intervals for different modalities of preventive care (e.g., blood pressure monitoring every 1–2 years vs. fasting lipid profile every 5 years)
- A varying time schedule for the same test depending upon a patient's risk (e.g., fasting lipid profile every 5 years for a patient with no risk of heart disease vs. annually for a diabetic patient)
- The multiple choice of tests with different time schedules and risk/benefit ratios for the same screening objective (e.g., annual fecal occult blood testing vs. colonoscopy every 10 years for colorectal cancer screening)

- Discussion of preventive healthcare services in a dedicated, scheduled health maintenance visit or opportunistically during an acute visit (e.g., offering tetanus prophylaxis to an overdue patient who came presented for an acute ankle sprain) [3]
- The dilemma of whether or not certain preventive healthcare options should be offered at all (e.g., digital rectal examination and prostate-specific antigen test for prostate cancer screening)

Unfortunately, considerable evidence exists from surveys of both patients and physicians demonstrating that physicians fall short of providing all of the necessary preventive care for their patients. In a population-based telephone survey of 13,275 adult patients and physicians in 12 metropolitan areas in the USA, only 54.9 % and 52.2 % reported receiving preventive healthcare and screening, respectively, determined by RAND's Quality Assessment Tools system [4]. In a self-report survey of 3881 primary care physicians randomly sampled from the professional associations representing family medicine, internal medicine, pediatrics, and obstetrics/gynecology, the percentage of physicians who provided adequate clinical preventive service (defined as providing the service to more than 80 % of their patients who were indicated to receive them) varied from 60.2 to 87.2 % for screening, 26.6–44.7 % for immunizations, and 21.3–47.7 % for counseling [5].

A recent review performed by the Centers for Disease Control and Prevention (CDC) showed little improvement in the provision of preventive services up to the year 2010, with 62.7 % of adults aged 18 years and over being screened for tobacco abuse, 64.5 % of adults aged 50–75 years being screened for colorectal cancer, and just 28 % of adults aged 18–64 years receiving seasonal influenza vaccine [6]. Even when the initial preventive service is implemented appropriately, one study found that fewer than 75 % of patients receive adequate follow-up care [7]. From the findings of these and other related studies, deficiencies in the provision of preventive care are classified predominantly as underutilization, although overutilization (e.g., performing screening testicular examination in asymptomatic men) and inappropriate utilization (e.g., performing a digital rectal examination to assess for fecal occult blood in lieu of three take-home fecal occult blood test cards [8]) could also occur.

The various reasons as to why clinical preventive services are not implemented as well as those for why they should be are both numerous and complex. Physicians may not adhere to recommended clinical practice guidelines due to lack of awareness, lack of familiarity, disagreement with the recommendation, lack of self-efficacy (e.g., belief that they could effectively perform the recommended service), lack of outcome expectancy (e.g., belief that the performance of the recommended service will lead to the desired outcome), inertia of previous practice, and external barriers including lack of adequate time, resources, and reimbursement [9]. A physician's level of experience may affect how much of the recommended guidelines he or she performs [10]. External barriers arising from the complexity of the healthcare delivery system, such as lack of continuity of care and breakdown in communication, may be bigger factors than the individual physician attributes [11]. The vagaries of each practice may be a particularly relevant issue in the USA, where preventive service delivery is dependent upon individual patient and physician interactions and not through centrally organized programs as seen in Europe and Japan, which increase the potential for variability in implementation and follow-up [12].

Challenges Unique to Men

Common issues regarding preventive healthcare have been shown to be both unique to male patients as well as more amplified. A survey by Sandman et al. determined that [13]:

- One of four men (24 %) did not see a physician within the past year, three times the rate found in women (8 %)
- 33 % of men do not have a definable "regular doctor," compared to 19 % of women
- 41 % of men did not receive preventive services in the past year, compared to 16 % of women

Other studies have also shown that men do not utilize preventive services as much as women. A recent review cited nine studies ranging in published year from 1989 to 2007 that showed men were less likely to endorse and engage in preventive services than women [14]. A Canadian study showed that men were less likely to be screened for colorectal cancer, diabetes, and hyperlipidemia compared to women [15].

Various adverse health outcomes that are more prevalent in men include [16, 17]:

- Higher mortality from heart disease
- Higher mortality from cancer
- Shorter average expectation of life
- Higher rates of injury and death from accidents, including industrial and motor vehicle injury
- Higher suicide rates
- Higher homicide rates
- Higher rates of smoking
- Higher rates of alcohol abuse
- Higher rates of substance abuse

More recent studies conducted in other countries in North America, Europe, and Asia confirm the poorer health outcomes among men [18–20]. The gender gap illustrated above is even greater among men aged below 30 years, men in minority groups, and men in lower socioeconomic class. Fortunately, this gender gap virtually disappears once men are aged 65 years or older.

It is important to note that not all gender differences are statistically disadvantageous to men. For example, more men have been found to exercise three or more days per week than women (51 % vs. 39 %, respectively) [17]. Provision of smoking cessation counseling (30 % men vs. 31 % women), diet (44 % vs. 49 %), exercise (46 % vs. 52 %), alcohol and illicit drug abuse (22 % vs. 24 %), safety (6 % vs. 9 %), and sexually transmitted infections (STIs) (14 % vs. 17 %) is unacceptably low for both men and women [17].

Some studies have looked at social and behavioral determinants that may lead to underutilization of preventive healthcare services by men. Frequently cited determinants include lack of knowledge, fear of finding a disease, lack of time, low perceived risk, and negative perceptions about the screening procedure such as pain, discomfort, and embarrassment [21, 22]. A feature unique to men is their concept of masculinity and how it negatively impacts health-seeking behavior. Men have reported that they may regard seeking healthcare as showing vulnerability, lacking self-reliance, and being feminine [23, 24]. In particular, screening procedures involving the rectum such as colonoscopy and the digital rectal examination are regarded as threats to their masculinity.

Adhering to Current Age- and Risk Factor-Appropriate Guidelines for Preventive Care in Men

Several conclusions may be drawn from the data trends regarding provision of preventive services to men. Many, if not most, primary care physicians' offices fall short of providing appropriate preventive care to all of their patients. Second, data supports the difficulty of organizing appropriate preventive care for all patients in primary care physicians' offices; the barriers include lack of adequate time during an office visit, complexity of the recommendations, complexity of the healthcare delivery system, and physician beliefs and behaviors. Third, men have health behavior characteristics that place them at an increased risk for morbidity and mortality from a variety of conditions, and their greater lack of adequate preventive care compounds the situation. Lastly, organizing preventive care for men in the physician's practice will entail organizing the care for all patients in the practice.

Recent evidence from the literature supports a set of preventive services tailored to an individual's age, gender, and risk factors, rather than a one-size-fits-all battery of examinations and screening tests [25, 26]. With this in mind, one of the challenges toward implementing appropriate preventive care is the seemingly constant changes in guidelines. Fortunately the USPSTF, considered by many primary healthcare professionals to be the most authoritative of the guidelines for preventive services, has a Web site that is frequently updated with the most current evidence-based recommendations [25]. Other organizations that have Web sites that are regularly updated for provision of preventive services include the American Academy of Family Physicians (AAFP) [27] and the National Guideline Clearinghouse (NGC) [28]. A particularly useful Web site for vaccination recommendation updates is that of the CDC, which highlights the updated immunization guidelines from the Advisory Committee on Immunization Practices (ACIP) [29].

Implementing Preventive Healthcare Services for Men in the Office

Many studies have been performed with the outcome goal of finding ways to improve the rate of providing preventive healthcare in the ambulatory care setting. Extrapolation of data from these study findings to design an effective strategy for other physician practices has been difficult to interpret. One reason is that the complexity of each practice creates unique barriers that defy straightforward implementation of tools, even if they showed efficacy in other settings [30, 31]. Another reason is that many successful studies rely on external assistance through funding during the course of the research project, and once the study ends and the funded external assistance is removed, the implemented systems tend to disappear [32].

Nevertheless, several excellent reviews have arrived at similar conclusions in terms of effective interventions in the delivery of preventive healthcare services [33–36]. Patient and physician reminder systems have been shown to be effective tools. While these reminders do not need to be electronic, computer-generated prompting and reminding has the advantage of both efficiency and responsiveness [37, 38]. The availability of a complete electronic health record (EHR) system has the additional benefit of a lower incidence of missing clinical information relevant to patient care [39]. However, overall results are mixed on the performance of EHR on improving preventive healthcare outcomes. EHRs may better capture services not captured by medical claims in patients intermittently covered by health insurance [40].

EHRs with clinical decision support system (CDSS) have led to modest improvements in actual provision of preventive care, such as screening for abdominal aortic aneurysm [41]. EHRs that combined point-of-care recommendations, disease registry capabilities, and continuous performance feedback for physicians have led to modest increases in completion of a variety of preventive care services [42]. However, while a systematic review of electronic CDSS in primary care practices noted small improvements in processes of care, the authors noted that "there is wide variation and interpretation in CDSS implementation, and most studies can truly speak only to the effectiveness of a particular CDSS product used in a particular setting" [43, 44]. Use of the copy-and-paste practice in EHRs may lead to documentation of activities that did not occur, such as lifestyle counseling in diabetics, leading to spuriously low effectiveness of preventive care services [45].

A number of studies have assessed interventions targeting men to improve preventive care. However, the vast majority of these dealt with sex-specific issues (e.g., prostate cancer screening, testicular cancer screening) and did not address the social and behavioral attributes more prevalent in men to guide the intervention. Indeed, the authors in a 2008 review concluded that they cannot say targeting men works better than improving the delivery of the clinical service to both men and women. They concluded: "There is little published evidence on how to improve men's uptake of services and it remains unclear whether it is more effective to provide different services or the same services in a different way" [46]. An intriguing prospect is incorporating the man's partner in promoting care. Men do recognize their wives and partners as facilitating their adherence to clinical service uptake. Evidence does indicate that the partner could play a significant facilitating role in improving preventive service uptake, especially when combined with physician reminders [47].

Shared decision making, where the patient and physician discuss the pros and cons of each test or treatment option when more than one viable option is available and a decision for a particular option is achieved only after exploration and validation of the patient's values and preferences, has been proposed to be an integral part of patient-centered care [48]. Decision aids are tools that help facilitate this process and have shown to improve patient's knowledge, reduce their decisional conflict, increase the likelihood of greater involvement by the patient in decision making, and improve patient-physician communication [49]. Thus, these tools may be useful for addressing preference-sensitive clinical topics such as prostate cancer screening. Unfortunately, adoption of these tools outside the research setting is limited due to time constraints and physician's lack of awareness [50].

Interventions geared toward organizational change have been shown to be effective. These include the use of separate clinics devoted solely to prevention, the use of a planned care visit for prevention (e.g., delivering the services during health maintenance/periodic health examinations rather than opportunistically during acute or chronic visits), and the designation of nonphysician staff to conduct specific prevention activities. The importance of being cognizant of the organizational characteristics of the physician practice when effecting a change cannot be overestimated, and the evaluation of the organizational structure and culture is now recognized to be the key step prior to implementing any such intervention [51]. A large practice network-based study that assessed the effect of interventions to improve preventive care concluded that the organizational composition of the practice, defined as teamwork and tenacity, was more important than the actual tools being utilized to effect change [52].

Indeed, the organizational milieu of the practice may be more important than the actual tools used (e.g., EHR, CDSS) to foster patient-centered care and clinical service improvement [53]. Implementation of the Patient-Centered Medical Home (PCMH) model to primary care practices may have beneficial effects on preventive care through improved patient access and communication, availability of readily usable health risk assessments, institutions of periodic preventive health examinations, use of registries that store risk information and screening history, ability to track and follow up on tests and referrals, and feedback on performance. However, the optimal implementation of these features would require a novel payment model that rewards preventive care [54].

Based upon a systematic review of the literature, several steps can be envisioned in organizing preventive healthcare in men. The steps are consistent with the quality improvement models utilizing the Plan-Do-Study-Act cycle [55] and are necessarily abstract to accommodate the uniqueness of each practice:

- Set a clear goal among the healthcare team, comprised of physicians, midlevel providers, and support staff, in that organizing and improving preventive healthcare among the practice patients is of paramount importance.
- Take an inventory of the current workflow and preventive service implementation in the practice and determine the areas for improvement. The series of steps reviewed in the early section of this chapter, as well as the list of recommended services and priorities, may serve as a useful guide.
- Specify the roles that each team member will play in organizing the preventive healthcare service.

- Consider allocating dedicated health maintenance visits for each patient. This is particularly important for men who underutilize healthcare services.
- Have a contingency plan for those men who come in only for acute visits to also implement preventive care at the time of the visit.
- If the practice does not have a reminder system in its EHR or uses paper chart system, create or utilize the reminder tools available through professional organizations such as the AAFP. These can be either electronic [56] or manual flow sheets [57].
- Ensure that an appropriate follow-up process is in place.
- After a trial period, reassess how well the process has been implemented and adjust accordingly.

Conclusion

In organizing preventive healthcare for men, the key is to implement a system for the entire practice encompassing all patients, not just men. Emphasis should be placed on organizational change and reminders. For men, enticing them to actually come in for healthcare visits is crucial. Proactively scheduling health maintenance examinations and having a contingency plan for implementing preventive care at the time of the acute visits are also possible solutions. A follow-up plan should be incorporated into practices to ensure that the preventive services are maximally effective.

References

1. Jaen CR, Stange KC, Nutting PA. The competing demands of primary care: a model for the delivery of clinical preventive services. J Fam Pract. 1994;38:166–71.
2. Yarnall KSH, Pollack KI, Ostbye T, Krause KM, Michener JL. Primary care: is there enough time for prevention? Am J Public Health. 2003;93(4):635–41.
3. Flocke SA, Stange KC, Goodwin MA. Patient and visit characteristics associated with opportunistic preventive services delivery. J Fam Pract. 1998;47:202–8.
4. McGlynn EA, Asch SM, Adams J, Keesey J, Hicks J, DeCristofaro A, et al. The quality of health care delivered to adults in the United States. N Eng J Med. 2003;348(26):2635–45.
5. Ewing GB, Selassie AW, Lopez CH, McCutcheon EP. Self-report of delivery of clinical preventive services by U.S. physicians. Am J Prev Med. 1999;17(1):62–72.
6. MMWR. Use of selected clinical preventive services among adults – United States, 2007–2010. 2012; 61 Supplement: 1–79.
7. Bastani R, Yabroff KR, Myers RE, Glenn B. Interventions to improve follow-up of abnormal findings in cancer screening. Cancer. 2004;101(5 Suppl):1188–200.
8. Nadel MR, Shapiro JA, Klabunde CN, Seeff LC, Uhler R, Smith RA, et al. A national survey of primary care physicians' methods for screening for fecal occult blood. Ann Intern Med. 2005;142(2):86–94.
9. Cabana MD, Rand CS, Powe NR, Wu AW, Wilson MH, Abboud P-AC, et al. Why don't physicians follow clinical practice guidelines? JAMA. 1999;282(15):1458–65.

10. McKinlay JB, Link CL, Freund KM, et al. Sources of variation in physician adherence with clinical guidelines: results from a factorial experiment. J Gen Intern Med. 2007;22:289–96.
11. Crabtree BF. Individual attitudes are no match for complex systems. J Fam Pract. 1997;44(5):447–8.
12. Miles A, Cockburn J, Smith RA, Wardle J. A perspective from countries using organized screening programs. Cancer. 2004;101(5 Suppl):1201–13.
13. Sandman D, Simantov E, An C. Out of touch: American men and the health care system. Commonwealth Fund Men's and Women's Health Survey Findings March 2000. Available from: http://www.cmwf.org/usr_doc/sandman_outoftouch_374.pdf.
14. Dryden R, Williams B, McCowan C, et al. What do we know about who does and does not attend general health checks? Findings from a narrative scoping review. BMC Public Health. 2012;12:723.
15. Borkhoff C, Saskin R, Rabeneck L, et al. Disparities in receipt of screening tests for cancer, diabetes and high cholesterol in Ontario, Canada: a population-based study using area-based methods. Can J Public Health. 2013;104:e284–90.
16. Schofield T, Connell RW, Walker L, Wood JF, Butland DL. Understanding men's health and illness: a gender-relations approach to policy, research, and practice. J Am Coll Health. 2000;48:247–56.
17. Williams DR. The health of men: structured inequalities and opportunities. Am J Public Health. 2003;93(5):724–31.
18. Bilsker D, Goldenberg L, Davison J. A roadmap to men's health: current status, research, policy & practice. Vancouver: Men's Health Initiative of British Columbia; 2010. Available from: http://aboutmen.ca/application/www.aboutmen.ca/asset/upload/tiny_mce/page/link/A--Roadmap-to-Mens-Health-May-17-2010.pdf.
19. White A, De Sousa B, De Visser R, et al. Men's health in Europe. J Men's Health. 2010;8:192–201.
20. Ng C, Teo CH, Ho CC, et al. The status of men's health in Asia. Prev Med. 2014;67C:295–302.
21. Elnicki DM, Morris DK, Shockcor WT. Patient-perceived barriers to preventive health care among indigent, rural Appalachian patients. Arch Intern Med. 1995;155:421–4.
22. Tudiver F, Talbot Y. Why don't men seek help? Family physicians' perspectives on help-seeking behavior in men. J Fam Pract. 1999;48:47–52.
23. Evans J, Frank B, Oliffe JL, Gregory D. Health, Illness, Men and Masculinities (HIMM): a theoretical framework for understanding men and their health. J Men Health. 2011;8:7–15.
24. Courtenay WH. Constructions of masculinity and their influence on men's well-being: a theory of gender and health. Soc Sci Med. 2000;50:1385–401.
25. US Preventive Services Task Force. Available from: http://www.uspreventiveservicestaskforce.org/.
26. Han PKJ. Historical changes in the objectives of the periodic health examination. Ann Intern Med. 1997;127(19):910–17.
27. American Academy of Family Physicians. Recommendations by type: clinical preventive services. Available from: http://www.aafp.org/patient-care/clinical-recommendations/cps.html.
28. National Guideline Clearinghouse. Available from: http://www.guideline.gov/.
29. Centers for Disease Control and Prevention. Advisory Committee on Immunization Practices. Available from: http://www.cdc.gov/vaccines/acip/.
30. Stange KC. One size doesn't fit all: multimethod research yields new insights into interventions to increase prevention in family practice [editorial]. J Fam Pract. 1996;43:358–60.
31. McVea K, Crabtree BC, Medder JD, Susman JL, Lukas L, McIlvain E, et al. An ounce of prevention? Evaluation of the "Put Prevention into Practice" program. J Fam Pract. 1996;43:361–9.
32. Solberg LI, Kottke TE, Brekke ML. Will primary care clinics organize themselves to improve the delivery of preventive services? A randomized controlled trial. Prev Med. 1998;27:623–31.

33. Stone EG, Morton SC, Hulscher ME, Maglione MA, Roth EA, Grimshaw JM, et al. Interventions that increase use of adult immunization and cancer screening services: a meta-analysis. Ann Intern Med. 2002;136:641–51.
34. Smith WR. Evidence for the effectiveness of techniques to change physician behavior. Chest. 2000;118:8S–17S.
35. Grimshaw JM, Shirran L, Thomas R, Mowatt G, Fraser C, Bero L, et al. Changing provider behavior: an overview of systematic reviews of interventions. Med Care. 2001;39:II-2–II-45.
36. Garg AX, Adhikari NKJ, McDonald H, Rosas-Arellano MP, Devereaux PJ, Beyene J. Effects of computerized clinical decision support systems on practitioner performance and patient outcomes: a systematic review. JAMA. 2005;293:1223–38.
37. Nease Jr DE, Green LA. ClinfoTracker: a generalizable prompting tool for primary care. J Am Board Fam Pract. 2003;16(2):115–23.
38. Souza NM, Sebaldt RJ, Mackay JA, et al. Computerized clinical decision support systems for primary preventive care: a decision-maker researcher partnership systematic review of effects on process of care and patient outcomes. Implement Sci. 2011;6:87.
39. Smith PC, Araya-Guerra R, Bublitz C, Parnes B, Dickinson LM, Van Horst R, et al. Missing clinical information during primary care visits. JAMA. 2005;293(5):565–71.
40. DeVoe JE, Gold R, McIntire P, et al. Electronic health records vs. Medicaid claims: completeness of diabetes preventive care data in community health centers. Ann Fam Med. 2011;9:351–8.
41. Chaudhry R, Tulledge-Scheitel SM, Parks DA, et al. Use of a Web-based clinical decision support system to improve abdominal aortic aneurysm screening in a primary care practice. J Eval Clin Pract. 2012;18:666–70.
42. Zhou YY, Unitan R, Wang JJ, et al. Improving population care with an integrated electronic panel support tool. Popul Health Manag. 2011;14:3–9.
43. Bryan C, Boren SA. The use and effectiveness of electronic clinical decision support tools in the ambulatory/primary care setting: a systematic review of the literature. Inform Prim Care. 2008;16:79–91.
44. Lin KW. Do electronic health records improve processes and outcomes of preventive care? Am Fam Physician. 2012;85:956–7.
45. Turchin A, Goldberg SI, Breydo E, Shubina M, Einbinder JS. Copy/paste documentation of lifestyle counseling and glycemic control in patients with diabetes: true to form? Arch Intern Med. 2011;171:1393–4.
46. Robertson LM, Douglas F, Ludbrook A, et al. What works with men? A systematic review of health promoting interventions targeting men. BMC Health Serv Res. 2008;8:141.
47. Holland DJ. Sending men the message about preventive care: an evaluation of communication strategies. Int J Men's Health. 2005;4:97–114.
48. Barry MJ, Edgman-Levitan S. Shared decision making – the pinnacle of patient-centered care. N Engl J Med. 2012;366:780–1.
49. Stacey D, Légaré F, Col NF, et al. Decision aids for people facing health treatment or screening decisions. Cochrane Database of Syst Rev; 2014, Issue 1. Art. No.: CD001431. doi: 10.1002/14651858.CD001431.pub4.
50. Jimbo M, Rana GK, Hawley S, Holmes-Rovner M, Kelly-Blake K, Nease Jr DE, Ruffin MTIV. What is lacking in current decision aids on cancer screening? CA Cancer J Clin. 2013;63:193–214.
51. Wears RL, Berg M. Computer technology and clinical work: still waiting for Godot [editorial]. JAMA. 2005;293(10):1261–3.
52. Carpiano RM, Flocke SA, Frank SH, Stange KC. Tools, teamwork, and tenacity: an examination of family practice office system influences on preventive service delivery. Prev Med. 2003;36:131–40.
53. Nease Jr DE, Ruffin 4th MT, Klinkman MS, et al. Impact of a generalizable reminder system on colorectal cancer screening in diverse primary care practices: a report from the prompting and reminding at encounters for prevention project. Med Care. 2008;46:S68–73.

54. Sarfaty M, Wender R, Smith R. Promoting cancer screening within the patient centered home. CA Cancer J Clin. 2011;61:397–408.
55. Coleman MT, Endsley S. Quality improvement: first steps. Fam Pract Manag. 1999;6(3):23–7. Available from: http://www.aafp.org/fpm/990300fm/23.html.
56. Lewis M. Using your Palm-Top's date book as a reminder system. Fam Pract Manag. 2001;8(5):50–1. Available from: http://www.aafp.org/fpm/20010500/50usin.html.
57. Moser SE, Goering TL. Implementing preventive care flow sheets. Fam Pract Manag. 2001;8(2):51–6. Available from: http://www.aafp.org/fpm/20010200/51impl.html.

Chapter 5
The Evidence-Based Physical Examination of the Child and Adolescent Male

David A. Levine and Makia E. Powers

The Well-Child Examination for Children and Adolescents/Young Adults

The well visit for children and adolescents is paramount in promoting overall physical, social, and emotional health and preventing disease. The physical examination is an important component of the overall well-child or adolescent visit. The purpose of the physical examination is to identify any abnormalities that require further investigation. Healthy People 2020 objective states the importance of increasing the proportion of adolescents who have had a wellness check-up in the past 12 months [1]. The child and adolescent male examination has unique aspects that will be discussed in this chapter.

There are different approaches to the physical examinations described in the literature. The hypothesis-driven physical examination requires the healthcare provider to determine the appropriate physical examination components to be performed, based on the patient's chief complaint and presenting symptoms [2]. This type of physical exam is best used in scenarios in which a patient presents in an acute care setting with a chief complaint or for a chronic illness visit. The "full body" physical examination is taught to all medical students for the purpose of learning the components of all organ systems. For the purposes of the routine healthcare maintenance visit, a full examination is recommended, with special focus on specific components based on the age of the patient.

The American Academy of Pediatrics (AAP) publishes the Guidelines for Health Supervision of Infants, Children, and Adolescents, also known as "Bright Futures."

D.A. Levine, MD (✉) • M.E. Powers, MD, MPH
Department of Pediatrics, Morehouse School of Medicine,
720 Westview Drive, SW, Atlanta, GA 30310, USA
e-mail: dlevine@msm.edu; mpowers@msm.edu

© Springer International Publishing Switzerland 2016
J.J. Heidelbaugh (ed.), *Men's Health in Primary Care*, Current Clinical Practice,
DOI 10.1007/978-3-319-26091-4_5

Bright Futures contains evidence-based recommendations for key components and screening examinations that should be performed at each age-based visit [3]. Bright Futures is currently undergoing revisions based on the 2014 4th edition of the AAP Recommendations for Preventive Pediatric Health Care [4]. In 2010, the Patient Protection and Affordable Care Act (PPACA) included a provision that all children enrolled in insurance plans, Medicaid, and the Children's Health Insurance Program (CHIP) should receive preventive care screenings and services as recommended by Bright Futures.

Other organizations, such as the United States Preventive Services Task Force (USPSTF) and American Academy of Family Physicians (AAFP), also have screening recommendations for the child and adolescent well-examination visits. The AAFP Strength of Recommendation Taxonomy (SORT) evidence rating scale was created to evaluate the quality, quantity, and consistency of evidence as it relates to applying recommendations into clinical practice [5]. The purpose of this chapter is to describe the physical examination and to provide a summary of evidence from a variety of organizations and task forces.

Child Examination

When preparing to perform an examination of the male child, a healthcare provider should first strive to build rapport and partner with the child and his parent/guardian(s). It is important to make the child feel comfortable during the exam. The provider may ask the parent to hold the child in parent's lap and perform some of the noninvasive physical examination findings first (i.e., heart and lung examinations). The order of the examination of the child is commonly not performed in a head-to-toe order. Rather, the most invasive components of the examination (e.g., the ears, mouth, and nose) are performed last. Some medical educators talk about this method as being "central to peripheral." The physical examination of the male child consists of the early childhood (ages 1–4 years) and middle childhood (ages 5–10 years) periods. See Table 5.1 for more information on the important physical examination elements by age.

Weight for Length/Body Mass Index

One Healthy People 2020 objective seeks to increase the proportion of primary care physicians who regularly measure and interpret the body mass index (BMI) of their patients. Approximately 17 % of children and adolescents aged 2–19 years are considered obese. Obesity is more prevalent in older children and adolescents compared to younger children (8.4 % in 2–5 year olds, 17.7 % in 6–11 year olds, and 20.5 % in 12–19 year olds) [6]. Bright Futures recommends measuring weight, length, and height and plotting the weight-for-length for supine children (generally 2 years of age and under) and BMI for standing children (validated for 2 years of

Table 5.1 Key physical examination components in childhood and adolescence well examinations from Bright Futures

	Blood pressure	Weight for length/BMI	Eyes	Mouth	Neuro	GU	Skin	MSK	Spine	Chest
12 months		•	•	•	•	•				
15 months		•	•	•	•					
18 months		•	•	•	•		•			
2 years		•	•	•	•					
2 ½ years		•	•	•	•					
3 years	•	•	•	•	•					
4 years	•	•	•	•	•					
5–6 years	•	•	•	•	•					
7–8 years	•	•		•		•		•		
9–10 years	•	•				•	•		•	
11–17 years	•	•				•	•		•	•
18–21 years	•	•				•	•	•		

*Bright Futures recommends a comprehensive physical examination, with concentration on key components for specific age groups

age and older). These parameters should be calculated at every scheduled well visit. Body mass index greater than 85th percentile is considered overweight and greater than 95th percentile, obese [7]. These children and their parents should receive specific and detailed counseling on how to promote healthy lifestyles—centered on healthy diet and daily exercise—in order to decrease risk factors for developing future cardiovascular disease and diabetes mellitus. The USPSTF, AAFP, and American Diabetes Association (ADA) also recommend routine BMI screening. The ADA and Bright Futures recommend that testing for prediabetes should be considered in children and adolescents who are overweight or obese and have two or more risk factors for diabetes. Relevant risk factors include a family history of type 2 diabetes mellitus or gestational diabetes in first-degree relatives, high-risk racial/ethnic group (e.g., African-American, American Indian), signs of insulin resistance (e.g., acanthosis nigricans, hypertension, or dyslipidemia), or prior small-for-gestational age birth weight. Prediabetes testing would include a fasting blood sugar, hemoglobin A1C, total cholesterol, and in some circumstances an oral glucose tolerance test [4, 8].

Blood Pressure

The fourth report of the National High Blood Pressure Education Program (and Bright Futures) recommends routine annual blood pressure screening starting at age 3 years and continuing through childhood and adolescence. Blood pressure percentile charts—based on age, gender, and height—should be used for children and adolescents ages 3–18. Please see Table 5.2 [9].

Table 5.2 Blood pressure norms for boys by age and height percentile [9]

Age (year)	BP percentile	Systolic BP (mm Hg) ← Percentile of height →							Diastolic BP (mm Hg) ← Percentile of height →						
		5th	10th	25th	50th	75th	90th	95th	5th	10th	25th	50th	75th	90th	95th
1	50th	80	81	83	85	87	88	89	34	35	36	37	38	39	39
	90th	94	95	97	99	100	102	103	49	50	51	52	53	53	54
	95th	98	99	101	103	104	106	106	54	54	55	56	57	58	58
	99th	105	106	108	110	112	113	114	61	62	63	64	65	66	66
2	50th	84	85	87	88	90	92	92	39	40	41	42	43	44	44
	90th	97	99	100	102	104	105	106	54	55	56	57	58	58	59
	95th	101	102	104	106	108	109	110	59	59	60	61	62	63	63
	99th	109	110	111	113	115	117	117	66	67	68	69	70	71	71
3	50th	86	87	89	91	93	94	95	44	44	45	46	47	48	48
	90th	100	101	103	105	107	108	109	59	59	60	61	62	63	63
	95th	104	105	107	109	110	112	113	63	63	64	65	66	67	67
	99th	111	112	114	116	118	119	120	71	71	72	73	74	75	75
4	50th	88	89	91	93	95	96	97	47	48	49	50	51	51	52
	90th	102	103	105	107	109	110	111	62	63	64	65	66	66	67
	95th	106	107	109	111	112	114	115	66	67	68	69	70	71	71
	99th	113	114	116	118	120	121	122	74	75	76	77	78	78	79
5	50th	90	91	93	95	96	98	98	50	51	52	53	54	55	55
	90th	104	105	106	108	110	111	112	65	66	67	68	69	69	70
	95th	108	109	110	112	114	115	116	69	70	71	72	73	74	74
	99th	115	116	118	120	121	123	123	77	78	79	80	81	81	82
6	50th	91	92	94	96	98	99	100	53	53	54	55	56	57	57
	90th	105	106	108	110	111	113	113	68	68	69	70	71	72	72
	95th	109	110	112	114	115	117	117	72	72	73	74	75	76	76
	99th	116	117	119	121	123	124	125	80	80	81	82	83	84	84

Age	BP percentile	SBP							DBP						
7	50th	92	94	95	97	99	100	101	55	55	56	57	58	59	59
	90th	106	107	109	111	113	114	115	70	70	71	72	73	74	74
	95th	110	111	113	115	117	118	119	74	74	75	76	77	78	78
	99th	117	118	120	122	124	125	126	82	82	83	84	85	86	86
8	50th	94	95	97	99	100	102	102	56	57	58	59	60	60	61
	90th	107	109	110	112	114	115	116	71	72	72	73	74	75	76
	95th	111	112	114	116	118	119	120	75	76	77	78	79	79	80
	99th	119	120	122	123	125	127	127	83	84	85	86	87	87	88
9	50th	95	96	98	100	102	103	104	57	58	59	60	61	61	62
	90th	109	110	112	114	115	117	118	72	73	74	75	76	76	77
	95th	113	114	116	118	119	121	121	76	77	78	79	80	81	81
	99th	120	121	123	125	127	128	129	84	85	86	87	88	88	89
10	50th	97	98	100	102	103	105	106	58	59	60	61	61	62	63
	90th	111	112	114	115	117	119	119	73	73	74	75	76	77	78
	95th	115	116	117	119	121	122	123	77	78	79	80	81	81	82
	99th	122	123	125	127	128	130	130	85	86	86	88	88	89	90
11	50th	99	100	102	104	105	107	107	59	59	60	61	62	63	63
	90th	113	114	115	117	119	120	121	74	74	75	76	77	78	78
	95th	117	118	119	121	123	124	125	78	78	79	80	81	82	82
	99th	124	125	127	129	130	132	132	86	86	86	88	89	90	90
12	50th	101	102	104	106	108	109	110	59	60	61	62	63	63	63
	90th	115	116	118	120	121	123	123	74	75	75	76	77	78	78
	95th	119	120	122	123	125	127	127	78	79	80	81	82	82	82
	99th	126	127	129	131	133	134	135	86	87	88	89	90	90	90
13	50th	104	105	106	108	110	111	112	60	60	61	62	63	64	64
	90th	117	118	120	122	124	125	126	75	75	76	77	78	79	79
	95th	121	122	124	126	128	129	130	79	79	80	81	82	83	83
	99th	128	130	131	133	135	136	137	87	87	88	89	90	91	91

(continued)

Table 5.2 (continued)

Age (year)	BP percentile ↓	Systolic BP (mm Hg) ← Percentile of height →							Diastolic BP (mm Hg) ← Percentile of height →						
		5th	10th	25th	50th	75th	90th	95th	5th	10th	25th	50th	75th	90th	95th
14	50th	106	107	109	111	113	114	115	60	61	62	63	64	65	65
	90th	120	121	123	125	126	128	128	75	76	77	78	79	79	80
	95th	124	125	127	128	130	132	132	80	80	81	82	83	84	84
	99th	131	132	134	136	138	139	140	87	88	89	90	91	92	92
15	50th	109	110	112	113	115	117	117	61	62	63	64	65	66	66
	90th	122	124	125	127	129	130	131	76	77	78	79	80	80	81
	95th	126	127	129	131	133	134	135	81	81	82	83	84	85	85
	99th	134	135	136	138	140	142	142	88	89	90	91	92	93	93
16	50th	111	112	114	116	118	119	120	63	63	64	65	66	67	67
	90th	125	126	128	130	131	133	134	78	78	79	80	81	82	82
	95th	129	130	132	134	135	137	137	82	83	83	84	85	86	87
	99th	136	137	139	141	143	144	145	90	90	91	92	93	94	94
17	50th	114	115	116	118	120	121	122	65	66	66	67	68	69	70
	90th	127	128	130	132	134	135	136	80	80	81	82	83	84	84
	95th	131	132	134	136	138	139	140	84	85	86	87	87	88	89
	99th	139	140	141	143	145	146	147	92	93	93	94	95	96	97

BP, blood pressure

[a]The 90th percentile is 1.28 SD, the 95th percentile is 1.645 SD, and the 99th percentile is 2.326 SD over the mean
For research purposes, the standard deviations in Appendix Table B-1 allow one to compute BP Z-scores and percentiles for boys with height percentiles given in Table 5.3 (i.e., the 5th, 10th, 25th, 50th, 75th, 90th, and 95th percentiles). These height percentiles must be converted to height Z-scores given by (5 % = −1.645; 10 % = −1.28; 25 % = −0.68; 50 % = 0; 75 % = 0.68; 90 % = 1.28 %; 95 % = 1.645) and then computed according to the methodology in steps 2–4 described in Appendix B. For children with height percentiles other than these, follow steps 1–4 as described in Appendix B

Normal blood pressures are considered to be systolic blood pressure (SBP) and diastolic blood pressure (DBP) less than the 90th percentile; prehypertension is defined as SBP/DBP measured between the 90th and 95th percentiles; stage 1 hypertension is SBP or DBP between 95th percentile and 5 mm Hg above the 99th percentile; and stage 2 hypertension is SBP/DBP greater than 99th percentile plus 5 mm Hg. Abnormal blood pressure measurements should be repeated, ensuring it is performed manually and using an appropriate-sized cuff.

If repeated blood pressure readings are still considered prehypertension, then weight management and healthy lifestyle guidance are recommended, and blood pressure measurement should be repeated in 6 months. If the repeated blood pressures are between the 95th and 99th percentiles, then blood pressure measurement should be rechecked within 1–2 weeks, and the provider considers a workup to decide between essential and secondary hypertension (full medical history, family history, physical examination, CBC, renal panel, UA, lipids, glucose, and renal/cardiac ultrasound may be indicated). If there are concerns for secondary hypertension, then the child should be referred to the appropriate specialists (i.e., cardiologists, nephrologists, endocrinologists, or rheumatologists) [10]. Infants under age 3 years with preexisting conditions (e.g., renal, cardiac, or endocrine systems) should also be evaluated [3].

Eyes

In the young child ages 12–30 months, Bright Futures recommends examination of the eyes, and screening for eye problems including strabismus, and other rare, yet severe conditions (e.g., retinoblastoma and congenital cataracts). To evaluate for retinal diseases, the healthcare provider will shine an ophthalmoscope in each eye and observe the orange/brown tint of the retina (the so-called red reflex). If the red reflex is absent, providers should refer the child to a pediatric ophthalmologist for further evaluation.

The cover/uncover test is used to evaluate conjugate eye movement. To perform the cover/uncover test, the provider places a hand or an eye obstructer over one eye, while the child is looking straight ahead at an object. One eye is rapidly covered while observing the uncovered eye for any movement. Repeat with the other eye as needed. The Hirschberg light reflex is also used via shining any light in the eye and observing for the reflection in the child's pupils. If the reflection is symmetrical or just to the medial side of the pupil bilaterally, then the eye is considered to be normal. Any abnormalities in these physical examination maneuvers are concerning for strabismus or other disconjugate eye disorders, and patients should be referred urgently to a pediatric ophthalmologist [10].

Mouth

Dental caries is the most common pediatric chronic disease in the USA [11]. Twenty percent of children aged 2–11 years have untreated dental caries [12, 13]. Primary care providers play an important role in assessing risk of dental caries at well-child examinations [13–15]. The medical provider should also perform a visual inspection and refer to a dentist if there are any concerns. The dentition should be fully examined starting at the 12-month visit and continued periodically throughout childhood to observe for signs of dental caries until age 8 years, according to Bright Futures. During the oral exam, the healthcare provider should inspect for any visual signs of tooth decay (e.g., brown spots, holes in teeth, visible plaque, or teeth missing due to caries). In addition, the healthcare provider should observe for any signs of gingival inflammation or malocclusion.

The American Dental Association and the American Academy of Pediatrics Section on Oral Health recommend performing dental risk assessments to determine a child's risk of dental caries [16]. The dental risk assessment is a series of questions that determines if a child is at low or high risk for dental caries. Please see Fig. 5.1. If not performed in a child's dental home, then pediatricians have been recommended to apply dental varnish to children's primary teeth [15]. USPSTF also recommends that if not done in the dental home or if there is poor access to pediatric dental care, primary care clinicians apply fluoride varnish to the primary teeth of all infants and children starting at the age of primary tooth eruption (B recommendation). Bright Futures recommends the following online training modules on fluoride varnish application for primary care providers (www.smilesforlifeoralhealth.org) [3, 17].

Neurologic/Developmental

The purpose of the neurologic examination in children is to observe the higher cortical functions, language development, gait, and strength at key milestone visits. During the 12-month visit, the healthcare provider should observe the gait of the child by paying particular attention to the position and orientation of the feet. The 15-month-old child may demonstrate signs of stranger avoidance during the examination, which is within normal limits for this age. The 18-month-old child should be more mobile, and the provider can observe gait (specifically running, walking), hand control, and arm/spine movement.

At age 2 years, the healthcare provider should observe running, scribbling, socialization, and ability to follow commands as well as an assessment of language acquisition and clarity. At 2 ½ years, the healthcare provider should observe coordination, language acquisition, clarity, and socialization as well as an assessment of vocalization. At age 3 years, observe language acquisition and speech clarity and note adult–child interaction. At age 4 years, the healthcare provider should observe fine and gross motor skills and assess language acquisition, speech fluency and clarity, thought content, and abstraction. At ages 5–6 years, the healthcare provider

Oral Health Risk Assessment Tool

The American Academy of Pediatrics (AAP) has developed this tool to aid in the implementation of oral health risk assessment during health supervision visits. This tool has been subsequently reviewed and endorsed by the National Interprofessional Initiative on Oral Health.

Instructions for Use

This tool is intended for documenting caries risk of the child, however, two risk factors are based on the mother or primary caregiver's oral health. All other factors and findings should be documented based on the child.

The child is at an absolute high risk for caries if any risk factors or clinical findings, marked with a ⚠ sign, are documented yes. In the absence of ⚠ risk factors or clinical findings, the clinician may determine the child is at high risk of caries based on one or more positive responses to other risk factors or clinical findings. Answering yes to protective factors should be taken into account with risk factors/clinical findings in determining low versus high risk.

Patient Name:_____ Date of Birth:_____ Date:_____

Visit: ☐6 month ☐9 month ☐12 month ☐15 month ☐18 month ☐24 month ☐30 month ☐3 year
☐4 year ☐5 year ☐6 year ☐Other_____

RISK FACTORS	PROTECTIVE FACTORS	CLINICAL FINDINGS
⚠ Mother or primary caregiver had active decay in the past 12 months ☐Yes ☐No	● Existing dental home ☐Yes ☐No ● Drinks fluoridated water or takes fluoride supplements ☐Yes ☐No ● Fluoride varnish in the last 6 months ☐Yes ☐No ● Has teeth brushed twice daily ☐Yes ☐No	⚠ White spots or visible decalcifications in the past 12 months ☐Yes ☐No ⚠ Obvious decay ☐Yes ☐No ⚠ Restorations (fillings) present ☐Yes ☐No
● Mother or primary caregiver does not have a dentist ☐Yes ☐No		● Visible plaque accumulation ☐Yes ☐No
● Continual bottle/sippy cup use with fluid other than water ☐Yes ☐No ● Frequent snacking ☐Yes ☐No ● Special health care needs ☐Yes ☐No ● Medicaid eligible ☐Yes ☐No		● Gingivitis (swollen/bleeding gums) ☐Yes ☐No ● Teeth present ☐Yes ☐No ● Healthy teeth ☐Yes ☐No

ASSESSMENT/PLAN			
Caries Risk: ☐Low ☐High **Completed:** ☐Anticipatory Guidance ☐Fluoride Varnish ☐Dental Referral	**Self Management Goals:** ☐Regular dental visits ☐Dental treatment for parents ☐Brush twice daily ☐Use fluoride toothpaste	☐Wean off bottle ☐Less/No juice ☐Only water in sippy cup ☐Drink tap water	☐Healthy snacks ☐Less/No junk food or candy ☐No soda ☐Xylitol

---

Treatment of High Risk Children

If appropriate, high-risk children should receive professionally applied fluoride varnish and have their teeth brushed twice daily with an age-appropriate amount of fluoridated toothpaste. Referral to a pediatric dentist or a dentist comfortable caring for children should be made with follow-up to ensure that the child is being cared for in the dental home.

Adapted from Ramos-Gomez FJ, Crystal YO, Ng MW, Crall JJ, Featherstone JD. Pediatric dental care: prevention and management protocols based on caries risk assessment. *J Calif Dent Assoc.* 2010;38(10):746–761; American Academy of Pediatrics Section on Pediatric Dentistry and Oral Health. Preventive oral health intervention for pediatricians. *Pediatrics.* 2003; 122(6):1387–1394; and American Academy of Pediatrics Section on Pediatric Dentistry. Oral health risk assessment timing and establishment of the dental home. *Pediatrics.* 2003;111(5):1113–1116.

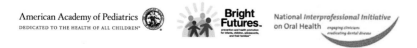

American Academy of Pediatrics
DEDICATED TO THE HEALTH OF ALL CHILDREN™

Bright Futures.
prevention and health promotion
for infants, children, adolescents,
and their families™

National *Interprofessional Initiative*
on Oral Health *engaging clinicians*
eradicating dental disease

Fig. 5.1 AAP oral risk assessment tool [3, 4]

Oral Health Risk Assessment Tool Guidance

Timing of Risk Assessment

The Bright Futures/AAP "Recommendations for Preventive Pediatric Health Care," (ie, Periodicity Schedule) recommends all children receive a risk assessment at the 6- and 9-month visits. For the 12-, 18-, 24-, 30-month, and the 3- and 6-year visits, risk assessment should continue if a dental home has not been established. View the Bright Futures/AAP Periodicity Schedule—http://brightfutures. aap.org/clinical_practice.html.

Risk Factors

⚠ Maternal Oral Health

Studies have shown that children with mothers or primary caregivers who have had active decay in the past 12 months are at greater risk to develop caries. **This child is high risk.**

Maternal Access to Dental Care

Studies have shown that children with mothers or primary caregivers who do not have a regular source of dental care are at a greater risk to develop caries. A follow-up question may be if the child has a dentist.

Continual Bottle/Sippy Cup Use

Children who drink juice, soda, and other liquids that are not water, from a bottle or sippy cup continually throughout the day or at night are at an increased risk of caries. The frequent intake of sugar does not allow for the acid it produces to be neutralized or washed away by saliva. Parents of children with this risk factor need to be counseled on how to reduce the frequency of sugar-containing beverages in the child's diet.

Frequent Snacking

Children who snack frequently are at an increased risk of caries. The frequent intake of sugar/refined carbohydrates does not allow for the acid it produces to be neutralized or washed away by saliva. Parents of children with this risk factor need to be counseled on how to reduce frequent snacking and choose healthy snacks such as cheese, vegetables, and fruit.

Special Health Care Needs

Children with special health care needs are at an increased risk for caries due to their diet, xerostomia (dryness of the mouth, sometimes due to asthma or allergy medication use), difficulty performing oral hygiene, seizures, gastroesophageal reflux disease and vomiting, attention deficit hyperactivity disorder, and gingival hyperplasia or overcrowding of teeth. Premature babies also may experience enamel hypoplasia.

Protective Factors

Dental Home

According to the American Academy of Pediatric Dentistry (AAPD), the dental home is oral health care for the child that is delivered in a comprehensive, continuously accessible, coordinated and family-centered way by a licensed dentist. The AAP and the AAPD recommend that a dental home be established by age 1. Communication between the dental and medical homes should be ongoing to appropriately coordinate care for the child. If a dental home is not available, the primary care clinician should continue to do oral health risk assessment at every well-child visit.

Fluoridated Water/Supplements

Drinking fluoridated water provides a child with systemic and topical fluoride exposure, a proven caries reduction intervention. Fluoride supplements may be prescribed by the primary care clinician or dentist if needed. View fluoride resources on the Oral Health Practice Tools Web Page http://aap.org/oralhealth/PracticeTools.html.

Fluoride Varnish in the Last 6 Months

Applying fluoride varnish provides a child with highly concentrated fluoride to protect against caries. Fluoride varnish may be professionally applied and is now recommended by the United States Preventive Services Task Force as a preventive service in the primary care setting for all children through age 5 http://www.uspreventiveservicestaskforce.org/Page/Topic/recommendation-summary/dental-caries-in-children-from-birth-through-age-5-years-screening. For online fluoride varnish training, access the Caries Risk Assessment, Fluoride Varnish, and Counseling Module in the Smiles for Life National Oral Health Curriculum, www.smilesforlifeoralhealth.org.

Tooth Brushing and Oral Hygiene

Primary care clinicians can reinforce good oral hygiene by teaching parents and children simple practices. Infants should have their mouths cleaned after feedings with a wet soft washcloth. Once teeth erupt it is recommended that children have their teeth brushed twice a day. For children under the age of 3 (until 3rd birthday) it is appropriate to recommend brushing with a smear (grain of rice amount) of fluoridated toothpaste twice per day. Children 3 years of age and older should use a pea-sized amount of fluoridated toothpaste twice a day. View the AAP Clinical Report on the use of fluoride in the primary care setting for more information http://pediatrics.aappublications.org/content/early/2014/08/19/peds.2014-1699.

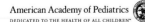   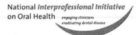

Fig. 5.1 (continued)

Clinical Findings

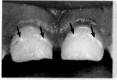

⚠ **White Spots/Decalcifications**
This child is high risk.
White spot decalcifications present—immediately place the child in the high-risk category.

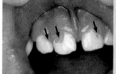

⚠ **Obvious Decay**
This child is high risk.
Obvious decay present—immediately place the child in the high-risk category.

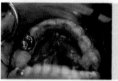

⚠ **Restorations (Fillings) Present**
This child is high risk.
Restorations (Fillings) present—immediately place the child in the high-risk category.

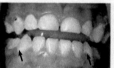

Visible Plaque Accumulation
Plaque is the soft and sticky substance that accumulates on the teeth from food debris and bacteria. Primary care clinicians can teach parents how to remove plaque from the child's teeth by brushing and flossing.

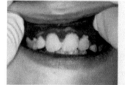

Gingivitis
Gingivitis is the inflamation of the gums. Primary care clinicians can teach parents good oral hygiene skills to reduce the inflammation.

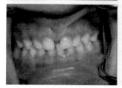

Healthy Teeth
Children with healthy teeth have no signs of early childhood caries and no other clinical findings. They are also experiencing normal tooth and mouth development and spacing.

For more information about the AAP's oral health activities email oralhealth@aap.org or visit www.aap.org/oralhealth.

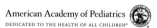

American Academy of Pediatrics
DEDICATED TO THE HEALTH OF ALL CHILDREN™

Bright Futures.
prevention and health promotion for infants, children, adolescents, and their families™

National *Interprofessional Initiative* on Oral Health *engaging clinicians eradicating dental disease*

Fig. 5.1 (continued)

should observe fine motor and gross motor skills, including gait, and assess language acquisition, speech fluency and clarity, thought content, and ability to understand abstract thinking. After age 6 years, development is commonly assessed by school performance [3, 10].

Skin

Bright Futures recommends targeted skin examinations at two key ages in childhood: the 18-month visit and the 9–10-year well visit. Providers may choose to perform full skin examinations at each visit, but these are the primary age groups targeted to observe for any signs of onset of genetic disease, such as neurofibromatosis, and to look for any signs of self-injury. During the 18-month well visit, it is important to inspect the skin for any abnormal lesions or changes in previously noted birthmarks and to observe for nevi, café au lait spots, birthmarks, or bruising. At 9–10 years of age, the healthcare provider should observe for tattoos, piercings, signs of abuse/self-inflicted injuries; inspect nevi or birthmarks; and note any changes to previous conditions or findings [3, 10].

Musculoskeletal

The musculoskeletal examination at the well-child visit is usually normal. Bright Futures recommends a targeted age of 7–8 years to make sure to observe hip, knee, and ankle function. A cursory exam, with observation of function, is commonly done at every health maintenance exam [3, 10]. It is during this age range that many children begin to have increased hours participating in sports and outdoor activities. The purpose of the musculoskeletal examination during the pre-participation physical examination is to observe for any gross abnormalities in the major joints (the hip, knee, and ankle). The AAP pre-participation physical examination form provides detailed components of the musculoskeletal elements to be examined. The forms and resources are available from the AAP [18]. For more details, see the section below on the pre-participation physical in the adolescent.

Spine

At ages 9–10 years, examine the back for any obvious signs of scoliosis [3, 10]. There is a considerable controversy between the American Academy of Pediatrics and USPSTF recommendation on scoliosis screening in childhood. See the section below on scoliosis screening in the adolescent.

GU Exams

Infancy and Early Childhood

Arguably the most important, genitourinary physical examination at any age is the newborn physical exam. Bright Futures notes that the healthcare provider must determine that the anatomic structures appear normal and that there are no penile anomalies and no evidence of any ambiguous genitalia. Location of the urethral meatus should be noted relative to the distal tip of the penis. Testes should be assessed to ensure that they are descended and if a congenital hydrocele or inguinal hernia is present. The anus should be examined for patency [3].

To detect a congenital hydrocele, the newborn's scrotum and testes should be examined by inspection, palpation, and confirmatory transillumination. The healthcare provider should inspect for any swelling of the scrotum that might suggest a hydrocele or hernia. The scrotum should be palpated for any swelling around the testes. With a hydrocele, there will usually be a palpable testis with an area of surrounding swelling. If a hydrocele is suspected, then transillumination is an effective confirmatory physical examination technique. A light source such as an otoscope is applied to the side of the scrotum to look for transmission of light; a red glow is a positive test [10] (see Fig. 5.11, below).

After the newborn exam, unless a parent presents with a question or concern, the male genitalia will only require inspections until the 12-month visit. Parents may have concerns related to possible hernia or other condition. At the 12-month visit, it is important to reexamine for hydrocele [3].

Parents may have questions related to circumcision outcome if they have elected to have this procedure performed. In 2012, task force comprising of CDC, AAP, AAFP, and American Congress of Obstetricians and Gynecologists (ACOG) published a technical report on male circumcision This report stated that the benefits of circumcision, such as fewer urinary tract infections, less HIV/STI, and reduced risk of penile cancer prevention, outweigh the risk of the procedure. The evidence-based synthesis also found no evidence of penile sexual dysfunction, sensitivity, or sexual dissatisfaction among circumcised men. They recommend that parents receive factually correct, non-biased information from which to make their decisions [19].

After the 12-month visit, visual inspection for any signs of puberty is warranted. The next prioritized age in the Bright Futures guidelines is age 7 years when children should be examined for early signs of puberty. Precocious puberty is a rare condition (1 in 5000 children) in which secondary sexual characteristics appear before age 9 years in boys. This should be contrasted with premature adrenarche, when the child may have early appearance of secondary sexual hair but without testicular enlargement, which is the first sign of puberty (see below) [20]. Boys should be examined annually with a genitourinary exam after age 7 [3].

A rectal exam is seldom indicated for infants and children, unless there is a symptomatic complaint. Such complaints as acute abdominal pain, or anal pain, bleeding, or trauma would warrant a gentle, patient, and rectal exam in a child. Many examiners recommend using the fifth digit to allow for as little discomfort as possible for the rectal examination of the young child [10].

Later Childhood

As noted above, once the male child reaches age 7 years, he should have a partial
genitourinary exam annually until age 10 years, focusing on sexual maturity rating
(formerly known as Tanner staging). In this case, the goal is to ensure that the child
has not yet had any signs or symptoms of precocious puberty and is maintaining
sexual maturity rating of 1 (Fig. 5.3, below). Testicular enlargement is the first sign
of puberty in boys, yet this may be very difficult for the child to notice as the changes
are slow, and most preadolescent boys are not cognitively able to have full abstract
reasoning to notice the changes. With that in mind, it is the pubic hair pattern that
should be observed. A complete genitourinary exam (including palpation) would
only be performed on a male child if there were complaints such as testicular pain,
penile pain, rash, or groin pain (hypothesis-driven physical exam).

Children develop modesty at different ages. The examiner should use gloves for
the genitourinary examination for any technique other than simple inspection if
beyond the newborn period. It is also proper to ask the child if they would like other
persons in the room (siblings, family members other than parent/guardian) to either
turn their heads or to leave the exam room. For children under age 11 years, it is the
policy of the American Academy of Pediatrics for the parent to stay in the examination room due to the nature of the examination [3].

The Adolescent

The physical examination of the adolescent male is a key component of the well-
preventive visit. Adolescence is defined as persons aged 11–14 (early adolescents),
15–17 (middle adolescents), and 18–21 (late adolescents). There is limited evidence
on the value of the full physical examination and modest evidence on certain components of the physical examination. Bright Futures is the only evidence-based
document that provides a comprehensive approach to the adolescent physical
examination.

The Bright Futures recommendations state to perform a complete physical
examination at each annual health supervision visit but to pay special attention to
the following key components [3] (see Table 5.1, above):

- Blood pressure
- Height
- Weight
- Body mass index (BMI)
- General survey
- Dermatologic
- Spine
- Genitalia

General Approach to Engaging Adolescent Men in the Office

Many adolescents present to their healthcare provider for routine preventative visits or sport physicals. Providers should explain the principle of confidentiality and the format of the adolescent visit to the parents and adolescent at the beginning of the visit. It is essential for all adolescents to have time spent alone with the provider and to explain this reason fully to the parents. During the time alone, providers should elicit a comprehensive social history. It is important to build rapport with the adolescent during the first portion of the visit while obtaining the medical history and confidential adolescent psychosocial history (aka HEEADDSSS) [21]. The HEEADDSSS examination includes social history about the "home," "environment," "education/employment," "activities," "drug use," "diet," "safety," "sexuality," and "suicidality." It is essential to approach the HEEADDSSS examination as a conversation rather than a list of questions [18].

Vital Signs

Anthropometric Measures Each adolescent should have height and weight measured and plotted on standard male growth curves at each well-preventive visit. See Fig. 5.2 for the current CDC growth charts. Healthy People 2020 NWS 10.3 states to reduce the proportion of adolescents age 12–19 who are considered obese. The body mass index (BMI) should be calculated, plotted, and interpreted at each visit. Bright Futures, AAP, USPSTF, Centers for Disease Control and Prevention (CDC), and American Diabetes Associations recommend measuring BMI yearly [1, 3, 8].

Blood Pressure The prevalence of prehypertension among young adolescents is approximately 16 % [23]. Research studies have shown that adolescents with prehypertension are more likely to develop hypertension within a few years, compared to adolescents with normal blood pressure [24]. Adolescents with hypertension have been shown to have early signs of target organ damage, such as increased carotid intima–media thickness [25] and increased left ventricular mass [26]. For these reasons, the National Blood Pressure Education Program Working Group on High Blood Pressure in Children and Adolescents added prehypertension as a designation. Blood pressure should be measured annually in all male children and adolescents starting at age 3. For early and middle adolescents, providers should use the percentile charts (see Table 5.2 for the blood pressure percentile chart). Prehypertension is considered percentiles greater than 85th percentile, and hypertension is greater than the 99th percentile for height and age. Late adolescents, ages 18–21, can be screened using the adult criteria for prehypertension (SPB 121–139/DBP 81–89) and hypertension (SBP $\geq$140 and DBP $\geq$90) [3, 10].

2 to 20 years: Boys
Body mass index-for-age percentiles

NAME _____

RECORD # _____

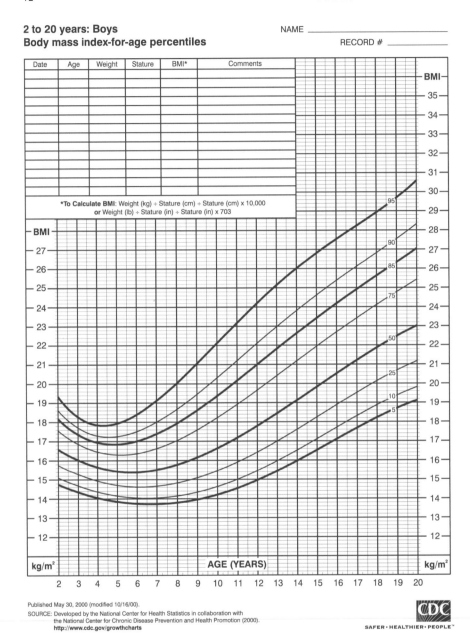

Published May 30, 2000 (modified 10/16/00).
SOURCE: Developed by the National Center for Health Statistics in collaboration with
the National Center for Chronic Disease Prevention and Health Promotion (2000).
http://www.cdc.gov/growthcharts

Fig. 5.2 CDC growth charts [22]

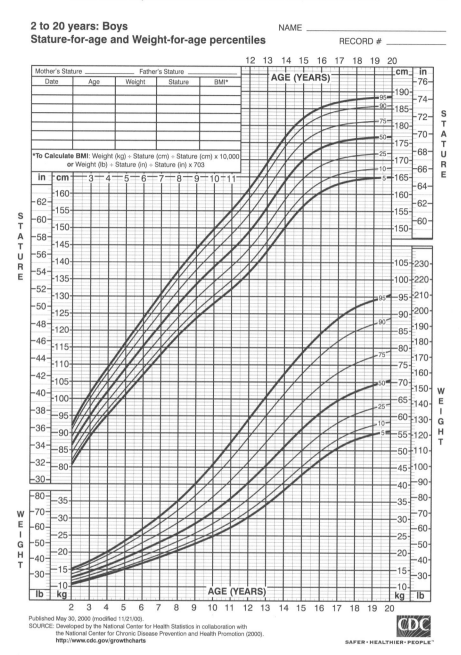

2 to 20 years: Boys
Stature-for-age and Weight-for-age percentiles

NAME _____

RECORD # _____

Fig. 5.2 (continued)

General Appearance The general examination of the adolescent visit focuses on the overall appearance of the adolescent. Observe the adolescents' voice and facial hair to determine if they are appropriate to the patient's age. Does the patient appear slender, emaciated, or obese? Note his dress, grooming, and personal hygiene and any odors from the body or breath. Observe to see if he appears disheveled or has torn/tattered clothes, which could indicate potential social concerns [3].

Vision The Snellen vision chart should be used to test visual acuity. The following organizations recommend Snellen vision screening at least once during adolescence: the American Academy of Pediatrics Committee on Practice and Ambulatory Medicine, the American Association of Certified Orthoptists, the American Association for Pediatric Ophthalmology and Strabismus, and the American Academy of Ophthalmology. Bright Futures recommends testing at ages 12, 15, and 18 years. (For younger children, it is recommended annually from ages 3 to 8 and then every other year until age 12.) Testing at other ages would be only if there was a patient or parent concern. If the vision on the Snellen chart is 20/40 or worse or if there are any significant eye complaints, the patient is referred to the pediatric ophthalmologist, if available, or general ophthalmologists or optometrists, depending on the community [3, 10].

Hearing According to Bright Futures, hearing should be tested only if there is a concern raised by patient or family. (For younger children, testing starts at age 4 and annually to age 6 and then every other year until age 10) [3, 4].

Dermatologic Exam

The healthcare provider should thoroughly inspect the skin, specifically for abnormal lesions, acne, and moisture content. The skin should be evaluated and characterized if overly dry or oily. Children and adolescents may have atopic dermatitis or eczema, which may appear as erythematous or hyperpigmented patches, with or without excoriations, commonly on flexor surfaces of the extremities. The face and facial hair should be inspected for any signs of acne, hyperpigmentation, or inflamed papules in the beard area which may indicate pseudofolliculitis barbae, commonly encountered in older African-American adolescent males. Evidence of acne vulgaris may appear as closed or open comedones, papules, pustules, and cystic or nodular lesions on the face, neck, chest, and/or back [10].

The healthcare provider should examine the male child for any signs of abuse or self-inflected injuries, such as abnormal bruising, ligature markings, or cutting [27, 28]. Signs of substance abuse may include track marks from intravenous drug use or perioral blisters from inhalant use [29]. The skin should be inspected for any tattoos or piercings [30].

Breast Exam

A breast exam should be performed on early and middle adolescent males, via inspection of the chest and observation for unilateral or bilateral breast enlargement, signifying gynecomastia. For these adolescents with gynecomastia, breasts should be palpated for glandular tissue and masses, noting the location, symmetry, and any tenderness to palpation [10].

Back/Spine

There are conflicting guidelines across organizations on the value of examining the back and spine in the child and adolescent male. Bright Futures recommends examining the spine during the annual routine health supervision visits. However, the USPSTF and AAFP recommend against routine screening of asymptomatic adolescents for adolescent idiopathic scoliosis (AIS). AIS is met by the following criteria: (1) age greater than 10 years of age, (2) curvature of the spine with Cobb angle greater than 10°, and (3) the absence of other etiologies of scoliosis, such as congenital or neuromuscular diseases [3, 5].

The young man is inspected with his back facing the examiner, to detect any obvious curvature of the spine. The patient should flex forward at the waist to accentuate any lateral curvature. If scoliosis is present, the level of the scapulae will be noticeably different. Finally, the young man is inspected from the lateral side for any apparent kyphosis [10].

Genitourinary

According to Bright Futures, beginning at age 11 and annually thereafter, each young man should have a complete genitourinary examination. This includes visual inspection for sexual maturity rating, observation for signs of sexually transmitted infections (STIs), and palpation of the testes for hydrocele, hernias, varicocele, or masses [3].

Inspection

Inspection may be performed with the male either lying or standing. However, males must stand for the palpation portion of the exam or the examiner may not detect varicoceles. For that reason, many examiners will have the patient stand with the examiner sitting for the entire genitourinary exam. The first part of inspection is a determination of the sexual maturity rating, mostly relying on the public hair pattern (Table 5.3).

Table 5.3 Sexual maturity rating

	Pubic hair	Genitalia	
		Testes/scrotum	Penis
SMR 1	No pubic hair	Same proportion of size since childhood	Same proportion of size since childhood
SMR 2	Sparse growth of long, downy, and mostly straight (some curl at the base) hair	Testes are larger, and the scrotum may have increased pigment and altered in texture	Slight or no enlargement
SMR 3	Darker, coarser, and curly hair but sparsely in the pubic area	Testes further enlarged	Longer and larger
SMR 4	Coarse, curly, adult pattern, over the entire pubic area	Testes further enlarged, and scrotal skin increased pigmentation	Further enlarged in length and width; glans may have further development
SMR 5	Adult pattern, coarse and curly hair over the pubic area, inner thighs, and in a triangle up toward the umbilicus	Adult in size and shape	Adult in size and shape

Adapted from Bickley, 11th Edition [10]

Figures 5.1, 5.2, 5.3, 5.4, and 5.5 highlight a pictorial representation of the sexual maturity ratings for males. Once staged, it is possible to counsel the young man on when to expect his most rapid physical growth as well as when it is predicted that his genitalia have reached the ultimate adult size and structure. The most rapid growth phase usually occurs between SMR 4 and SMR 5. Once the young male has achieved SMR 5, growth velocity slows significantly, and many men have stopped maturing completely. Similarly, the penis and testes are usually finished growing and maturing once the young male has achieved SMR 5. In general, puberty in males starts at ages 9–13.5 years and finishes from ages 13.5 to 17 years [9, 31] (Figs. 5.6 and 5.7).

The genitalia should be inspected for any congenital anomalies that were not discovered on previous physical examinations. The next part of inspection includes looking for any signs of lesions consistent with STIs. The penis should first be inspected for any clear or cloudy discharge (note, sometimes, even when queried, adolescents will deny a discharge, but it may be noted on physical examination). The genitalia should be inspected for vesicles of herpes simplex infection or genital warts of human papillomavirus infections (condyloma acuminata). The examiner should also inspect the pubic hair for any evidence of pediculosis pubis (crab lice). While not nearly as common, patients may also have the condylomata lata rash of secondary syphilis. The CDC website has open access materials defining and describing each of these lesions which serve as excellent teaching tools for both clinicians and patients. The materials are at http://www.cdc.gov/std/default.htm [32]. Benign pearly penile papules are a common and normal finding in adolescent men that may cause anxiety in the patient, with concern that they represent an STI (Fig. 5.8).

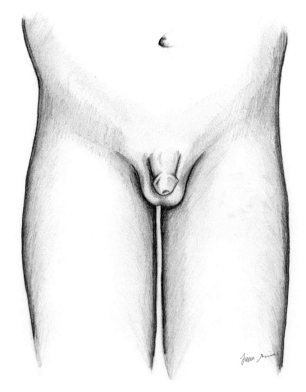

Fig. 5.3 Sexual maturity rating (Tanner stages) 1. Original artwork by Tierra Smith, MSM MD Class of 2017

Pearly penile papules are angiofibromata of the glans and corona of the penis. They have no symptoms, and often the adolescent will not even note them to the examiner. They are a physiologic variant of the normal penis and should not be treated [33].

Palpation

After inspection, the next part of the male genital exam is palpation for hernia, hydrocele, spermatocele, varicocele, any other palpable anomalies and to further examine for penile discharge. Adolescent men may experience spontaneous and unintended erections during the examination, and palpation of the glans penis during the genital exam can cause embarrassment for both the patient and for the provider. Thus, palpation of the glans should be kept to an essential minimum. Many examiners, especially those with teen clinics for adolescent men follow the palpation of the male genitalia should begin with examination of any potential inguinal hernia. The gloved examiner should gently insert a finger into the scrotum and invaginate scrotal skin proximally to the inguinal canal until encroaching upon the

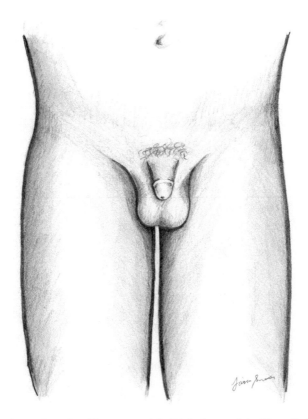

Fig. 5.4 Sexual maturity rating (Tanner stages) 2. Original artwork by Tierra Smith, MSM MD Class of 2017

external inguinal ring; sometimes the finger might enter the inguinal canal. The patient should be asked to perform a Valsalva maneuver (ask the patient to "bear down" or "cough") and detect if any portion of the intestine abuts the finger that was inserted [9, 31] (Fig. 5.9).

The next part of palpation in the male genital examination is the testicular examination. Each testicle should be palpated from the top to the bottom between the thumb and first 1–2 digits. The examiner should note the shape, size, any tenderness, and any masses. In general, in adults the testes are 4–5 cm long and 3 cm wide; the left testicle commonly hangs lower than the right [31] (Fig. 5.10).

Sometimes, hydroceles may be missed in early childhood and may persist until adolescence, as the hydrocele would cover the entire anterior surface of the testis. Transillumination may be used to confirm a clinical suspicion (Fig. 5.11). Varicoceles are more apparent when the patient is standing upright. They are a dilated venous plexus and feel like "a bag of worms" when palpated. Spermatoceles are firm palpable masses separate from and superior to the testes within the spermatic cords. While not usually required for diagnosis, they would also transilluminate [31]. At

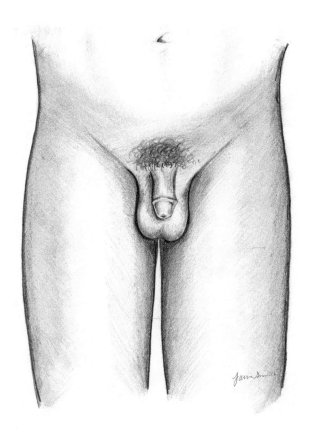

Fig. 5.5 Sexual maturity rating (Tanner stages) 3. Original artwork by Tierra Smith, MSM MD Class of 2017

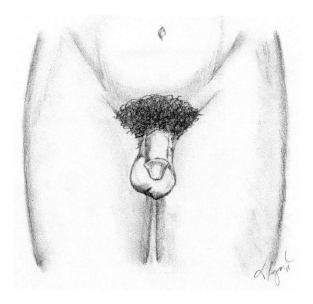

Fig. 5.6 Sexual maturity ratings (Tanner stages) 4. Original artwork by Tasaday Lynch, MSM MD Class of 2018

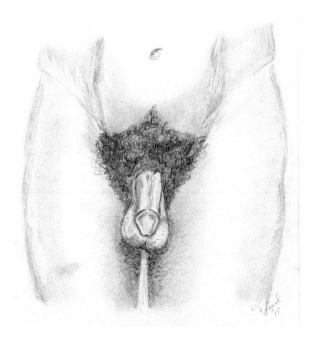

Fig. 5.7 Sexual maturity ratings (Tanner stages) 5. Original artwork by Tasaday Lynch, MSM MD Class of 2018

Fig. 5.8 Pearly penile papules. Reproduced with permission of Physicians for Reproductive Health, "Male Adolescent Reproductive and Sexual Health." Available at http://prh.org/wp-content/uploads/Male-Adolescent-SRH-Care.pptx [31]

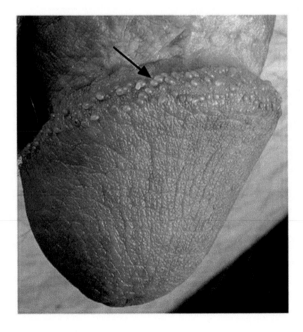

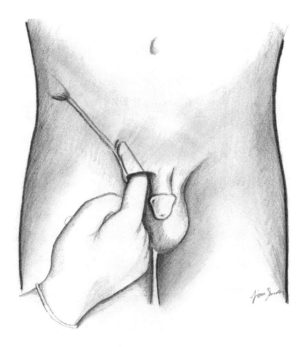

Fig. 5.9 Inguinal hernia physical examination original artwork by Tierra Smith, MSM MD Class of 2017

the same location, the examiner also might detect an epididymal cyst. Both spermatoceles and epididymal cysts are normal variants and require no intervention unless rapidly enlarging or significantly tender [10].

There is a discrepancy between organizations regarding palpation of the testes for detection of masses. Bright Futures recommends annual testicular exams starting at age 11 years. If there is a firm mass that cannot be separated from the testis, suggestive of a testicular tumor, then a scrotal ultrasound should be obtained. Testicular cancers are very uncommon conditions with high rate of survival (incidence is 5.6 per 100,000, 95.3 % 5-year survival rate [34]). However, according to the USPSTF, the testicular examination is not recommended as part of the routine physical examination, and instruction in testicular self-examination is also no longer recommended. The USPSTF gives this screening a grade of "D" with the instruction, "do not screen," as it may cause potential harms, such as false-positive results, anxiety, and harms from diagnostic tests or procedures. Due to the high cure rate regardless of stage, there is inadequate evidence to suggest that early detection by the examiner or self-examination improves outcomes [35]. Of course, if the clinician is examining for hydrocele and detects a hard mass that will not separate from the testis, then elaborated testing and intervention are necessary.

The final part of the palpation section is the gentle palpation of the remainder of the penis. With the adolescent standing, the examiner has an optimal view of the dorsal surface. The examiner should raise the penis and examine the ventral surface,

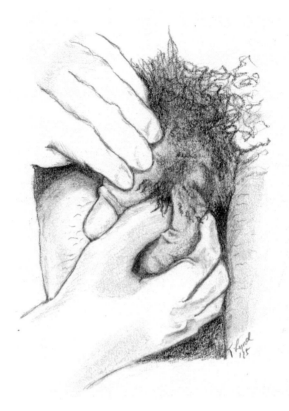

Fig. 5.10 Testicular palpation original artwork by Tasaday Lynch, MSM MD Class of 2018

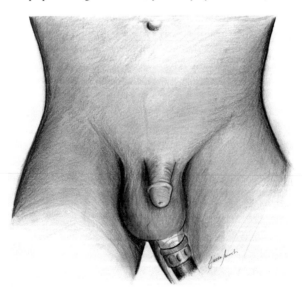

Fig. 5.11 Transillumination original artwork by Tierra Smith, MSM MD Class of 2017

again inspecting for any lesions suggestive of HSV, HPV, or other lesions. While holding the penis, looking discretely at the urethral opening will allow the examiner to inspect for any discharge, inflammation, or lesions at the urethra [10].

Rectal examinations are not a part of the routine adolescent physical examination. However, if the provider obtains a sexual history of anal-receptive intercourse, it is prudent to examine the anus for any signs of STIs (discharge, inflammation, discomfort, vesicles, or genital warts). As part of the examination, a rectal swab for nucleic acid amplification test (NAAT) for chlamydia and gonorrhea is warranted. While urine testing for STIs is warranted for any penile symptoms or testing, swabs must be used for anal or oral symptoms or testing. Please see Chap. 10 on Sexually Transmitted Infections in men [36].

Pre-Participation Physicals

A common reason that adolescents present to the primary care provider is for sports or other vigorous activity pre-participation evaluations (PPEs). While alternative locations such as doing sport physicals for an entire team at the school may be attractive to the athlete, parent, and coach, it may be the only time that the adolescent has a primary care visit in that year. Ideally, the sport PPE, like all service to the adolescent, should be conducted in the medical home [37, 38]. In the medical home, the adolescent should have a full history and physical evaluation conducted annually with added history and physical relevant to the PPE. While there is limited data evaluating the efficacy of the PPE, all student athletes are mandated by states to have such an evaluation prior to practice or sport participation.

In essence, the sports/other activity PPE requires elaborated history related to cardiovascular risks (e.g., including a personal history of cardiovascular conditions, murmurs, chest pain, or a family history of heart disease before age 50 years or of sudden death), neurologic risks (e.g., prior concussion, seizures), any other relevant medical conditions, and a history of orthopedic or soft tissue injuries. The adolescent should have a careful cardiac evaluation conducted in a room that allows auscultating even subtle heart murmurs. The adolescent in a PPE should also have a brief screening orthopedic evaluation of all the extremities, the back, and the neck [18]. These examination components can be found on the PPE examination forms. Should any abnormal conditions be detected, further evaluation is required prior to approving participation [39, 40].

Screening Office Procedures in the Well-Child/Adolescent Visits

Bright Futures mandates certain screening procedures and tests at certain key ages and also mandates risk screening based on history. There is variable evidence for the individual tests recommended. Evidence appraisal from USPSTF and AAFP is in

Table 5.4 Selected screening recommendations for child/adolescent male

	Bright Futures from AAP[a]	AAFP/USPSTF[b]
Vision	Ages 3–6 years, 8,10, 12, 15, 1 8 years	No routine screening
Hearing	Ages 4–6 years, 8, 10 year	No routine screening
Obesity screening	Annual BMI screening starting age 2 years	Routine BMI screening (B)
Hypertension	Routine BP screening starting at age 3 years	Routine screening (I)
Dental caries	Periodic screening: 12–30-month visits; 3 years, and 6 years; dental referral for a visit every 6 months	• No routine screening (I) • Prescribe oral fluoride supplementation (B) • PCP to apply fluoride varnish to teeth (B)
Genital herpes screening	No routine screening	No routine screening (D)
HIV screening	Risk screening starting at age 11 years	Routine screening starting at age 15 (A)
Chlamydia and gonorrhea screening	Screen if adolescent is sexually active per CDC STD treatment guidelines, endorsed by AAP	I (adolescent men)
Depression screening	Annually starting at age 11 year	B (ages 12–18)
I (ages 7–11)		

[a]AAP does not offer appraisal evaluation in Bright Futures
[b]AAFP follows the USPTF guidelines: A, recommends this service; B, recommends; C, recommends selectively providing this service; D, recommends against this service; I, current evidence is insufficient to make recommendation

Table 5.4; selected Bright Futures recommendations are also highlighted in Table 5.3 on the issues appraised by USPSTF and AAFP, but AAP does not rate the evidence.

Office procedures and testing are included in the 2014 Recommendations for Pediatric Preventive Health Care. Newborns have some required testing, such as hearing, metabolic screening, and pulse oximetry. Hearing is assessed in the newborn nursery, but if not completed, the test will need to be arranged in a center equipped to perform the newborn hearing screen. The newborn metabolic and genetic screening test is critical, and results must be documented before the infant is 6 weeks of age. Formerly known as the phenylketonuria (PKU) test (PKU was the first test), the number of tests in the newborn screen depends upon the individual state; it is now 20–25 different metabolic/genetic tests. Recently, critical congenital heart defect screening via pulse oximetry was added as a routine screen in the newborn nursery. Again, if the test was not performed in the newborn nursery, it should be obtained at the first office visit. Any detected abnormalities should be followed by echocardiography and pediatric cardiology consultation [4].

Bright Futures also recommends office testing for developmental and behavioral problems. Developmental screening is required at ages 9, 18, and 30 months using a validated screening test; autism screening is required at 24 and 30 months. Depression screening with a validated tool is required at age 11 and annually afterward. Bright Futures has freely distributed autism and depression screening tests; developmental screening tests are inexpensive and available from the authors and their organizations. See Table 5.3 [4].

Table 5.3: Developmental and Behavioral Screening Tests

For office laboratory testing, there are limited recommended screening tests in Bright Futures. Hemoglobin testing is required at 12 months, with risk screening (e.g., poor diet, poverty, alternative diets) at 4 months and then at each office visit after 12 months. Lead screening is still required in most communities; it is required at 12 and 24 months, but risk assessment should be conducted at each visit from 6 months to 6 years with extra testing if there are risk factors. Risks include living in an older building with cracked or peeling patient, parent industrial exposures, lead poisoning in the community or family and others. Tuberculosis risk should be assessed at 1 month, 6 months, and then 12 and 24 months and subsequent annual visits. Risks include exposure to someone with active TB (coughing, losing weight), someone with a positive PPD, a personal history of international travel to a high-risk area, contact with someone who has been incarcerated, and other risks. PPD testing should be performed with any positive screening question [4].

Dyslipidemia risk (e.g., family history of heart disease, stroke, sudden death, hypercholesterolemia, or personal measurement with the interpretation of obese) should be assessed at 24 months and again every 2 years. If there are any risk factors noted, a fasting lipid panel should be obtained. Additionally, according to the AAP, one lipid profile should be performed regardless of risk between ages 9–11 and 18–21 years. At these ages, the lipid profiles do not need to be fasting in order to facilitate universal screening. If there are abnormalities on the random (non-fasting) lipid panel, then the child would be brought back for a fasting panel [4].

There is some disagreement between the AAP and the CDC as to STI/HIV (chlamydia and gonorrhea tests, HIV test, and syphilis test in areas of high endemic rates) screening and testing. The AAP/Bright Futures mandates screening sometime between ages 16 and 18 [4], but the CDC has more specific guidelines [36]. The USPSTF has noted there were insufficient data from which to make a recommendation related to STI screening in adolescent males. Please see Chap. 10 for more information.

Acknowledgments We are indebted to two Morehouse School of Medicine medical students. Ms. Tasaday Lynch and Ms. Tierra Smith are current students and contributed the original artwork to this chapter.

References

1. Office of Disease Prevention and Healthy Promotion, US. Department of Health and Human Services, "Healthy People 2020." Available at http://www.healthypeople.gov/2020/default.aspx. Retrieved on August 1, 2015.
2. Yudkowsky R, Otaki J, Lowenstein T, Riddle J, Nishigori H, Bordage G. A hypothesis-driven physical examination learning and assessment procedure for medical students: initial validity evidence. Med Educ. 2009;43:729–40.

3. Hagan JF, Shaw JS, Duncan PM. Guidelines for health supervision of infants, children and adolescents. 3rd ed. Elk Grove Village, IL: American Academy of Pediatrics; 2008.
4. Committee on Practice and Ambulatory Medicine, Bright Futures Periodicity Schedule Workgroup. 2014 Recommendations for Pediatric Preventive Health Care. Policy Statement. Pediatrics. 2014;13(3):568–70.
5. Ebell MH, Siwek J, Weiss BD, Woolf SH, Susman J, Ewigman B, et al. Strength of recommendation taxonomy (SORT): a patient-centered approach to grading evidence in the medical literature. J Am Board Fam Pract. 2004;17(1):59–67.
6. Ogden CL et al. Prevalence of childhood and adult obesity in the United States, 2011-2012. JAMA. 2014;311:806–14.
7. Barlow SE. Expert committee recommendations regarding the prevention, assessment, and treatment of child and adolescent overweight and obesity: summary report. Pediatrics. 2007;120 Suppl 4:S164–92.
8. American Diabetes Association. Standards of Medical Care in Diabetes – 2015. Diabetes Care. 2015;38(S1):S1–S99.
9. The fourth report on the diagnosis, evaluation, and treatment of high blood pressure in children and adolescents. Pediatrics. 2004;114(2 Suppl):555–76.
10. Bickley L. Bates' guide to physical examination and history taking. 11th ed. Philadelphia, PA: Wolters Kluwer Health/Lippincott Williams and Wilkins; 2013.
11. National Center for Health Statistics. Health, United States 2013: With Special Feature on Prescription Drugs. 2014. Hyattsville, MD.
12. Dye BA, Li X, Beltran-Aguilar ED. Selected oral health indicators in the United States, 2005–2008. NCHS Data Brief. 2012;96:1–8.
13. Dye BA, Tan S, Smith V, Lewis BG, Barker LK, Thornton-Evans G, et al. Trends in oral health status: United States, 1988–1994 and 1999–2004. Vital Health Stat. 2007;11(248):1–92.
14. Kagihara LE, Niederhauser VP, Stark M. Assessment, management, and prevention of early childhood caries. J Am Acad Nurse Pract. 2009;21(1):1–10.
15. Section on Oral Health. Maintaining and improving the oral health of young children. Pediatrics. 2014;134(6):1224–9.
16. American Academy of Pediatric Dentistry. Guideline on caries-risk assessment and management for infants, children and adolescents. Clin Guidel. 2014;36(6):127–34.
17. STFM Group on Oral Health. Smiles for life: a national oral health curriculum. http://www.smilesforlifeoralhealth.org. Retrieved 30 Jul 2015.
18. Council on Sports Medicine and Fitness, American Academy of Pediatrics. "Preparticipation Physical Evaluation." https://www.aap.org/en-us/about-the-aap/Committees-Councils-Sections/Council-on-sports-medicine-and-fitness/Pages/PPE.aspx. Retrieved 30 Jul 2015.
19. AAP Task Force on Circumcision. Circumcision policy statement. Pediatrics. 2012;130(3):585–6.
20. Kaplowitz P. Clinical characteristics of 104 children referred for evaluation of precocious puberty. J Clin Endocrinol Metab. 2004;89:3644–50.
21. Klein DA, Goldenring JM, Adelman WP. HEEADSSS 3.0: The psychosocial interview for adolescents updated for a new century fueled by media. Contemp Pediatr. 2014: 16–28.
22. National Center for Health Statistics in collaboration with the National Center for Chronic Disease Prevention and Health Promotion, "CDC Growth Charts." 2000. http://www.cdc.gov/growthcharts. Retrieved 30 Jul 2015.
23. McNiece KL et al. Prevalence of hypertension and pre-hypertension among adolescents. J Pediatr. 2007;150(6):640–4. 644.e1.
24. Redwine KM et al. Development of hypertension in adolescents with pre-hypertension. J Pediatr. 2012;160(1):98–103.
25. Lande MB et al. Effects of childhood primary hypertension on carotid intima media thickness: a matched controlled study. Hypertension. 2006;48(1):40–4.
26. Lande MB et al. Left ventricular mass index in children with white coat hypertension. J Pediatr. 2008;153(1):50–4.

27. Shain B, the Committee on Adolescence. Suicide and suicide attempts in adolescents: a clinical report. Pediatrics. 2007;120(3):669–76.
28. Barrocas AL, Hankin BL, Young JF, Abela JRZ. Rates of nonsuicidal self-injury in youth: age, sex, and behavioral methods in a community sample. Pediatrics. 2012;130(1):39–45.
29. Levy SJL, Kokotailo PK, the Committee on Substance Abuse. Substance use screening, brief intervention, and referral to treatment for pediatricians: a policy statement. Pediatrics. 2011;128(5):e1330–40.
30. Braverman PK. Body art: piercing, tattooing, and scarification. Adolesc Med. 2006;17: 505–19.
31. Physicians for Reproductive Health. "Male Adolescent Reproductive and Sexual Health." http://prh.org/wp-content/uploads/Male-Adolescent-SRH-Care.pptx. 2015. Freely accessible and retrieved 22 Apr 2015.
32. CDC website: Retrieved from http://www.cdc.gov/std/default.htm on April 23, 2015.
33. Hogewoning CJA et al. Pearly penile papules: still no reason for uneasiness. J Am Acad Dermatol. 2003;49:50–4.
34. Surveillance, Epidemiology, and End Results Program, National Cancer Institute. "SEER Stat Fact Sheets: Testis Cancer." http://seer.cancer.gov/statfacts/html/testis.html. Retrieved 22 Apr 2015.
35. United States Preventive Task Force. "Clinical Summary: Testicular Cancer: Screening." 2011. Retrieved April 22, 2015 from http://www.uspreventiveservicestaskforce.org/Page/Document/ClinicalSummaryFinal/testicular-cancer-screening.
36. Centers for Disease Control and Prevention. Sexually Transmitted Diseases Treatment Guidelines, 2010. MMWR. 2010;59(RR12):1–114.
37. Medical Home Initiatives for Children with Special Needs Project Advisory Committee. The Medical Home: A Policy Statement. Pediatrics. 2002;110(1):184–6.
38. American College of Sports Medicine. ACSM information on pre-participation physical examinations. 2011. Retrieved on April 30, 2015 from https://www.acsm.org/docs/brochures/pre-participation-physical-examinations.pdf.
39. Rice S, and the Council on Sports Medicine and Fitness. Medical conditions affecting sports participation: a clinical report. Pediatrics. 2008;121(4):841–8.
40. American Academy of Family Physicians, American College of Sports Medicine, American Medical Society for Sports Medicine, American Academy of Pediatrics. PPE Preparticipation Physical Evaluation. 4th ed. Elk Grove Village, IL: American Academy of Pediatrics; 2010.

Chapter 6
Caring for the Adolescent Male

Cullen N. Conway, Samuel Cohen-Tanugi, Dennis J. Barbour, and David L. Bell

Introduction

Older adolescent and young adult (AYA) males have traditionally been left out/ignored in our healthcare system that primarily focuses on tertiary care [1]. AYA males are commonly defined as males between the ages of 10 and 24 [2]. As our healthcare system embarks on tasks of early prevention and improving the health of populations, greater attention will need to be paid to the "state of complete physical, mental, and social well-being and not merely the absence of disease or infirmity" as defined by the World Health Organization [3]. This holistic definition extends beyond the scope of the traditional pathology-focused Western tradition of medicine. For AYA males, social well-being and disease are, in fact, inseparable. The first half of this chapter will provide an overview of the major causes of mortality and morbidity in AYA males, discuss the barriers AYA males face in seeking and utilizing healthcare, and discuss the interplay of masculinity, health, and healthcare utilization. In the second half of this chapter, we will address ways of engaging males, despite these barriers, by constructing a vision of "AYA male-centered healthcare."

C.N. Conway, MPH (✉) • S. Cohen-Tanugi • D.L. Bell, MD, MPH
Columbia University Medical Center, New York, NY, USA
e-mail: conway@ohsu.edu

D.J. Barbour, Esq
Partnership for Male Youth, Washington, DC, USA

© Springer International Publishing Switzerland 2016
J.J. Heidelbaugh (ed.), *Men's Health in Primary Care*, Current Clinical Practice,
DOI 10.1007/978-3-319-26091-4_6

Mortality

Mortality increases rapidly across adolescence. The United States of America (USA) has the sixth highest adolescent male mortality rate among high-income countries [4, 5]. Compared with females, males in high-income countries such as the USA are more likely to die of all major causes of mortality. The dominant cause of injury deaths among young men was transport injuries worldwide [5]. Although males have seen marked improvements in healthcare outcomes over the past 20 years, their mortality remains unacceptably high [5]. In the USA, the top three causes of death for males 10–24 years old are caused by unintentional injuries, homicide, and suicide [6]. Unintentional injury alone, which includes motor vehicle injuries, unintentional poisoning and drug overdose, drowning, and unintentional discharge of a firearm, account for 75 % of all mortality. Motor vehicle injuries account for the majority (71 %) of all unintentional injuries [4].

Morbidity

Chronic Illness

Reducing preventable chronic diseases is dependent on reducing alcohol, drug, and tobacco abuse, decreasing obesity, and increasing physical activity. Forty-six percent of high school males report having ever smoked a cigarette versus 43 % of high school females, and 12 % of males started smoking before age 13 versus 8 % of females [7]. The prevalence of obesity is 20 % among high school males and is rising compared to a stabilized rate of 17 % among high school females [8]. However, 38.8 % of males report 60 min of daily exercise compared to only 18.5 % of females [9].

Mental Health

AYA males are at high risk for depression. According to the 2013 Youth Risk Behavior Survey (YRBS), 30 % of high school students experienced some disruption of daily activity due to feeling sad or hopeless continuously for 2 or more weeks in a row. Among other mental health disorders that affect young males are anxiety disorders, attention deficit hyperactivity disorder (ADHD), psychotic disorders, bipolar and related disorders, obsessive compulsive disorder, and oppositional defiant disorder [10]. Although rates of depression and suicidal ideation are higher among females than males in adolescence and young adulthood, males are more likely to complete suicide. Depression is twice as common in women [11]. Men are three times more likely to die by suicide than women [12].

Substance Use

AYA males have higher substance abuse rates than females, and boys under 17 drink alcohol more heavily than any other population group. Among high school males, 39.5 % report any alcohol use in the past 30 days, and 23.8 % report consuming more than 5 drinks [13]. In 2011, among 9th through 12th grade students, males were more likely than females to use ecstasy, heroin, methamphetamines, hallucinogenic drugs, anabolic steroids, or illegal needle-injected drugs. Males were also more likely to be offered, sold, or given an illegal drug on school property. Drug use is exceedingly common, with 25.9 % reporting marijuana use in the past 30 days, 10.5 % inhalant use, and 9.8 % ecstasy use. Males are more likely to use cocaine than females, with 7.9 % of males reporting having ever used cocaine, as compared to 5.7 % of females. Current use of cocaine (used once or more in the past 30 days) is higher among males (4.1 %) than females (1.8 %). Males are more likely to use heroin than females, with 3.9 % of males reporting having ever used heroin, as compared to 1.8 % of females [7, 13]. In 2011, 21.5 % of adolescent males engaged in prescription drug use (e.g., oxycodone, hydrocodone, benzodiazepines) [14]. The majority (80 %) current heroin users report that their opioid use began with opioid pain relievers [15]. However, heroin users were far more likely to start with prior nonmedical pain reliever, according to one study [16].

Early substance use (before age 13 years) is common in males (23.3 % of males reporting early alcohol use and 10.4 % early marijuana use), with risk factors including low supervision and parental monitoring [17]. Similar behaviors by peers were the most powerful predictor of teen drug use [18].

Sexual Health Risks

In our risk-based health models based on pregnancy prevention, we traditionally begin our thoughts about sexual health risks (SHR) with the debut of heterosexual intercourse. Between 1998 and 2002, young males on average delayed their age of sexual debut. As of 2013, the median age has remained relatively consistent between 17 and 18 years of age since 2002 [19]. Current best estimates of sexual orientation in male youth reveal that 3 % of young males identify as homosexual or bisexual and 4 % report same-sex sexual behaviors [20]. While sexual behavior with same-sex partners can be an expression of sexual orientation (e.g., homosexual or bisexual), they are not equivalent [21]. Sexual encounters with same-sex partners, especially in adolescence and young adulthood, may represent experimentation and exploration.

There are documented risks associated with early sexual debut, unprotected sex, and sexual encounters with same-sex partners. A young age of onset of sexual behavior is associated with increased rates of sexually transmitted infections (STIs), early fatherhood, and sexual coercion. Early fatherhood is common, with 15 % of males fathering a child before age 20 [22]. AYA males also bear a disproportionate share of STIs relative to other age groups. In a national sample of 18- to 22-year-olds, 3.7 % were infected with *Chlamydia trachomatis*, 1.7 % with *Trichomonas*, and

0.4 % with *Neisseria gonorrhoeae* [23, 24]. Sexual behavior with same-sex partners is associated with higher sexual health risk.

Compared to men who have sex with women, rates of HIV and syphilis are higher among men who have sex with men (MSM) [25, 26]. MSM account for the largest numbers of new HIV infections, and African American MSM are the only group with increasing rates of HIV infection in the USA [27, 28]. Sexual orientation (e.g., identification with the LGBT ((lesbian, gay, bisexual, transgender) community) is associated with an increased risk for a much larger set of physical, mental, and social problems which impact health, including depression, suicidal ideation and behavior, homelessness, familial rejection, dropping out of school, substance abuse, STIs, and victimization [29]. Although equally important to understand the issues of LGBT youth, this chapter will focus on males, in general, inclusive, but not specific to MSM which will be covered in a later chapter.

Complexities and Barriers of Care for AYA Males

Many efforts toward prevention of disease do not require healthcare access. To date, we do not have proven in-office clinical interventions for many of the specific conditions that we aspire to prevent. The true value of the annual physical exam has also been questioned [30]. However, understanding how AYA males interact with the healthcare system currently, why they do and do not interact, and the reasons why we should and how we could strive to engage them in the healthcare system reveals a complex picture.

Lack of Health Service Infrastructure for Males

As boys transition out of childhood and into adolescence, their visits to primary care providers begin to decline. By mid to late adolescence, boys stop visiting their childhood physicians, which results in increasingly low rates of primary care visits [31]. In contrast, for girls, this transition is marked by their first visit to the gynecologist or primary care physician. This first visit traditionally involved their first annual Pap smears for cervical cancer screening. With newer guidelines emerging over the past decade that recommend initial Pap smears at the age of 21, we may start to see changing rates. However, without other policy or guideline changes, a broad range of services still exist that are specifically geared toward women's health, strengthening this connection of women to health services. Included among these are the US-centric physician-regulated pregnancy prevention services—access to contraception—as well as other SHR screening.

Males do not have a comparable connection to the health system that promotes utilization of services in this transitional period of their life. Among both male and female 12–17-year-olds, less than half receive the recommended yearly preventive care visits [32]. As compared to females, young adult males are less likely to have a usual source of healthcare (63 % vs. 78 %), are less likely to have visited a doctor in the past year (59 % vs. 81 %), and are less likely to have visited the emergency department within the last year (19 % vs. 27 %) [31, 33–35]. The lack of knowledgeable clinicians engaged in caring for the AYA males; the lack of clear clinical guidelines for AYA males, including routine STI screening as we have for women for chlamydia; and the common lack of insurance coverage for this age group are commonly stated systemic factors for low rates of preventive service utilization by AYA males [36–38]. We will discuss the latter two factors further.

Despite guidelines that include preventive services for AYA males—the American Medical Association's Guidelines for Adolescent Preventive Services (GAPS) [39] and Bright Futures [40]—the counseling of male teenagers, particularly around the prevention of sexually transmitted infections (STIs) or HIV infection, still warrant significant improvement [37, 41]. Primary care providers take male sexual histories three times less often than female sexual histories and counsel males two times less than females on the use of condoms [42]. The USPSTF does not recommend STI screening for men who are not at increased risk [43]. The USPSTF recommends HIV and syphilis screening for men engaging in high-risk sexual behavior. Additionally, because of significant geographic and community variation, physicians should consider the risk in the community and populations they serve when making decisions about screening men for syphilis [43]. Despite the fact that *Chlamydia* infections are common and curable, the clearest guidelines for the frequency of screening exist for heterosexual women, but not for heterosexual men [44].

Young adults represent the age group with lowest health insurance coverage rates, with young adult males having lower rates than their female counterparts [31, 33, 45, 46]. The passage of the Affordable Care Act in 2010 and the accompanying expansion of dependent coverage may lead to advances in AYA male coverage [46]. However, coverage rates and associated health service utilization rates among young males remain unacceptably low.

Masculinities

Masculinity may be defined as, "a set of culturally shared beliefs about how men should and should not present themselves" [47]. It is a complex and socially guided set of activities that represent what it means to be a man [48]. Dominant masculine norms tend to stress independence, strength, autonomy, and emotional stoicism [49]. Current scholars of masculinity suggest that masculine behaviors are "neither biologically determined nor unique," but, rather, learned through social interactions that begin early in life and continue through adult life [50–52]. Adolescent and young adult years offer increasingly salient opportunities to "try" masculine gender norms and incorporate them or challenge them [36, 48, 49, 53]. However, research on masculinity suggests that there may not be any one dominant or homogenous masculine gender norm, but instead a complex spectrum of masculinities [54].

Of considerable concern in adolescent male health is the frequent and increasing disconnect from healthcare associated with exposure to masculine gender norms over the period of adolescence [55]. Taken together, the dominant cultural view of masculinity and the individual expressions of masculinity make masculinity both a systemic and an individual factor in the health-seeking behaviors by males. Strong adherence to the dominant masculine ideals is associated with less care-seeking behaviors [53, 55]. With hegemonic masculine gender norms stressing autonomy, strength, and self-reliance, many young males see health-seeking behaviors as incongruent with what it means to be a man [36, 55]. This disconnect between young males and the healthcare system represents a missed opportunity to provide them with the support and care that they need during this transitional period of their lives [55]. Subscription to masculine beliefs among AYA males has been associated with poor sexual health outcomes, poorer mental health outcomes, and lower health service utilization [52, 53, 55, 56].

The relationship between the subscription to dominant masculine beliefs with poorer mental health outcomes must be underscored. Poor mental health outcomes are most likely related to increased subscription to anger, as the most commonly expressed emotion, which likely leads to injury, particularly violence to the other or to the self. In other words, it is likely that our top three causes of mortality are mediated through masculinity's emotional lens. Many young males use emotional stoicism and acting tough and stereotypical masculine feelings and behaviors, as the only coping strategy available to them. Furthermore compounding the issue, the proscribed stoicism limits adolescent and young males' willingness to share their concerns or seek social support or psychological support [57]. This results in many young males remaining or becoming disconnected from supportive and caring adults who are willing to listen to their concerns and offer support.

Frameworks for Engaging AYA Males

Trauma-Informed Care Framework

An AYA male-centered space creates an environment that is safe, welcoming, and inclusive. Adolescents, in general, and sometimes young adults, can evoke strong emotional responses and can make them vulnerable to our unconscious biases [58]. Similarly, many AYA males, particularly in groups, but sometimes as individuals, can evoke strong emotional responses, sometimes based on systemic factors such as unconscious racism or homophobia. The confines of the ideals of masculinity can create trauma, particularly as it relates to mental health [59–61]. The toxic effects of these and sometimes more obvious physically and emotionally traumatic experiences, such as overall aspects of poverty, arrests, and incarcerations can create a sense of powerlessness that in turn generates feelings of resentment and anger [60]. It is imperative that clinical environments, at a minimum, do not recreate these experiences.

A trauma-informed care framework can be one component in addressing these issues [59]. Trauma-informed care stresses the importance of providers and staff being sensitive, receptive, and understanding of the complex issues that AYA males face. This understanding must encompass the issues of masculinity, racism, discrimination, and poverty and the role these issues play on the physical and mental health of these young males. The presence of these issues also serves as barriers to healthcare access [59].

Providers must therefore develop an understanding of the issues faced by young males, recognize the symptoms of these issues, and respond in an appropriate manner. The most significant protective factor for adolescents and especially those who have experienced trauma is a healthy relationship with at least one caring adult [59, 60]. Developing and maintaining a supportive and trusting relationship with a young man may directly benefit their health. In this way healthcare providers are in a unique position to offer the support and healthy relationship that many AYA males need.

Positive Youth Development and Strength-Based Frameworks

The foundation of a Positive Youth Development (PYD) framework is assessing and building on the strengths of AYA male patients, rather than focusing on problems [62]. The PYD framework includes three basic assumptions:

1. Focus on strengths and assets rather than deficits and problems.
2. Strengths and assets are usually acquired through positive relationships, especially with pro-social and caring adults.
3. The development of youth assets occurs in multiple contexts and environments [62].

Many of our young males, particularly minority and other marginalized youth, receive messages that they are troublesome, even dangerous. These messages can diminish the possibility of ultimate positive development. Strength-based practice reframes the toxic messages that our AYA males endure [63]. One can use strength-based messaging while simultaneously challenging false assumptions. The use of strength-based communication strategies creates opportunities to:

1. Teach youth to recognize and capitalize on their strengths
2. Make suggestions to boost strength areas that are lacking or deficient
3. Engage youth in a discussion about needed behavioral change
4. Have structured discussions about behavioral change (e.g., motivational interviewing/health coaching) [64]

When these principles are applied to the sphere of primary care, providers gain the opportunity to facilitate the development of skills and assets among AYA males.

Engaging AYA Males in Healthcare

Structure Discussions and Relationships for Behavioral Change

Overall there is a lack of evidence to support the benefits of an annual health mainte-nance examination on asymptomatic adults [30, 65]. In the traditional tertiary health-care sense, AYA males are healthy. However, an "AYA-centered" model would support healthy behaviors and engage young males in behavioral change early. Services focused on healthy lifestyle behaviors would address those issues related to the pre-vention of early mortality and morbidity in adolescence and young adulthood as well as issues related to morbidity and mortality in older males in later adulthood. This model goes beyond an imparting of knowledge, beyond the basics of knowing one's anatomy, and beyond ruling out pathology. It would truly engage the individual in a patient-centered way to encourage physical and mental health behaviors that help to prevent the top three causes of mortality. Most of our current office-based interven-tions do not take this patient-centered approach. Structured discussions, called moti-vational interviewing (MI) or health coaching, are promising techniques to encourage healthier lifestyles among AYA males.

Motivational Interviewing

Motivational interviewing (MI) and health coaching are terms for the same skill set [65]. MI is effective regardless of gender, i.e., gender neutral. However, it has been validated to help patients achieve behavioral change in a number of different areas. Among the validated behavioral targets that are particularly relevant to AYA males are improving diet, enhancing exercise, pedometer use, weight loss, alcohol cessa-tion, smoking cessation, promoting condom use, and decreasing risky sexual behav-iors [57, 58, 66].

Motivational interviewing is a complex skill set that can be learned and mastered [67]. It honors patient autonomy to make choices regarding when and how to change [63, 67]. The motivational interviewing approach is often most effective with clients who are resistant to change. From a psychological perspective and using the stages of change model, these patients may not be actively contemplating behavioral change, i.e., in "precontemplation" [68]. Thus, it is important that providers "roll with the resistance" while redirecting ambivalent feelings toward a motivation for change [67]. Motivational interviewing is effective in working with patients to identify, understand, and aspire to positive behavioral change, regardless of where they are in their stage of change. In using this framework effectively, the provider becomes an ally in promot-ing positive behavioral change, rather than an expert, authority, or lecturer.

MI is a patient-centered style of counseling built on collaborative principles and has two primary elements. The first is the spirit of unconditional acceptance—meeting the patient where they are in the moment. This includes a foundation of empathy, non-judgment, and reception throughout discussions. The second element focuses on eliciting change talk. Together, these two elements create a nuanced balance of effective motivational interviewing.

MI incorporates valued behaviors of supportive and empathetic listening and reflection [67]. In MI, providers engage the patient at whatever behavioral change they would like to engage. Key to MI is the notion that all of the options and strategies for behavioral change come from the patient. This process is built on the understanding that the provider is accepting the patient where they are, not judging or berating their behaviors. MI helps the patient explore the costs and benefits of potential behaviors. Providers elicit and listen carefully to clients' readiness to change—"change talk." Throughout discussion, providers focus on eliciting, reflecting on, and reinforcing change talk. In doing so, patient ambivalence is resolved, by focusing on positive and proactive behaviors that promote the patient's self-chosen goals [67].

The Physician's Office Staff

The physician's office staff is a central element of a safe and welcoming environment for AYA males. Young males will engage when they know that the staff and their clinicians genuinely care about them. As with all patients, but particularly with "hard to reach" and "difficult to engage" populations, it is largely about relationships—connections [36, 61]. Lessons learned from the LGBT experience of healthcare reveal the importance of having all staff members on board with the clinic's vision. Over 95 % of surveyed LGBT patients reported having monitored healthcare providers' behavior for signs of acceptance [69]. The human context in a visit makes it meaningful and acceptable. Understanding that they, as AYA males, are genuinely listened to and that they matter is of utmost importance [70]. Implicit is the recognition that the medical staff are knowledgeable and can address their health needs [36, 71]. However this connection must extend beyond the patient's clinician. Having an engaging staff from the beginning of registration and throughout is important. Successful LGBT clinics stress the importance of training receptionists, medical assistants, nurses, and physicians to deal respectfully with LGBT patients. Although the need is particularly important for vulnerable populations such as the LGBT population, the same holds true for non-LGBT AYA males.

Clinical Resources

A number of the referenced sources in this chapter contain practical information that is directly applicable to clinical practice. Most of these focus on sexual and reproductive health issues and the AYA males (see, e.g., Bell, Marcell). However, until recently little practical guidance existed to assist clinicians in their interactions with the AYA male patient in areas outside of sexual and reproductive health. In response to this need, the Partnership for Male Youth released the Health Provider Toolkit for Adolescent and Young Adult Males in 2014. The Toolkit contains a database of all the known scientific literature on the healthcare needs of AYA males in six domains: healthy eating and physical activity, sexual and reproductive health, trauma, substance use disorders, mental health, and the physical examination and immunizations. That database also includes clinical recommendations and some practical guidance applicable to the AYA male visit that has been released in recent years by medical- and health-related organizations. In 2015, the work of the Partnership for Male Youth is expanding on the Health Provider Toolkit by developing resources and tools specific to AYA male clinical visit. These include an AYA male patient self-assessment tool on healthy sexuality and immunizations, together with a clinician guide on the subjects, which was released mid-2015. Additional clinical resources are under development and will continue to be released in subsequent years. For further and current information visit: The Partnership for Male Youth (http://www.partnershipformaleyouth.org).

Conclusion

AYA males continue to face a unique and specific set of risk factors and causes of mortality and morbidity. Young males face many and create some barriers between themselves and the health system, including issues such as masculine gender norms and gender nonconformity. This disconnection between AYA males and the health system has hindered our ability to provide these young males necessary services. In order to better serve AYA males and their health needs, we must adopt ways to be more accessible to and inclusive of them. This process begins with building male friendly clinical environments that welcome males and demonstrate that health seeking is congruent with being a healthy and responsible man. Working collaboratively with AYA males on their health issues can decrease current risk behaviors while acknowledging their strengths, as well as proactively working toward lifelong behavioral changes that can hopefully decrease early morbidities and mortality.

References

1. Barrett AE, White HR. Trajectories of gender role orientations in adolescence and early adulthood: a prospective study of the mental health effects of masculinity and femininity. J Health Soc Behav. 2002;43(4):451–68.
2. Adolescent & Young Adult Health Program. (n.d.). Retrieved November 18, 2015, from http://mchb.hrsa.gov/programs/adolescents/.
3. Grad FP. The preamble of the constitution of the world health organization. Bull World Health Organ. 2002;80:981–84.
4. Singh GK, Azuine RE, Siahpush M, Kogan MD. All-cause and cause-specific mortality among US youth: socioeconomic and rural-urban disparities and international patterns. J Urban Health. 2013;90:388–405.

5. Viner RM, Coffey C, Mathers C, et al. 50-year mortality trends in children and young people: a study of 50 low-income, middle-income, and high-income countries. Lancet. 2011;377:1162–74.
6. Kann L, Kinchen S, Shanklin SL, et al. Youth risk behavior surveillance—United States, 2013. MMWR Surveill Summ. 2014;63:1–168.
7. Eaton DK, Kann L, Kinchen S, et al. Youth risk behavior surveillance-United States, 2011. Morbidity and mortality weekly report Surveillance summaries (Washington, DC: 2002) 2012;61:1–162.
8. Ogden CL, Statistics NCfH. Prevalence of obesity in the United States, 2009–2010. US Department of Health and Human Services, Centers for Disease Control and Prevention, National Center for Health Statistics; 2012.
9. Physical Activity Facts; 2012. Accessed May 14, 2015, from www.cdc.gov/healthyyouth/physicalactivity/facts.htm.
10. American Academy of Psychiatry. Highlights of Changes from DSM-IV-TR to DSM-5; 2013.
11. Broh BA. Gender and the body. The Wiley Blackwell Encyclopedia of Health, Illness, Behavior, and Society; 2014.
12. Wylie C, Platt S, Brownie J, Chandler A. Men, suicide and society. London: Samaritans; 2012.
13. Centers for Disease Control and Prevention. Youth Risk Behavior Surveillance System: Selected 2011 National Health Risk Behaviors and Health Outcomes by Sex; 2012;5:5.0–6.7.
14. Likely M, Males T. Youth Risk Behavior Surveillance System: Selected 2011 National Health Risk Behaviors and Health Outcomes by Sex. Suicide; 5:5.0–6.7
15. Kolodny A, Courtwright DT, Hwang CS, et al. The prescription opioid and heroin crisis: a public health approach to an epidemic of addiction. Annu Rev Public Health. 2015;36:559–74.
16. Muhuri PK, Gfroerer JC, Davies MC. Associations of nonmedical pain reliever use and initiation of heroin use in the United States. The CBHSQ Data Review; 2013.
17. Flannery DJ, Williams LL, Vazsonyi AT. Who are they with and what are they doing? Delinquent behavior, substance use, and early adolescents' after-school time. Am J Orthopsychiatry. 1999;69:247–53.
18. Garnier HE, Stein JA. An 18-year model of family and peer effects on adolescent drug use and delinquency. J Youth Adolesc. 2002;31:45–56.
19. Finer LB, Philbin JM. Sexual initiation, contraceptive use, and pregnancy among young adolescents. Pediatrics. 2013;131(5):886–91.
20. Chandra A. Sexual behavior, sexual attraction, and sexual identity in the United States: data from the 2006–2008 National Survey of Family Growth: Citeseer; 2011.
21. Coker TR, Austin SB, Schuster MA. The health and health care of lesbian, gay, and bisexual adolescents. Annu Rev Public Health. 2010;31:457–77.
22. Martinez G, Daniels K, Chandra A. Fertility of men and women aged 15–44 years in the United States: National Survey of Family Growth. Natl Health Stat Rep. 2010;2006:1–28.
23. Miller WC, Ford CA, Morris M, et al. Prevalence of chlamydial and gonococcal infections among young adults in the United States. JAMA. 2004;291:2229–36.
24. Miller WC, Swygard H, Hobbs MM, et al. The prevalence of trichomoniasis in young adults in the United States. Sex Transm Dis. 2005;32:593–8.
25. Xu F, Sternberg MR, Markowitz LE. Men who have sex with men in the United States: demographic and behavioral characteristics and prevalence of HIV and HSV-2 infection: results from National Health and Nutrition Examination Survey 2001–2006. Sex Transm Dis. 2010;37:399–405.
26. Mimiaga MJ, Helms DJ, Reisner SL, et al. Gonococcal, chlamydia, and syphilis infection positivity among MSM attending a large primary care clinic, Boston, 2003 to 2004. Sex Transm Dis. 2009;36:507–11.
27. Prejean J, Song R, Hernandez A, et al. Estimated HIV incidence in the United States, 2006–2009. PLoS One. 2011;6, e17502.
28. Ard K, Harvey J, Makadon J. Improving the health care of lesbian, gay, bisexual and transgender people: Understanding and eliminating health disparities. The National LGBT Health Education Center, The Fenway Institute, Brigham and Women's Hospital; 2012.
29. Kitts RL. Barriers to optimal care between physicians and lesbian, gay, bisexual, transgender, and questioning adolescent patients. J Homosex. 2010;57:730–47.

30. Prochazka AV, Lundahl K, Pearson W, Oboler SK, Anderson RJ. Support of evidence-based guidelines for the annual physical examination: a survey of primary care providers. Arch Intern Med. 2005;165:1347–52.
31. Kirzinger WK, Cohen RA, Gindi RM. Health care access and utilization among young adults aged 19–25: early release of estimates from the National Health Interview Survey, January–September 2011. Centers for Disease Control and Health. Atlanta, GA: Centers for Disease Control and Prevention; 2012:1–10.
32. Irwin CE, Adams SH, Park MJ, Newacheck PW. Preventive care for adolescents: few get visits and fewer get services. Pediatrics. 2009;123:e565–e72.
33. Adams SH, Newacheck PW, Park MJ, Brindis CD, Irwin CE. Health insurance across vulnerable ages: patterns and disparities from adolescence to the early 30s. Pediatrics. 2007;119:e1033–e9.
34. Bonhomme JJ. Men's health: impact on women, children and society. J Men's Health Gend. 2007;4:124–30.
35. Marcell AV, Klein JD, Fischer I, Allan MJ, Kokotailo PK. Male adolescent use of health care services: where are the boys? J Adolesc Health. 2002;30:35–43.
36. Armstrong B, Cohall A. Health promotion with adolescent and young adult males: an empowerment approach. Adolesc Med State Art Rev. 2011;22:544–80. xii.
37. Marcell AV, Bell DL, Lindberg LD, Takruri A. Prevalence of sexually transmitted infection/human immunodeficiency virus counseling services received by teen males, 1995–2002. J Adolesc Health. 2010;46:553–9.
38. Sonenstein FL. Young men's sexual and reproductive health: toward a national strategy (getting started); 2000.
39. American Medical Association. Guidelines for adolescent preventive services (GAPS): recommendations monograph: American Medical Association, Department of Adolescent Health; 1995.
40. Green M. Bright futures: guidelines for health supervision of infants, children, and adolescents: ERIC; 1994
41. Ma J, Wang Y, Stafford RS. US adolescents receive suboptimal preventive counseling during ambulatory care. J Adolesc Health. 2005;36:441. e1–e7.
42. Lafferty WE, Downey L, Holan CM, et al. Provision of sexual health services to adolescent enrollees in medicaid managed care. Am J Public Health. 2002;92:1779–83.
43. Meyers D, Wolff T, Gregory K, et al. USPSTF recommendations for STI screening. Am Fam Physician. 2008;77:819–24.
44. Workowski KA, Bolan G. Sexually transmitted diseases treatment guidelines. MMWR Recomm Rep. 2015;64:1–140.
45. Callahan ST, Harris SK, Austin SB, Woods ER. Who is at risk of being uninsured among 19–24 year olds? J Adolesc Health. 2002;30:104.
46. Sommers BD, Buchmueller T, Decker SL, Carey C, Kronick R. The Affordable Care Act has led to significant gains in health insurance and access to care for young adults. Health Aff. 2013;32:165–74.
47. Bell DL, Rosenberger JG, Ott MA. Masculinity in adolescent males' early romantic and sexual heterosexual relationships. Am J Men's Health. 2015;9(3):201–8.
48. West C, Zimmerman DH. Doing gender. Gend Soc. 1987;1:125–51.
49. Courtenay WH. Constructions of masculinity and their influence on men's well-being: a theory of gender and health. Soc Sci Med. 2000;50:1385–401.
50. Brody LR. The socialization of gender differences in emotional expression: display rules, infant temperament, and differentiation. Gender and emotion: social psychological perspectives 2000:24–47.
51. Chodorow NJ. The reproduction of mothering: psychoanalysis and the sociology of gender. Berkeley, CA: University of California Press; 1999.
52. Pleck JH, Sonenstein FL, Ku LC. Masculinity ideology: its impact on adolescent males' heterosexual relationships. J Soc Issues. 1993;49:11–29.
53. Tyler RE, Williams S. Masculinity in young men's health: exploring health, help-seeking and health service use in an online environment. J Health Psychol. 2014;19:457–70.

54. Connell RW, Messerschmidt JW. Hegemonic masculinity rethinking the concept. Gend Soc. 2005;19:829–59.
55. Marcell AV, Ford CA, Pleck JH, Sonenstein FL. Masculine beliefs, parental communication, and male adolescents' health care use. Pediatrics. 2007;119:e966–e75.
56. Vogel DL, Heimerdinger-Edwards SR, Hammer JH, Hubbard A. "Boys don't cry": examination of the links between endorsement of masculine norms, self-stigma, and help-seeking attitudes for men from diverse backgrounds. J Couns Psychol. 2011;58:368.
57. Addis ME, Mahalik JR. Men, masculinity, and the contexts of help seeking. Am Psychol. 2003;58:5.
58. Lerman A. Examining our unconscious biases. In: Ginsburg KR, Kinsman SB, editors. Reaching teens: strength-based communication strategies to build resilience and support healthy adolescent development. Elk Grove Village, IL: American Academy of Pediatrics; 2014. p. 165–9.
59. Rich J, Corbin T, Bloom S, Rich L, Evans S, Wilson A. Healing the hurt: trauma-informed approaches to the health of boys and young men of color. Center for Nonviolence and Social Justice, Drexel University School of Public Health and Department of Emergency Medicine 2009:9.
60. Ginsburg KR. Wisdom from model strength-based programs That work with youth who are traditionally labeled "at risk". In: Ginsburg KR, Kinsman SB, editors. Reaching teens: strength-based communication strategies to build resilience and support healthy adolescent development. Elk Grove Village, IL: American Academy of Pediatrics; 2014. p. 9–17.
61. Lewis VJ, Campbell K, Diaz A, Dowshen NL, Ginsburg KR, Jenkins R. Cultural humility. In: Ginsburg KR, Kinsman SB, editors. Reaching teens: strength-based communication strategies to build resilience and support healthy adolescent development. Elk Grove Village, IL: American Academy of Pediatrics; 2014. p. 145–9.
62. Butts J, Mayer S, Ruth G. Focusing juvenile justice on positive youth development: Chapin Hall Center for Children at the University of Chicago, Chicago; 2005.
63. Ginsburg KR. The journey from risk-focused attention to strength-based care. In: Ginsburg KR, Kinsman SB, editors. Reaching teens: strength-based communication strategies to build resilience and support healthy adolescent development. Elk Grove Village, IL: American Academy of Pediatrics; 2014. p. 9–17.
64. Frankowski BL, Leader IC, Duncan PM. Strength-based interviewing. Adolesc Med State Art Rev. 2009;20:22–40. vii–viii.
65. Huffman M. Health coaching: a new and exciting technique to enhance patient self-management and improve outcomes. Home Healthc Nurse. 2007;25:271–4.
66. Douaihy A, Kelly TM, Gold M, editors. Motivational interviewing: a guide for medical trainees. New York: Oxford University Press; 2014.
67. Hettema J, Steele J, Miller WR. Motivational interviewing. Annu Rev Clin Psychol. 2005;1:91–111.
68. Remafedi G, French S, Story M, Resnick MD, Blum R. The relationship between suicide risk and sexual orientation: results of a population-based study. Am J Public Health. 1998;88:57–60.
69. Eliason MJ, Schope R. Original research: does "don't ask don't tell" apply to health care? Lesbian, gay, and bisexual people's disclosure to health care providers. J Gay Lesbian Med Assoc. 2001;5:125–34.
70. Ginsburg KR. Body language. In: Ginsburg KR, Kinsman SB, editors. Reaching teens: strength-based communication strategies to build resilience and support healthy adolescent development. Elk Grove Village, IL: American Academy of Pediatrics; 2014. p. 111–7.
71. Kapphahn CJ, Wilson KM, Klein JD. Adolescent girls' and boys' preferences for provider gender and confidentiality in their health care. J Adolesc Health. 1999;25:131–42.

Chapter 7
The Evidence-Based Well Male Examination in Adult Men

Mark J. Flynn

Introduction

There are approximately 154 million men of all ages in the United States (USA), with approximately 75 % of those being age 18 years and over [1]. There are more than 44.4 million periodic adult preventive health visits annually in the USA [2]. There are a variety of reasons such visits continue to be recommended by physicians and desired by patients, but the adult preventive health examination has drawn increasing attention with regard to utility and benefit, not to mention cost-effectiveness and outcomes. If one considers the leading causes of death in men in the USA (Table 7.1), a reasonable argument could be made to focus efforts in prevention for these conditions, where such ability exists [3].

Health insurance and access to care are strong determinants of utilization of primary care [4]. Between 2002 and 2012, in adults aged 18–44 years, the percentage of private coverage with insurance fell from 68.7 % to 61.4 %, while the percentage with Medicaid coverage increased from 7.1 % to 11.6 % [4]. According to data from the National Health Interview Survey, adults aged 25–34 years (23.4 %) were the most likely to lack health insurance coverage. Among persons under age 65 years, adults aged 45–64 years (71.1 %) were the most likely to have private coverage. Among adults in age groups 18–24 years, 25–34 years, and 35–44 years, men were more likely than women to lack health insurance coverage [5].

Many of the recommendations for guiding preventive health care come from the US Preventive Services Task Force (USPSTF). The USPSTF was created in 1984 as an "independent, volunteer panel of national experts in prevention and evidence-based medicine… (that) works to improve the health of all Americans by making evidence-based recommendations about clinical preventive services such as screenings,

M.J. Flynn (✉)
Family Medicine Residency, Naval Hospital Camp Pendleton, Camp Pendleton, CA, USA
e-mail: navyfpdoc@gmail.com

© Springer International Publishing Switzerland 2016
J.J. Heidelbaugh (ed.), *Men's Health in Primary Care*, Current Clinical Practice,
DOI 10.1007/978-3-319-26091-4_7

Table 7.1 Leading causes of
death in males, USA, 2011

Cause	Percent
Heart disease	24.6
Cancer	24.1
Unintentional injuries	6.3
Chronic lower respiratory diseases	5.4
Stroke	4.2
Diabetes	3.1
Suicide	2.5
Alzheimer's disease	2.0
Influenza and pneumonia	2.0
Kidney disease	1.8

Centers for Disease Control and Prevention. Leading Causes of Death in Males United States, 2011. http://www.cdc.gov/men/lcod/2011/index.htm. Accessed 05 May 2015

Table 7.2 What the US Preventive Services Task Force grades mean and suggestions for practice

Grade	Definition	Suggestion for practice
A	Recommended service	Offer to provide
B	Recommended service	Offer to provide
C	Not routinely recommended; net benefit likely small	Offer to provide if other considerations support offering
D	Recommended against	Discourage use
I	Evidence insufficient for or against	Ensure patient understanding regarding uncertainty about risk vs. benefit

US Preventive Services Task Force. http://www.uspreventiveservicestaskforce.org. Accessed 03 May 2015

counseling services, and preventive medicine" [6]. Each recommendation from the USPSTF carries a letter grade dictated by the strength of evidence and the balance of harms compared to risks of a given service (Table 7.2). Currently, there are up to 20 level A or B recommendations for adult men [7]. Not all will be covered in this chapter, but as a basis for performing an annual health review or checkup, clinicians should consider performing the level A and B services, avoiding most level D services yet discussing them so as to offer shared decision-making, and discussing the risk versus benefit ratio for level C or I services across individual men.

History

The essential components of the history for the adult male are the past medical and surgical histories, current medications and allergies, as well as family and social histories. Any lifestyle risk factors should be addressed including diet and exercise

Table 7.3   CAGE questionnaire

Have you ever felt you should **C**ut down on your drinking?
Have people **A**nnoyed you by criticizing your drinking?
Have you ever felt bad or **G**uilty about your drinking?
Have you ever had a drink first thing in the morning to steady your nerves or get rid of a hangover (**E**ye opener)?

Ewing JA. Detecting Alcoholism: The CAGE Questionnaire. JAMA 252: 1905–1907, 1984.

patterns; obesity; substance use or abuse including tobacco, alcohol, prescription controlled substances, and illicit drugs; sexual practices; and personal and family history of mood disorders.

Risk Factor Assessment

All adults should be screened for alcohol misuse, and anyone engaged in hazardous or risky drinking be offered behavioral counseling interventions (grade B) [8]. It is estimated that 30 % of the US population is involved in alcohol misuse, resulting in more than 85,000 deaths per year [9]. Risky drinking is defined by consumption of more than four drinks on any day or more than 14 in a week. However, in men over 65 years of age, the acceptable amounts drop to three per day and seven per week [10]. The CAGE questionnaire remains a viable tool to use in the clinical setting in the assessment of alcohol use (Table 7.3) [11]. Each item is scored a 0 or a 1; a total score of 2 or higher is considered clinically significant [8].

Tobacco use continues to be a prevalent risk factor and remains the leading preventable cause of death in the USA [12]. Twenty-one percent of adult men are current smokers, while 55 % have never smoked. Social and ethnic differences apply as well. When considered by race without consideration of ethnicity, 10 % of Asian adults were active smokers, compared to 19 % of American Indian or Alaska Natives, 17 % of black adults, and 19 % of white adults; 17 % of Hispanic men were smokers, compared with 22 % each for non-Hispanic white men and non-Hispanic black men. Other factors that were associated with a higher rate of tobacco use were unemployed status, being in a poor family, and lack private insurance or Medicaid [13]. As such, all men should be screened for current or past tobacco use and clinicians should provide tobacco cessation interventions for those who use tobacco products (grade A). The "5-A" behavioral counseling framework is a useful tool for discussion of tobacco use with patients:

1. **A**sk about tobacco use.
2. **A**dvise to quit through clear personalized messages.
3. **A**ssess willingness to quit.
4. **A**ssist to quit.
5. **A**rrange follow-up and support [12].

Recommendations of Others

The American Academy of Family Physicians (AAFP) concurs with the USPSTF statements on alcohol and tobacco screening [14]. The American College of Preventive Medicine recommends the following:

1. Tobacco usage history should be obtained at all visits.
2. Nonsmokers should be encouraged not to start.
3. Office and medical record systems that identify patients as tobacco users should be employed.
4. Physicians and other office staff should advise all tobacco users to quit.
5. Physicians and other office staff should identify and assist smokers who are willing to quit.
6. Physicians and other office staff should provide motivational interventions for smokers who are not willing to quit [15].

Sexually Transmitted Infections

The USPSTF has recommendation statements that apply for general counseling, as well as for screening for human immunodeficiency virus (HIV), hepatitis B and C, and syphilis.

Intensive behavioral counseling is recommended for all adults who are at increased risk for sexually transmitted infections (grade B). Risk groups that have been included in counseling studies include adults with current sexually transmitted infections (STIs) or other infections within the past year, adults who have multiple sexual partners, and men who do not consistently use condoms. Awareness of populations with increased risk of STIs should also help guide clinicians toward recommending counseling services. In particular, African Americans have the highest STI prevalence of any racial/ethnic group, and STI prevalence is higher in American Indians, Alaska Natives, and Latinos than in white persons.

Increased STI prevalence rates are also found in men who have sex with men (MSM), persons with low incomes living in urban settings, current or former inmates, military recruits, persons who exchange sex for money or drugs, persons with mental illness or a disability, current or former intravenous drug users, persons with a history of sexual abuse, and patients at public STI clinics. In general, the more time spent performing counseling, the better the evidence of benefit, with the best being intensive sessions lasting at least 2 h of contact time. Most successful approaches provided basic information about STIs and STI transmission, assessed the person's risk for transmission, and provided training in pertinent skills, such as condom use, communication about safe sex, problem solving, and goal setting [16].

Screening for HIV is recommended for all adults up to 65 years of age and for older adults who are at increased risk (grade A) [17]. Overall, about 36 % of all adults aged 18 and over have ever been tested for HIV, with women more likely than men

[13]. It is estimated that 20–25 % of individuals with HIV infection are unaware of their positive status, and there is clear benefit to early identification and treatment to markedly reduce the risk of progression to acquired immunodeficiency syndrome (AIDS), AIDS-related events, and death in individuals with immunologically advanced disease (defined as a CD4 count $< 0.200 \times 10^9$ cells/L) [17].

Men at high risk for infection with hepatitis B (HBV) should be screened (grade B). There are between 700,000 and 2.2 million people in the USA with chronic HBV. Persons considered at high risk for HBV infection include those from regions with a high prevalence of HBV infection (these include sub-Saharan Africa and Central and Southeast Asia), HIV-positive persons, intravenous drug users, household contacts of persons with HBV infection, and MSM. HBV infection carries the risk of long-term sequelae such as cirrhosis, hepatic decompensation, and hepatocellular carcinoma, thus testing and diagnosis are beneficial to determine candidacy for appropriate treatment and proper surveillance for other complicating conditions [18].

Screening for hepatitis C (HCV) is recommended for persons at high risk for infection, and one-time testing should be offered to any man born between 1945 and 1965 (grade B). HCV is the most common blood-borne pathogen in the USA and a leading cause of complications from chronic liver disease. It is estimated that 1.6 % of noninstitutionalized persons have the anti-HCV antibody. The most important risk factor for infection is past or present intravenous drug use, with a prevalence of 50 % or greater; others include sex with an injection drug user and having received a blood transfusion before 1992. Most patients with HCV were born between 1945 and 1965, hence the current recommendation for one-time testing in that defined group [19].

Screening for syphilis is recommended for all men at increased risk for infection (grade A), but the USPSTF recommends against routine screening on asymptomatic persons who are not at increased risk (grade D). At-risk populations include MSM and those who engage in high-risk sexual behavior, commercial sex workers, persons who exchange sex for drugs, and men in adult correctional facilities. There is no specific recommendation on frequency of testing in these groups. Of note, men diagnosed with other STIs may be more likely to engage in high-risk behaviors, placing them at greater risk for syphilis, but there is no evidence that supports routine screening of men with another diagnosed STI for syphilis [20].

Depression

As one of the leading causes of disability, depression affects individuals, families, businesses, and society [21]. It is estimated that 8 % of adult males have symptoms of depression, compared to 12 % of adult females [13]. All adults over the age of 18 should be screened for depression when support systems are in place to assure accurate diagnosis, effective treatment, and follow-up (grade B); when such supports are not in place, it is recommended that no such screening be performed (grade C) [21]. Other factors increase the likelihood of experiencing symptoms of depression including being unemployed, poverty, Medicaid status for those under age 65 years, and having both Medicare and Medicaid for those over 65 years of age [13]. A variety of screening tools exist that have been found to have good sensitivity, however, with only fair specificity. Such tools include the Zung Self-Rating Depression Scale, Beck Depression Inventory, General Health Questionnaire, Center for Epidemiologic Studies Depression Scale, SelfCARE (D), and the Geriatric Depression Scale [21]. All positive screening tests should lead to subsequent full diagnostic evaluation and assessment of severity.

Physical Examination

There are few interventions in the physical examination that demonstrate improved outcomes in healthy, asymptomatic individuals. The focus of the exam should be toward those pertinent areas in relation to risk factors noted in the history, in follow-up to previously diagnosed conditions, or addressing specific concerns or complaints of the patient. Two elements that are of proven benefit are the blood pressure measurement and assessment of body mass index (BMI) [22].

Blood Pressure Assessment

All adults over 18 years of age should be screened for high blood pressure as a method of identifying adults at risk for cardiovascular disease (grade A). For this recommendation, hypertension was defined as a systolic blood pressure (SBP) of 140 mm Hg or higher, while the diastolic blood pressure (DBP) was 90 mm Hg or higher, and these measurements should be obtained on two occasions at least 1 week apart. There was no specific recommendation regarding frequency of measurements, due to lack of evidence. Rather than setting a cutoff point to implement treatment, clinicians are recommended to consider the man's overall cardiovascular risk profile when making decisions [23].

Recommendations of Other Groups

The most recent report from the Eighth Joint National Committee (JNC 8) reinforced the definition of hypertension as noted above (systolic blood pressure of 140 mm Hg or greater and diastolic blood pressure of 90 mm Hg or greater). It stratified recommendations for adults based on age. For those 60 years or older, JNC 8 recommended initiating therapy for an $SBP \geq 150$ mm Hg or $DBP \geq 90$ mm Hg. For adults less than 60 years of age, the same DBP goal is recommended, but a more aggressive SBP goal of 140 mm Hg is advised [24].

Table 7.4 Body mass index (BMI) definitions

19–24.9 kg/m^2	Normal
25.0–29.9 kg/m^2	Overweight
30.0–39.9 kg/m^2	Obese
40.0 kg/m^2 or higher	Extreme obesity

US Preventive Services Task Force. Obesity in adults: screening and management. http://www.uspreventiveservicestaskforce.org/Page/Topic/recommendation-summary/obesity-in-adults-screening-and-management. Accessed 29 Apr 2015

The American Heart Association (AHA), in conjunction with the American Academy of Cardiology (ACC), released guidelines in 2013 recommending a comprehensive overall cardiovascular risk assessment starting at age 20 years [25].

Obesity/Body Mass Index

Obesity rates in the USA are high, currently exceeding 30 % for all adults [26]. Data from the 2011–2012 National Health And Nutrition Examination Survey (NHANES) further show that 33.9 % of US adults 20 years of age and over are overweight, 35.1 % are obese, and 6.4 % are extremely obese [27]. These conditions are associated with other chronic health problems, such as coronary heart disease (CHD) and type 2 diabetes mellitus. Conversely, weight loss is associated with lower incidence of overall health problems and mortality. Therefore, all men should be screened for obesity, and those with a body mass index (BMI) of 30 kg/m^2 or higher should be offered referral to intensive, multicomponent behavioral interventions (grade B) [26] (Table 7.4). BMI is a calculation from measured height and weight, and therefore these should be obtained during the clinic visit. The USPSTF does not recommend a frequency of or interval between BMI measurements [26]. Abdominal waist circumference measurement should also be considered, as its relationship to outcomes in cardiometabolic syndrome has great significance.

Of note, Fryar and colleagues made this statement in regard to Asian adults: "The prevalence of obesity as measured by BMI among non-Hispanic Asian adults was much lower than that reported for non-Hispanic white, non-Hispanic black, and Hispanic adults. Although BMI is widely used as a measure of body fat, at a given BMI level body fat percentage and location may vary by gender, age, and race, and Hispanic origin. In particular, research suggests that Asian persons may have greater body fat percentages than white persons, especially at lower BMIs, and that significant health risks may begin at a lower BMI among Asian persons compared with others." [27]

Chronic Disease Screening

Abdominal Aortic Aneurysm

Abdominal aortic aneurysm (AAA) is estimated to occur between 3.9 % and 7.2 % of men over the age of 50 years. Risk factors include male gender, age greater than 60 years, cigarette smoking, hypertension, white or Native American ethnicity, obesity, family history of AAA, and underlying cardiovascular disease [28]. As such, the USPSTF recommends a one-time screening for AAA via ultrasonography for men ages 65–75 years who ever smoked (grade B) [29]. In a large trial with an AAA prevalence of 5 %, screening led to an absolute risk reduction in AAA death of 1.4 per 1000 men [30]. Offering screening to men who have never smoked is a grade C recommendation, based on other relevant risk factors [29].

Diabetes Mellitus

Diabetes mellitus is estimated to be present in 13.2 % of the adult male population over the age of 20 years, and among those diagnosed by a physician with the condition, 26.2 % have a hemoglobin A1c greater than 9 %. Undiagnosed diabetics are thought to represent 4.2 % of all adult men [31]. The American Diabetes Association (ADA) notes that traditional diagnoses of type 2 diabetes (DM2) occurring only in adults and type 1 diabetes (DM1) only in children is no longer accurate, as both can be found in either group. It is possible for DM2 patients to present in diabetic keto-acidosis, so clinicians must be aware of this possibility. Diagnostic tests for diabetes mellitus include a hemoglobin A1c of 6.5 % or higher, a fasting plasma glucose of 126 mg/dL (7.0 mmol/L) or higher, a 2-hour postprandial glucose of 200 mg/dL (11.1 mmol/L) or higher following a 75 g glucose load, or a patient with classic symptoms of hyperglycemic crisis that has a random plasma glucose of 200 mg/dL (11.1 mmol/L) or higher. Testing for DM2 in asymptomatic individuals should be considered in adults who qualify as overweight (BMI 25 kg/m^2 or higher or 23 kg/m^2 in Asian Americans) who have one or more risk factors for diabetes, starting at age 45 years and repeated every 3 years [32].

The USPSTF recommends screening for DM2 in asymptomatic individuals with a sustained blood pressure greater than 135/80 (grade B) and has insufficient evidence to make a recommendation in screening anyone with a blood pressure below that cutoff (grade I). The rationale for the USPSTF recommendation being different from the ADA was based on adequate evidence that lowering blood pressure in those with diabetes reduces the incidence of cardiovascular events and mortality [33].

Dyslipidemia

Approximately 11 % of adults aged 18 and over have cardiovascular disease, which accounts for nearly half of all deaths in the USA [13, 34]. Nearly one-third of coronary heart disease (CHD) events are attributable to total cholesterol levels greater than 200 mg/dL. In addition, high low density lipoprotein cholesterol (LDL-C) and low high-density lipoprotein cholesterol (HDL-C) are risk factors for developing coronary artery disease (CAD), and the risk for coronary events and deaths increases with increasing levels of total cholesterol and LDL and declining levels of HDL. Other risk factors include diabetes mellitus, previous personal history of CHD or noncoronary atherosclerosis, family history of CVD before the age of 50 years in male relatives or 60 years in female relatives, tobacco use, hypertension, and obesity (BMI of 30 or higher). The USPSTF strongly recommends screening men aged 35 years and older for lipid disorders (grade A) and men aged 20–35 years if they are at increased risk for CHD (grade B). There is no recommendation for men aged 20–35 years who are not at increased risk for CHD (grade C) [34].

The ACC and AHA released guidelines in 2013 that make comprehensive recommendations on initiation of statin therapy across a spectrum of ages and lipid disorders, including other medical comorbidities [35].

The USPSTF recommends against screening with either resting or exercise electrocardiography (ECG) for the prediction of CAD in asymptomatic adults at low risk for CHD events (grade D). They concluded there was insufficient evidence to make a recommendation of ECG testing in asymptomatic adults at intermediate or high risk for CHD events (grade I) [36].

Osteoporosis

Approximately 1 in 5 men are at risk for an osteoporosis-related fracture during their lifetime; however, evidence is limited on the benefits of screening. The USPSTF found insufficient evidence to make a recommendation (grade I) but found that clinicians should consider the following factors when discussing the role of testing with patients: potential preventable burden due to fractures and fracture-related illnesses, potential harms, and costs [37].

Other groups make more specific recommendations in favor of testing. The Endocrine Society recommends testing men with risk factors (those age 70 or greater or those age 50–69 with any of the following: low body weight; prior fracture as an adult; smoking or alcohol abuse; conditions such as delayed puberty, hypogonadism, hyperparathyroidism, hyperthyroidism, or COPD; and chronic use of glucocorticoids or GnRH agonists) with dual-energy X-ray absorptiometry (DEXA) [38]. The American College of Physicians (ACP) recommends that clinicians periodically perform individualized assessment of risk factors for osteoporosis in older men and that clinicians obtain dual-energy X-ray absorptiometry (DEXA) for men who are at increased risk for osteoporosis and are candidates for drug therapy [39]. The National Osteoporosis Foundation recommends screening all men age 70 years and older, men aged 50–69 years with risk factors, all adults over age 50 years with a fracture, and adults with a condition (e.g., rheumatoid arthritis) or taking a medication (e.g., glucocorticoids in a daily dose ≥5 mg prednisone or equivalent for ≥3 months) associated with low bone mass or bone loss [40].

Cancer Screening

The USPSTF has found sufficient evidence to favor screening for colorectal (grade A) [41] and lung cancers (grade B) [42] and for counseling about skin cancer (grade B) [43]. There are strong recommendations against screening (all grade D) for pancreatic, prostate, skin, and testicular cancers [44–47].

Colorectal

Colorectal cancer is the third most common type of cancer, with most cases diagnosed after age 55 years, and has a lifetime risk of 5.7 % for men. Factors associated with an increased risk include increased age, male gender, and black race. The USPSTF recommends screening for colorectal cancer using fecal occult blood testing, sigmoidoscopy, or colonoscopy in adults beginning at age 50 years and continuing to age 75 years (grade A). They recommend against routine screening in adults 76–85 years of age (grade C) and against screening in adults over 85 years (grade D) [41].

The American College of Gastroenterology recommends high-quality colonoscopy every 10 years; other methods include flexible sigmoidoscopy every 5–10 years or computed tomography colonography every 5 years. If these tests are not performed, consider the fecal immunochemical test (FIT) annually. Screening of average risk persons should begin at age 50, while African Americans should begin at age 45 [48].

Lung

Lung cancer is the third most common cancer and the leading cause of cancer death in the USA and is more common in men. Most cases occur after the age of 55 years, and the most important risk factor is smoking; age-adjusted rates vary according to the duration of and exposure to tobacco smoke. The USPSTF recommends annual screening for lung cancer with low-dose computed tomography (LDCT) in adults aged 55–80 years who have a 30 pack-year smoking history and currently smoke or who have quit within in the last 15 years. Screenings may be discontinued once an individual has not smoked for 15 years or develops a health problem that substantially limits life expectancy or the ability or willingness to have curative lung surgery (grade B) [42].

The American Cancer Society also recommends screening for lung cancer with LDCT in high-risk patients who are in relatively good health and meet criteria (persons aged 55–74 years who have a ≥30 pack-year smoking history and currently smoke or have quit in the past 15 years). It recommends against the use of chest radiography and strongly suggests that all adults who receive screening enter an organized screening program that has experience in LDCT [49].

Skin

Skin cancer is the most common type of cancer in the USA, and most deaths occur due to malignant melanoma. The main risk factor is exposure to ultraviolet radiation exposure from childhood through adulthood; other risks include being fair-skinned, having light hair and eye color or freckles, and those who sunburn easily. As such, the USPSTF recommends counseling young adults up to 24 years of age who have fair skin about minimizing their exposure to ultraviolet radiation to reduce the risk for skin cancer (grade B) [43]. However, there is currently insufficient evidence to assess the balance of risks and benefits for whole-body skin examination by a physician or patient skin self-examination for early detection of skin cancers (grade I) [46].

The American Academy of Dermatology recommends individuals perform a self-exam of the body annually and seek evaluation by a dermatologist for any changes, growing lesions, or bleeding [50].

Prostate

Prostate cancer screening continues to be a point of great debate, with varied recommendations from different specialties and groups. The average age of diagnosis is 67 years, with a median age of death from prostate cancer at age 80 years. The lifetime risk is 15.9 %, with a lifetime risk of dying of prostate cancer at 2.8 %. Autopsy studies have shown about a third of men between 40 and 60 years of age have evidence of prostate cancer, with as many as but most cases are well-differentiated lesions that would be considered unlikely to of clinical significance. Risk factors for developing prostate cancer include increased age, black race, and those with a family history of prostate cancer. Prostate-specific antigen (PSA) testing is the most common method of screening and has a conventional cutoff of 4.0 mcg/L, yet this value has limited predictability for detecting cancer. PSA testing at currently accepted ranges yield a false-positive rate of about 80 %, leading to additional and possibly unnecessary testing. With a concern for over diagnosis of prostate tumors, the USPSTF has recommended against PSA screening for prostate cancer (grade D) [45]. Their rationale is derived from potential harm in screening from ultimately leading to prostatectomy surgery that may yield urinary incontinence, impotence, and other complications that may outweigh the risk of watchful waiting.

The American Urological Association (AUA) recommends against PSA screening in men under age 40 years and does not recommend routine screening between ages 40–54 years in men with average risk. For men aged 55–69 years, the AUA strongly recommends shared decision-making for men considering PSA screening and proceeding based on an individual's preferences. Furthermore, they recommend screening interval of 2 years rather than annually to help reduce the rates of overdiagnosis and false positives. They do not recommend screening in men aged 70 years and older with a life expectancy of less than 10–15 years [51].

Testicular

The USPSTF recommends against screening for testicular cancer (grade D). It is a tumor of mostly younger men with a relatively low annual incidence rate that is most often discovered by the patient or a partner. In addition, because of the generally favorable outcomes of treatment, there is adequate evidence to suggest that screening offers little benefit. Screening by self-examination or clinician examination is unlikely to offer meaningful health benefits, given the very low incidence and high cure rate of even advanced testicular cancer.

Potential harms include false-positive results, anxiety, and harms from diagnostic tests or procedures [47].

Pancreatic

The USPSTF recommends against routine screening for pancreatic cancer in asymptomatic adults using abdominal palpation, ultrasonography, or serologic markers (grade D). There has been no convincing evidence that screening for pancreatic cancer decreases mortality, due to the poor prognosis of those who are diagnosed, and the USPSTF concluded that the harms of screening outweighed any potential benefits. There is a potential for significant harm due to the very low prevalence of pancreatic cancer, limited accuracy of available screening tests, the invasive nature of diagnostic tests, and the poor outcomes of treatment. As a result, the USPSTF concluded that the harms of screening for pancreatic cancer exceed any potential benefits [44].

Preventive Meds and Lifestyle

As debate persists regarding the value of the annual preventive health examination and data mounts that many previously valued tests fail to result in improved outcomes, there are still ways to make the visit valuable for the patient and the physician and fit as much benefit as possible into ever-shortening visits. With only a few true physical examination components found to be helpful, behavioral counseling should be done and tailored to the patient's situation, personal beliefs, and lifestyle. Moreover, key elements of preventive screening should be incorporated during acute and other health-care visits to maximize efficiency.

Cardiovascular disease (CVD) is a leading cause of death in the USA, and risk factors addressed above (e.g., diabetes, hyperlipidemia, hypertension, obesity, tobacco use) are exceedingly common. It has been shown that adults who follow appropriate guidelines for diet and exercise have improved cardiovascular morbidity and mortality compared to those who do not [52, 53]. Furthermore, most well adults can reap the potential benefits of improved nutrition, better eating behaviors, and enhanced physical activity [53].

The USPSTF recommends offering or referring adults who are overweight or obese and have additional CVD risk factors to intensive behavioral counseling interventions to promote a healthful diet and physical activity for CVD prevention (grade B) [54, 55].

Use of calculators to assess 10-year risk of a myocardial infarction is recommended. Such calculators take age, race, gender, lipid levels, tobacco use, diabetes history, current systolic blood pressure, and therapy for hypertension, based on recommendations from the ACC/AHA 2013 guidelines [35]. This gives a 10-year and lifetime risks for atherosclerotic cardiovascular disease (coronary death or nonfatal myocardial infarction, or fatal or nonfatal stroke). It is intended for use in those without ASCVD with a LDL cholesterol <190 mg/dL and is applicable to African American and non-Hispanic white men and women 40–79 years of age. Estimates of lifetime risk for ASCVD are provided for adults 20–59 years of age and are shown as the lifetime risk for ASCVD for a 50-year-old without ASCVD who has the risk factor values entered into the calculator. The estimates of lifetime risk are most directly applicable to non-Hispanic whites [56].

Aspirin Use

In addition to recommendations for obtaining an appropriate history, conducting a relevant exam, and applying proper screening, there is a role for preventive aspirin use. With the rates of cardiovascular disease in the USA as noted, risk assessment should be done with accepted tools based on risk factors of age, diabetes, serum lipid levels (including total cholesterol and high-density lipoprotein), blood pressure, and tobacco use [54]. Physicians should assess the overall risk for their patients and weigh that against the risk conferred by use of aspirin, specifically the risk of gastrointestinal (GI) bleeding and hemorrhagic strokes. The USPSTF recommends use of aspirin for men ages 45–79 years when the potential benefit due to reduction in myocardial infarctions outweighs the potential harm due to an increase in gastrointestinal bleeding (grade A); there is inadequate evidence to assess use in men age 80 years and older (grade I); and they recommend against routine use for myocardial infarction prevention in men younger than 45 years of age (grade D) [57]. In addition, the use of aspirin to prevent colorectal cancer is not recommended (grade D) [41].

Immunizations

Immunization recommendations come from the Centers for Disease Control and Prevention (CDC) Advisory Committee on Immunization Practices (ACIP) and are updated on a routine basis. Specific vaccinations for men vary based on age group and underlying medical conditions.

Influenza—Annual vaccination is recommended for all persons over the age of 6 months.

Tdap (Tetanus, diphtheria, and acellular pertussis)—Anyone aged 11 years and older should receive a dose of Tdap followed by tetanus and diphtheria (Td) boosters every 10 years following.

Varicella—All adults that do not show evidence of immunity to varicella should receive vaccination.

Human papillomavirus (HPV)—The current 4-valent vaccine (HPV4) series of three doses is recommended for males up to age 21, and males up to age 26 may also receive the vaccine series. HPV4 is also recommended for men who have sex with men (MSM) through the age of 26.

Zoster—A single dose of zoster vaccine is advised for adult men aged 60 years or older, whether or not they have had a prior shingles event.

Measles, mumps, rubella (MMR)—Any adult born in 1957 or later should have documentation of at least one dose of MMR vaccine. Unlike varicella, provider-diagnosed disease does not constitute acceptable evidence of immunity to these three conditions.

Pneumococcal—One dose of PCV13 is recommended for all adults 65 years of age or older who have not previously received the vaccine. A dose of PPSV23 should be given 6–12 months later. For adults 65 years and older who have already received one or more doses of PPSV23, the dose of PCV13 should be given at least 1 year after receiving the most recent dose of PPSV23.

Meningococcal—High-risk groups include college students, military recruits, those at occupational risk, and those at increased risk for infection (asplenic patients, persistent complement deficiencies).

Hepatitis A (HAV)—Any adult may seek HAV vaccination; those with increased risk include MSM, illicit drug users, those with occupational exposures, patients with chronic liver disease or receive clotting factor concentrates, travelers to endemic areas, and those with a close personal contact with anyone from an endemic area (such as adoptive parents of international children from endemic regions).

Hepatitis B (HBV)—Any adult may seek HBV vaccination; those with increased risk include sexually active individuals not in a monogamous relationship (specifically, more than one sex partner in the previous 6 months), those seeking evaluation or treatment for a sexually transmitted illness, current or recent injection drug users, MSM, those with potential occupational exposures, diabetics, those with end-stage renal disease, household contacts and sexual partners of HBV surface antigen-positive individuals, travelers to endemic areas, and adult residents of care facilities for any of the above listed conditions.

Haemophilus influenzae type b (Hib)—A single dose is recommended for asplenic adults, those with sickle cell disease, and those receiving a hematopoietic stem cell transplant.

Contraindications—Varicella, zoster, and MMW are contraindicated in those with immunocompromising conditions and in HIV with a CD4+ T lymphocyte count below 200 cells/microliter.

Clinicians should be familiar with current recommendations and refer to http://www.cdc.gov/vaccines/hcp/acip-recs/index.html when needed [58].

Insurance Coverage

Most insurance plans will cover, or may even mandate, an annual wellness or health maintenance visit, despite the relative lack of evidence that they improve outcomes. The current version of the Affordable Care Act (ACA) covers preventive services (Table 7.5) and closely resembles those recommended by the USPSTF and CDC [59]. Medicare Part B covers most outpatient screenings as well as additional services such as glaucoma testing, nutrition therapy services, and a yearly wellness visit [60].

With the advent of retail businesses now offering enhanced medical services, there are more options for obtaining routine preventive services and increasing competition for nation's health-care dollars. These are typically on a fee-for-service basis; as examples, Walgreens now offers physical exams that range from $79 to $122 and can increase based on the "length and complexity of the visit" [61]. Additional fees are added for immunizations, blood pressure screening and counseling, laboratory testing of any kind, and wound management, just to name several. Walmart offers "Get Well Stay Well" visits for up to $65, with nurse practitioners performing the care and has an itemized list of services and prices that range from point-of-care tests ($3–$15), external laboratory testing ($8–$36), and immunizations ($25 for the influenza vaccine, $214 for shingles) [62]. CVS MinuteClinic, also staffed by nurse practitioners and physician assistants, has a "comprehensive health screening" starting at $59 and follows a similar model of fee-for-service based on the need; this visit includes blood pressure assessment, height and weight (BMI), review of medical history, and glucose/A1c and lipid testing at an additional cost [63]. Services at such sites may be covered by private insurance. In short, these clinical services meet a need for access without necessarily achieving continuity but meet the basic need and allow patients to pick and choose what they want to have done.

The AAFP recommends that patients read their insurance policies and be aware of what services are covered and which ones are not and whether a co-pay will be required [64].

Table 7.5 Preventive care services covered under the Affordable Care Act (ACA)

Abdominal Aortic Aneurysm one-time screening
Alcohol misuse screening and counseling
Aspirin use for cardiovascular prevention
Blood pressure screening
Cholesterol screening
Colorectal cancer screening for adults over 50
Depression screening
Diabetes (type 2) screening for adults with hypertension
Diet counseling for adults at higher risk for chronic disease
HIV screening for everyone ages 15–65 and other ages at increased risk
Immunizations
Obesity screening and counseling for all adults
Sexually transmitted infection (STI) prevention counseling for adults at higher risk
Syphilis screening for all adults at higher risk
Tobacco use screening for all adults and cessation interventions for tobacco users
Your Medicare Coverage: Preventive visit & yearly wellness exams. http://www.Medicare.gov. Accessed 24 Feb 2015

Executive Physicals

At the other end of the provision-of-care spectrum resides what is referred to as the "executive physical." These exams are described as comprehensive exams often with extensive serologic and screening evaluations, and sometimes even "whole-body CT scans," on the pretext that such a thorough evaluation will find disease before it becomes a threat. Such visits can take a day or two to complete.

As Komaroff stated, "It makes good sense for companies to protect their top talent. Sometimes those who run the show can't find the time to mind their health.

That's where executive physicals come in. With an eye toward prevention, these 1- or 2-day examinations attempt to accommodate busy schedules while supporting the long-term wellness and productivity of a firm's key players" [65]. Many of the nation's most prominent hospitals and clinics offer programs that may cost up to $5000 [66] and find it is worth the expense both as a way to attract top candidates for positions and ensure annual health reviews for their most valued employees. The corporations see these as cost-effective ways for very busy executives to get "one-stop shopping" to address all of their health-care needs. However, very few of the tests performed during such physicals are recommended by the USPSTF, such as PSA, serum testosterone, uric acid, coronary artery calcium CT scoring, and carotid duplex ultrasonography [67].

Motivational Interviewing

Despite having very sound, evidence-based recommendations and clear guidelines for whom many of them apply, it can be challenging to convince some men about the value and need to make changes. The technique of motivational interviewing (MI) is not new, having first been used by Miller for patients with alcoholism [68]. It is fundamentally based on the physician–patient relationship, and the role of the physician is to stimulate a change that must begin with the patient and not be dictated by the former. This is accomplished by using open-ended questions, affirmations, and reflective listening [69]. For example, Ridner and colleagues found that residents' use of motivational interviewing techniques in tobacco cessation participants in the MI groups smoked fewer cigarettes, had higher self-efficacy, and had lower nicotine dependence scores [70]. More information can be found online (http://www.motivationalinterviewing.org) [71].

Effectiveness

Do regular preventive health visits improve outcomes in either morbidity or mortality? Overall, the answer is no. A Cochrane review found that general health checks did not decrease total, cardiovascular-related, or cancer-related mortality and morbidity. Furthermore, morbidity measures such as rates of stroke and cancer were also not affected. The number of new diagnoses did increase [72]. Other studies have shown positive outcomes; one systematic review found an increase in the number of patients receiving recommended preventive services, as well as a reduction in patient worry [73]. Another showed that periodic screening for elevated blood pressure and obesity were beneficial, but the routine complete physical examination was not [22].

Summary

The annual "physical exam" is, rightfully, due for a change in focus. The time physicians spend with patients during such visits is best suited for preventive health and basing recommendations for counseling, preventive health, and screening on evidence-based guidelines such as those provided by the USPSTF and CDC. While such guidelines are not prescriptive, they do rely greatly on shared decision-making between physician and patient and should foster important discussions on the appropriateness of preventive health services tailored for the individual.

References

1. Howden LM, Meyer JA. Age and sex composition: 2010. U.S. Census Bureau, May 2011. http://www.census.gov/prod/cen2010/briefs/c2010br-03.pdf. Accessed 05 May 2015.
2. Shires D, Stange K, et al. Prioritization of evidence-based preventive health services during periodic health examinations. Am J Prev Med. 2012;42(2):164–73.
3. Centers for Disease Control and Prevention. Leading Causes of Death in Males United States, 2011. http://www.cdc.gov/men/lcod/2011/index.htm. Accessed 05 May 2015.
4. Centers for Disease Control and Prevention. Men's Health FastStats. http://www.cdc.gov/nchs/fastats/mens-health.htm. Accessed 24 Apr 2015.
5. Martinez ME, Cohen RA. Health Insurance Coverage: Early Release of Estimates From the National Health Interview Survey, January–September 2014. National Center for Health Statistics; March 2015. http://www.cdc.gov/nchs/data/nhis/earlyrelease/insur201503.pdf.
6. U.S. Preventive Services Task Force. http://www.uspreventiveservicestaskforce.org. Accessed 03 May 2015.
7. U.S. Preventive Services Task Force A and B Recommendations for Adults. Accessed 24 Feb 2015.
8. U.S. Preventive Services Task Force. Alcohol misuse: screening and behavioral counseling interventions in primary care. http://www.uspreventiveservicestaskforce.org/Page/Topic/recommendation-summary/alcohol-misuse-screening-and-behavioral-counseling-interventions-in-primary-care. Accessed 29 Apr 2015.
9. Jonas DE, Garbutt JC, Amick HR, Brown JM, Brownley KA, Council CL, et al. Behavioral counseling after screening for alcohol misuse in primary care: a systematic review and meta-analysis for the U.S. Preventive Services Task Force. Ann Intern Med. 2012;157:645–54.
10. National Institute on Alcohol Abuse and Alcoholism. Rethinking Drinking: Alcohol and Your Health. Bethesda, MD: National Institute on Alcohol Abuse and Alcoholism; 2010. http://pubs.niaaa.nih.gov/publications/rethinkingdrinking/rethinking_drinking.pdf. Accessed 03 May 2015.
11. Ewing JA. Detecting alcoholism: the CAGE questionnaire. JAMA. 1984;252:1905–7.
12. U.S. Preventive Services Task Force. Tobacco use in adults and pregnant women: counseling and interventions. http://www.uspreventiveservicestaskforce.org/Page/Topic/recommendation-summary/tobacco-use-in-adults-and-pregnant-women-counseling-and-interventions. Accessed 05 May 2015.
13. Blackwell DL, Lucas JW, Clarke TC. Summary health statistics for U.S. adults: National Health Interview Survey, 2012. National Center for Health Statistics. Vital Health Stat 10(260); 2014. http://www.cdc.gov/nchs/data/series/sr_10/sr10_260.pdf. Accessed 05 May 2015.
14. American Academy of Family Physicians. Clinical Preventive Services. http://www.aafp.org/online/en/home/clinical/exam.html. Accessed 24 Feb 2015.
15. Kattapong VJ, Locher TL, Secker-Walker RH, Bell TA. American College of Preventive Medicine practice policy. Tobacco-cessation patient counseling. Am J Prev Med. 1998;15:160–2.

16. U.S. Preventive Services Task Force. Sexually transmitted infections: behavioral counseling. http://www.uspreventiveservicestaskforce.org/Page/Topic/recommendation-summary/ sexually-transmitted-infections-behavioral-counseling1. Accessed 29 Apr 2015.

17. U.S. Preventive Services Task Force. Human immunodeficiency virus (HIV) infection: screening. http://www.uspreventiveservicestaskforce.org/Page/Topic/recommendation-summary/human-immunodeficiency-virus-hiv-infection-screening. Accessed 29 Apr 2015.

18. U.S. Preventive Services Task Force. Hepatitis B virus infection: screening, 2014. http://www. uspreventiveservicestaskforce.org/Page/Topic/recommendation-summary/hepatitis-b-virus-infection-screening-2014. Accessed 29 Apr 2015.

19. U.S. Preventive Services Task Force. Hepatitis C: screening. http://www.uspreventiveser-vicestaskforce.org/Page/Topic/recommendation-summary/hepatitis-c-screening. Accessed 29 Apr 2015.

20. U.S. Preventive Services Task Force. Syphilis infection: screening. http://www.uspreventi-veservicestaskforce.org/Page/Topic/recommendation-summary/syphilis-infection-screening. Accessed 29 Apr 2015.

21. U.S. Preventive Services Task Force. Depression in adults: screening. http://www.uspreventi-veservicestaskforce.org/Page/Topic/recommendation-summary/depression-in-adults-screening. Accessed 29 Apr 2015.

22. Bloomfield HE, Wilt TJ. Evidence brief: role of the annual comprehensive physical examination in the asymptomatic adult. In: VA evidence-based synthesis program evidence briefs [internet]. Washington (DC): Department of Veterans Affairs (US); 2011. http://www.ncbi. nlm.nih.gov/books/NBK82767/.

23. U.S. Preventive Services Task Force. Blood pressure in adults (hypertension): screening. http://www.uspreventiveservicestaskforce.org/Page/Topic/recommendation-summary/blood-pressure-in-adults-hypertension-screening. Accessed 29 Apr 2015.

24. James PA, Oparil S, et al. Evidence-based guideline for the management of high blood pressure in adults. Report from the panel members appointed to the eighth Joint National Committee (JNC 8). JAMA. 2014;311(5):507–20. December 18, 2013. http://jama.jamanetwork.com/ article.aspx?articleid=1791497. Accessed 29 Apr 2015.

25. Goff Jr DC, Lloyd-Jones DM, Bennett G, Coady S, D'Agostino Sr RB, Gibbons R, Greenland P, Lackland DT, Levy D, O'Donnell CJ, Robinson JG, Schwartz JS, Shero ST, Smith Jr SC, Sorlie P, Stone NJ, Wilson PWF. 2013 ACC/AHA guideline on the assessment of cardiovascular risk: a report of the American College of Cardiology/American Heart Association Task Force on Practice Guidelines. Circulation. 2014;129 Suppl 2:S49–73.

26. U.S. Preventive Services Task Force. Obesity in adults: screening and management. http:// www.uspreventiveservicestaskforce.org/Page/Topic/recommendation-summary/obesity-in-adults-screening-and-management. Accessed 29 Apr 2015.

27. Fryar CD, Carroll MD, Ogden CL. Prevalence of overweight, obesity, and extreme obesity among adults: United States, 1960–1962 through 2011–12. National Heart, Lung, and Blood Institute, September 2014. http://www.cdc.gov/nchs/data/hestat/obesity_adult_11_12/obesity_adult_11_12.pdf. Accessed 03 May 2015.

28. Kent KC, Zwolak RM, Egorova NN, Riles TS, Manganaro A, Moskowitz AJ, Gelijns AC, Greco G. Analysis of risk factors for abdominal aortic aneurysm in a cohort of more than 3 million individuals. J Vasc Surg. 2010;52(3):539–48.

29. U.S. Preventive Services Task Force. Screening for abdominal aortic aneurysm. http://www. uspreventiveservicestaskforce.org/Page/Topic/recommendation-summary/abdominal-aortic-aneurysm-screening. Accessed 29 Apr 2015.

30. Thompson SG, Ashton HA, Gao L, Buxton MJ, Scott RA, Multicentre Aneurysm Screening Study (MASS) Group. Final follow-up of the Multicentre Aneurysm Screening Study (MASS) randomized trial of abdominal aortic aneurysm screening. Br J Surg. 2012;99(12):1649–56.

31. CDC Men's Health Data. http://www.cdc.gov/nchs/hus/men.htm#preventive. Accessed 05 May 2015.

32. American Diabetes Association. Standards of medical care in diabetes – 2015. Diabetes Care. 2015;38(Suppl 1):S8–16.

33. U.S. Preventive Services Task Force. Diabetes mellitus (type 2) in adults: screening. http://
www.uspreventiveservicestaskforce.org/Page/Topic/recommendation-summary/diabetes-
mellitus-type-2-in-adults-screening. Accessed 29 Apr 2015.
34. U.S. Preventive Services Task Force. Lipid disorders in adults (cholesterol, dyslipidemia): screening. http://www.uspreventiveservicestaskforce.org/Page/Topic/recommendation-summary/lipid-
disorders-in-adults-cholesterol-dyslipidemia-screening. Accessed 29 Apr 2015.
35. Stone NJ, Robinson J, Lichtenstein AH, Bairey Merz CN, Lloyd-Jones DM, Blum CB, McBride P,
Eckel RH, Schwartz JS, Goldberg AC, Shero ST, Gordon D, Smith Jr SC, Levy D, Watson K, Wilson
PWF. 2013 ACC/AHA guideline on the treatment of blood cholesterol to reduce atherosclerotic
cardiovascular risk in adults. J Am Coll Cardiol. 2014;63(25 Pt B):2889–934. doi:10.1016/j.jacc.
2013.11.002. https://www.joslin.org/docs/2013-ACC-AHA-Guideline-Treatment-of-Blood-
Cholestero-_to-Reduce-Atherosclerotic-Cardiovascular-Risk-in-Adults.pdf. Accessed 29 Apr
2015.
36. U.S. Preventive Services Task Force. Coronary heart disease: screening with electrocardiography. http://www.uspreventiveservicestaskforce.org/Page/Topic/recommendation-summary/
coronary-heart-disease-screening-with-electrocardiography. Accessed 29 Apr 2015.
37. U.S. Preventive Services Task Force. Osteoporosis: screening. http://www.uspreventiveser-
vicestaskforce.org/Page/Topic/recommendation-summary/osteoporosis-screening. Accessed
29 Apr 2015.
38. Watts NB, Adler RA, Bilezikian JP, Drake MT, Eastell R, Orwoll ES, Finkelstein
JS. Osteoporosis in men: an endocrine society clinical practice guideline. J Clin Endocrinol
Metab. 2012;97(6):1802–22.
39. Qaseem A, Snow V, Shekelle P, Hopkins R, Forciea MA, Owens DK, et al. Screening for
osteoporosis in men: a clinical practice guideline from the American College of Physicians.
Ann Intern Med. 2008;148:680–4.
40. National Osteoporosis Foundation. Clinician's guide to prevention and treatment of osteoporosis. http://nof.org/files/nof/public/content/file/344/upload/159.pdf. Accessed 12 May 2015.
41. U.S. Preventive Services Task Force. Colorectal cancer: screening. http://www.uspreventi-
veservicestaskforce.org/Page/Topic/recommendation-summary/colorectal-cancer-screening.
Accessed 29 Apr 2015.
42. U.S. Preventive Services Task Force. Lung cancer: screening. http://www.uspreventiveser-
vicestaskforce.org/Page/Topic/recommendation-summary/lung-cancer-screening. Accessed
29 Apr 2015.
43. U.S. Preventive Services Task Force. Skin cancer: counseling. http://www.uspreventiveser-
vicestaskforce.org/Page/Topic/recommendation-summary/skin-cancer-counseling. Accessed
29 Apr 2015.
44. U.S. Preventive Services Task Force. Pancreatic cancer: screening. http://www.uspreventi-
veservicestaskforce.org/Page/Topic/recommendation-summary/pancreatic-cancer-screening.
Accessed 14 May 2015.
45. U.S. Preventive Services Task Force. Prostate cancer: screening. http://www.uspreventiveser-
vicestaskforce.org/Page/Topic/recommendation-summary/prostate-cancer-screening.
Accessed 29 Apr 2015.
46. U.S. Preventive Services Task Force. Skin cancer: screening. http://www.uspreventiveser-
vicestaskforce.org/Page/Topic/recommendation-summary/skin-cancer-screening. Accessed
29 Apr 2015.
47. U.S. Preventive Services Task Force. Testicular cancer: screening. http://www.uspreventi-
veservicestaskforce.org/Page/Topic/recommendation-summary/testicular-cancer-screening.
Accessed 14 May 2015.
48. Rex DK, Johnson DA, Anderson JC, Schoenfeld PS, Burke CA, Inadomi JM. American College
of Gastroenterology guidelines for colorectal cancer screening 2008. Am J Gastroenterol.
2009;104:739–50. doi:10.1038/ajg.2009.104.
49. Smith RA, Manassaram-Baptiste D, Brooks D, Doroshenk M, Fedewa S, Saslow D, Brawley
OW, Wender R. Cancer screening in the United States, 2015: a review of current American

Cancer Society guidelines and current issues in cancer screening. CA Cancer J Clin. 2015;65(1):30–54. doi:10.3322/caac.21261. http://www.ncbi.nlm.nih.gov/pubmed/25581023. Accessed 12 Aug 2015.

50. American Academy of Dermatology. Prevent skin cancer. http://www.aad.org/spot-skin-cancer/learn-about-skin-cancer/prevent-skin-cancer. Accessed 11 Aug 2015.

51. Carter H, Albertsen P, et al. Early detection of prostate cancer: AUA guideline. American Urological Association; 2013.

52. U.S. Department of Health and Human Services, U.S. Department of Agriculture. Dietary Guidelines for Americans, 2010. 7th ed. Washington, DC: U.S. Government Printing Office; 2010.

53. U.S. Department of Health and Human Services. 2008 Physical Activity Guidelines for Americans. ODPHP Publication No. U0036. Washington, DC: U.S. Department of Health and Human Services; 2008.

54. U.S. Preventive Services Task Force. Healthful diet and physical activity for cardiovascular disease prevention in adults: behavioral counseling. http://www.uspreventiveservicestask-force.org/Page/Topic/recommendation-summary/healthful-diet-and-physical-activity-for-cardiovascular-disease-prevention-in-adults-behavioral-counseling. Accessed 14 May 2015.

55. U.S. Preventive Services Task Force. Healthful diet and physical activity for cardiovascular disease prevention in adults with cardiovascular risk factors: behavioral counseling. http://www.uspreventiveservicestaskforce.org/Page/Topic/recommendation-summary/healthy-diet-and-physical-activity-counseling-adults-with-high-risk-of-cvd. Accessed 29 Apr 2015.

56. ASCVD Risk Estimator. American College of Cardiology and the American Heart Association. http://tools.cardiosource.org/ASCVD-Risk-Estimator/. Accessed 14 May 2015.

57. U.S. Preventive Services Task Force. Aspirin for the prevention of cardiovascular disease: preventive medication. http://www.uspreventiveservicestaskforce.org/Page/Topic/recommendation-summary/aspirin-for-the-prevention-of-cardiovascular-disease-preventive-medication. Accessed 29 Apr 2015.

58. Centers for Disease Control and Prevention. ACIP Vaccine Recommendations, Advisory Committee for Immunization Practices. http://www.cdc.gov/vaccines/hcp/acip-recs/index.html. Accessed 17 Apr 2015.

59. Preventive services for adults: free preventive services. http://www.healthcare.gov. Accessed 26 Apr 2015.

60. Your Medicare Coverage: Preventive visit & yearly wellness exams. http://www.Medicare.gov. Accessed 24 Feb 2015.

61. Price Menu. http://www.walgreens.com. Accessed 17 Apr 2015.

62. The Clinic at Walmart. http://www.walmart.com/cp/Walmart-Clinics/1078904. Accessed 18 May 2015.

63. CVS MinuteClinic. http://www.cvs.com/minuteclinic. Accessed 18 May 2015.

64. Health Insurance: Understanding What It Covers. http://familydoctor.org/familydoctor/en/healthcare-management/insurance-bills/health-insurance-understanding-what-it-covers.html. Accessed 18 May 2015.

65. Komaroff AL. Executive physicals: what's the ROI? Harvard Business Review; September 2009

66. Langreth R. The $5000 Checkup: Are those deluxe executive exams worth it? http://www.forbes.com/forbes/2007/1224/074.html. Accessed 18 May 2015.

67. The Kelsey-Seybold Clinic Executive Health Assessment Program. https://www.kelsey-seybold.com/for-employers/houston-executive-health/documents/eha%20proposal-0115.pdf. Accessed 18 May 2015.

68. Miller WR. Motivational interviewing with problem drinkers. Behav Psychother. 1983;11: 147–72.

69. Stewart EE, Fox C. Encouraging patients to change unhealthy behaviors with motivational interviewing. Fam Pract Manag. 2011;18(3):21–5.

70. Ridner SL, Ostapchuk M, Cloud RN, Myers J, Jorayeva A, Ling J. Using motivational interviewing for smoking cessation in primary care. South Med J. 2014;107(5):314–9.

71. Motivational Interviewing Network of Trainers. http://www.motivationalinterviewing.org. Accessed 14 May 2015.
72. Krogsbøll LT, Jørgensen KJ, Grønhøj Larsen C. General health checks in adults for reducing morbidity and mortality from disease. Cochrane Database Syst Rev. 2012;10, CD009009.
73. Boulware LE, et al. Systematic review: the value of the periodic health evaluation. Ann Intern Med. 2007;146(4):289–300.

Chapter 8
Promoting Cardiovascular Health in Men

Michael Mendoza and Colleen Loo-Gross

Epidemiology/Disease Burden

Heart disease remains the leading cause of death in the United States (USA) and the leading cause of mortality in men, killing 307,384 men in 2010. Although the age-adjusted heart disease death rate decreased 30 % from 257.6 to 179.1 deaths per 100,000 population between 2000 and 2010, heart disease still accounts for approximately 1 in 4 deaths among males [1]. Heart disease is the leading cause of mortality for men across most racial/ethnic groups in the USA, including African Americans, American Indians or Alaska Natives, Hispanics, and whites. For Asian American or Pacific Islander men, heart disease is second only to cancer as the leading cause of mortality [2]. About 8.5 % of all white men, 7.9 % of black men, and 6.3 % of Mexican American men have coronary heart disease. Half of the men who die suddenly of coronary heart disease have no previous symptoms. It is thought that between 70 % and 89 % of sudden cardiac events occur in men [3]. High blood pressure, low-density lipoprotein (LDL) cholesterol, diabetes mellitus, and smoking are key risk factors for heart disease. About half of Americans (49 %) have at least one of these three risk factors [4].

M. Mendoza, MD, MPH, MS (✉)
Department of Family Medicine, University of Rochester—Highland Hospital, Rochester, NY, USA

Department Public Health Sciences, University of Rochester—Highland Hospital, Rochester, NY, USA
e-mail: Michael_mendoza@urmc.rochester.edu

C. Loo-Gross, MD, MPH
Department of Family Medicine, University of Rochester—Highland Hospital, Rochester, NY, USA
e-mail: colleen.loo@gmail.com

© Springer International Publishing Switzerland 2016
J.J. Heidelbaugh (ed.), *Men's Health in Primary Care*, Current Clinical Practice,
DOI 10.1007/978-3-319-26091-4_8

125

General Prevention

Risk Factors

Multiple factors are associated with an increased risk of cardiovascular disease. The greater the risk factor burden, the greater the lifetime risk for cardiovascular morbidity and mortality. Traditional risk factors include diabetes mellitus, smoking status, total serum cholesterol, and systolic blood pressure measurement [5]. Guidelines suggest cardiovascular screening with an assessment of traditional risk factors every 4–6 years for individuals aged 20–79 years [6].

The pooled cohort risk equations developed by the American College of Cardiology/American Heart Association (ACC/AHA) have led to a novel atherosclerotic cardiovascular disease (ASCVD) risk calculator, which estimates the 10-year risk of experiencing an initial atherosclerotic CVD event (defined as nonfatal myocardial infarction, coronary heart disease death, or nonfatal or fatal stroke). The risk calculator includes variables of age, gender, race, systolic blood pressure, total cholesterol and high-density lipoprotein (HDL) cholesterol levels, smoking status, use of antihypertensive medication, and diagnosis of diabetes mellitus. Recommendations support screening with assessment of 10-year ASCVD risk every 4–6 years for individuals aged 40–79 years with no prior ASCVD [6]. The ASCVD calculator can be accessed at http://tools.cardiosource.org/ASCVD-Risk-Estimator/.

Evaluation is ongoing for additional biomarkers that may further improve cardiovascular disease risk prediction. Examples include the use of measured high-sensitivity C-reactive protein (hs-CRP), apolipoprotein B (ApoB), creatinine or estimated glomerular filtration rate, and microalbuminuria. The 2013 ACC/AHA guidelines recommend consideration of hs-CRP assessment in select instances and provide no recommendations for or against assessment of ApoB, renal function, or albuminuria for the purposes of cardiovascular disease risk prediction [6].

Diet

A healthy diet is an important component of optimal cardiovascular health. Beneficial effects have been associated with increased fruit, vegetable, and fiber intake. Diets with less saturated fat have been shown to reduce cardiovascular morbidity. For example, the Mediterranean diet which contains a primarily plant-based diet has been shown to correlate with decreased development of cardiovascular disease as well as decreased cardiovascular disease events [7, 8]. Research has also suggested gender differences with regard to long-term benefits following nutritional intervention focused on the Mediterranean diet, with men showing greater decrease in consumption of red and processed meats, decrease in abdominal waist circumference, and more significant changes in lipid profiles [9]. This is notable as studies show a positive association of processed meat intake and less clearly of unprocessed red meat intake, with higher risk of cardiovascular disease morbidity and mortality

[10–12]. Furthermore, decreased dietary sodium intake has also been shown to lower risk of cardiovascular disease. Conversely, increased sodium consumption is associated with higher cardiovascular mortality [13].

In recent years, guidelines have also addressed the proposed use of vitamin and antioxidant supplements to improve cardiovascular health. Examples have included vitamin E, vitamin C, beta-carotene, vitamin D, folic acid, and omega-3. However, USPSTF recommendations indicate there is insufficient evidence available to evaluate the use of the multivitamin or other nutrient supplementations for primary prevention of cardiovascular disease, with the exception of beta-carotene and vitamin E, which should be avoided given evidence indicating no reduction in cardiovascular risk [14].

Obesity

Obesity is a well-established risk factor for cardiovascular disease. When compared to normal weight young men, those with obesity (defined as body mass index [BMI], greater than or equal to 30 kg/m^2) have a 30 % increased absolute risk for poorer health outcomes including hypertension, myocardial infarction, venous thrombo-embolism, and premature death, as well as type 2 diabetes mellitus [15]. Multiple studies have shown associations of elevated BMI with increased cardiovascular risk. This relationship persists independent of additional metabolic comorbidities often associated with obesity such as hypertension, impaired glucose tolerance, abdominal waist circumference greater than 40 inches, and dyslipidemia [16–18].

Improved nutrition and dietary modifications have been shown to be effective interventions in decreasing obesity, thereby improving cardiovascular health. Evidence suggests that a number of dietary approaches successfully lead to healthy weight loss, with the common factor being decreased caloric intake and ability for the individual to maintain the resultant weight loss [19]. Comprehensive interventions also include physical activity and behavior therapy and have shown the strongest benefit in sustained weight loss for obese men [20].

Exercise/Physical Activity

It is generally accepted that regular physical activity and exercise are associated with reduced mortality from cardiovascular causes. In large observational cohort studies, men aged 50 years and older who self-classified as participating in moderate physical activity had 1.3 more years of total life expectancy and 1.1 more years of life without CVD when compared to men in the low physical activity. When comparing high physical activity to low activity, that benefit grew to 3.7 and 3.2 years, respectively [21]. When comparing regular exercise with inactivity in prospective cohort studies, men and women aged 50–71 years who exercised vigorously more than 2 times a week had a 2.5 % mortality rate, whereas those who were inactive had a mortality rate of 4.8 % [22].

Smoking Cessation

Tobacco use is a major, modifiable contributor to morbidity and mortality associated with cardiovascular disease. Smoking confers a dose–response increased risk of stroke and coronary heart disease in both genders, although studies suggest a higher relative risk for female as compared to male smokers for reasons that are not yet clearly understood. Current smoking has been associated with 83 % (95 % CI, 1.58–2.12) increased risk of stroke in women and 67 % (95 % CI, 1.49–1.88) increased risk of stroke in men, compared to nonsmokers [23]. However, evidence suggests that cardiovascular morbidity and mortality significantly improve over time to nonsmoker risk levels with cessation of cigarette smoking, regardless of gender or age [23–25]. Clinicians should assess all individuals for tobacco use status and should advise cessation, as this practice alone may provide a small increase in cessation rates [26]. Cessation support should also be offered, including counseling and pharmacotherapy options including nicotine replacement therapy, both of which have been shown to be beneficial in improving and maintaining smoking cessation rates [26, 27].

Aspirin

The US Preventive Services Task Force (USPSTF) recommends aspirin for the primary prevention of cardiovascular disease in men when the benefits outweigh the risks, most notably gastrointestinal (GI) bleeding. In men, primary prevention studies of aspirin have found a 32 % relative risk reduction for myocardial infarction (MI) but no effect on stroke or all-cause mortality. For men aged 45–79 years, aspirin is recommended to reduce risk of MI, and it is not recommended in men less than 45 years of age. There is insufficient evidence for recommendation for men aged 80 years and older. The risk of GI complications varies with age for both men and men. For men less than 60 years of age, the risk of GI bleeding over 10 years is 8 per 1000. The risk increases to 24 per 1000 between men aged 60 and 70 years and to 36 per 1000 between aged 70 and 79 years [28].

Conditions

Hypertension

Strict control of blood pressure is paramount to optimal cardiovascular health. The risk of CVD rises continuously with increasing blood pressure values, roughly doubling for every 20 mm Hg systolic or 10 mm Hg diastolic increase in blood pressure measurement. Additionally, benefits of treating hypertension include both reduced cardiovascular morbidity and mortality, with 35–40 % decreased risk of stroke,

20–25 % decreased risk of myocardial infarction (MI), and 50 % decreased risk of congestive heart failure (CHF) [29, 30].

USPSTF guidelines recommend screening for hypertension (HTN) in men age 18 years and older, without specific recommendation for frequency, whereas the ACC/AHA guidelines recommend screening beginning at age 20 years, with a frequency of at least every 2 years for those without elevated blood pressure. The Joint National Committee on Prevention, Detection, Evaluation, and Treatment of Blood Pressure (JNC-7) guidelines further recommend at least annual screening for those with prehypertension [31–33]. Diagnosis of hypertension is established with at least 2 mean elevated blood pressure measurements obtained on separate visits, defined by systolic blood pressure at or above 140 mm Hg or diastolic blood pressure at or above 90 mm Hg [29].

For treatment of hypertension, healthy lifestyle modifications should be implemented, followed by pharmacotherapy if blood pressure remains above goal. Lifestyle changes include weight loss, modified diet with reduced sodium intake, increased physical activity, smoking cessation, and moderation of alcohol intake. When alternative options are available, consideration should also be given to avoid use of medications which are associated with high blood pressure, such as nonsteroidal anti-inflammatory drugs (NSAIDs) [29].

Based on guidelines established by panel members appointed to the Eighth Joint National Committee (JNC-8), hypertension treatment goals are to maintain blood pressure below 140/90 mm Hg for individuals younger than 60 years of age, including those with comorbidities of diabetes or chronic kidney disease. For individuals age 60 years and older, goal blood pressure would be below 150/90 mm Hg [34]. Monitoring of response to pharmacotherapy should occur monthly, with treatment modification until hypertension is controlled, at which time the follow-up interval may be increased as appropriate for the individual [34, 35].

Figure 8.1 summarizes the JNC-8 guidelines for the management of hypertension. For initial antihypertensive medication in the general population, appropriate options include a thiazide diuretic, calcium channel blocker (CCB), angiotensin-converting enzyme inhibitor (ACEI), or angiotensin receptor blocker (ARB). However, selection among antihypertensive treatment options may vary based on patient-specific factors, supported by clinical evidence and expert opinion. For the general African American population, preferred pharmacotherapy should include a thiazide diuretic or CCB. For all adults with chronic kidney disease, an ACEI or ARB would be initial recommended treatment options given the benefits of renal protection [34]. In most cases, medication doses should be maximized prior to consideration of adding another antihypertensive medication.

With regard to gender-specific management of hypertension, research has shown inconsistent results in achieving successful blood pressure control in men compared to women. However, one study further stratified groups by age category, with significant findings showing that while men less than age 65 years had worse blood pressure control, the gender difference then reversed for those aged 65 years and older [36]. Similar findings have been shown in the older population, with older men having better control of hypertension when compared to older women [37].

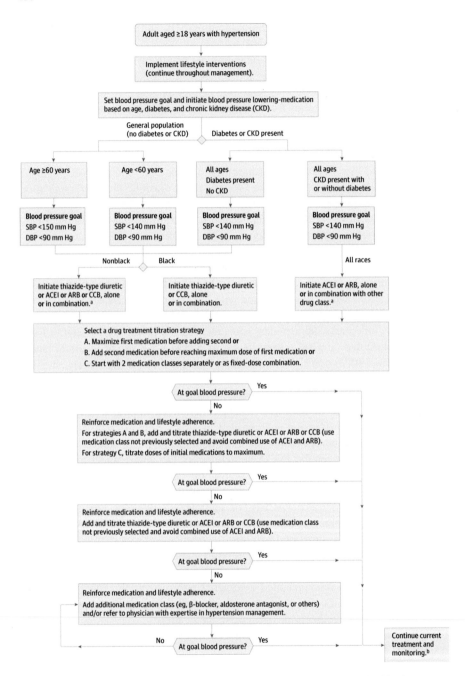

Fig. 8.1 2014 Hypertension Guideline Management Algorithm. *SBP* systolic blood pressure, *DBP* diastolic blood pressure, *ACEI* angiotensin-converting enzyme, *ARB* angiotensin receptor blocker, *CCB* calcium channel blocker. [a]ACEIs and ARBs should not be used in combination. [b]If blood pressure fails to be maintained at goal, reenter the algorithm where appropriate based on the current individual therapeutic plan. JAMA. 2014;311(5):507–520. doi:10.1001/jama.2013.284427

While further investigation is needed to better understand these gender and age group differences, the findings warrant consideration in the overall approach to management of hypertension.

Diabetes Mellitus

An estimated 19.7 million American adults struggle with type 2 diabetes mellitus [38]. Among adults, most studies and meta-analyses do not find significant male–female differences in the overall prevalence of type 2 diabetes [39–42]. It is thought, however, that undiagnosed diabetes is more common in men than in women, with men accounting for 5.3 million of the 8.2 million such cases. Type 2 diabetes is disproportionately more prevalent among underrepresented minorities: non-Hispanic whites (7.7 %), non-Hispanic blacks (13.5 %), and Mexican Americans (11.4 %) [38]. In subgroup analyses of specific demographic groups, however, when a significant male–female difference is found, it is usually greater in the males [43]. Several studies even report male gender as an independent risk factor for the incidence [44].

The approach to screening and diagnosis of diabetes is generally similar between men and women, with the glycosylated hemoglobin (HbA1c) slowly becoming the method of choice for screening, although fasting plasma glucose and 2-hour glucose tolerance tests remain common ways to screen for diabetes. HbA1c values above 6.5 % are considered to be diagnostic of diabetes, and levels between 5.7 and 6.4 % are considered to be in the prediabetic range where aggressive interventions should be pursued to address patients who are at significant risk for developing diabetes. Fasting plasma glucose levels of 126 mg/dL or greater are considered diagnostic, with levels between 100 and 126 mg/dL considered prediabetic [45, 46].

Overall, treatment goals should be individualized, but generally recommended glycemic targets include HbA1c <7 % in nonpregnant adults. A more stringent target of <6.5 % has been suggested for selected individual patients if this can be achieved without significant hypoglycemia or other adverse effects of treatment such as those who have a short duration of diabetes, type 2 diabetes treated with lifestyle or metformin only, long life expectancy, or no significant cardiovascular disease. Less stringent targets may be appropriate for patients with a history of severe hypoglycemia, limited life expectancy, advanced microvascular or macrovascular complications, extensive comorbid conditions, or long-standing diabetes in whom the general goal is difficult to attain [45, 46]. Blood pressure goals vary across guidelines but range from <130/80 mm Hg to <140/90 mm Hg. Antiplatelet treatment with aspirin 75–162 mg/day should be considered as primary prevention strategy for patients with diabetes at increased cardiovascular risk (such as most men >50 years old and women >60 years old with ≥1 additional major risk factor) but should not be recommended for patients with low cardiovascular risk. Lipid goals often include LDL cholesterol <100 mg/dL, and many suggest a target LDL of <70 mg/dL in patients with cardiovascular disease [45].

As with most chronic illnesses, diabetic care is enhanced when patients experience interprofessional, comprehensive patient-focused management plan in a continuity primary care setting. Initial visits for diabetes should address cardiovascular issues directly related to diabetes care, as well as related conditions that are more prevalent among patients with diabetes such as depression, obstructive sleep apnea, fatty liver disease, cancer, fractures, or periodontal disease. Based on a foundation of self-management education and support, over time patients acquire the knowledge and skill to manage this chronic condition [47]. Nutrition therapy, carbohydrate management, weight loss, and physical activity are all important components of the initial treatment strategy for any patient with diabetes. Smoking cessation is advised for all diabetic patients, as is screening for depression, which is a comorbid and complicated condition in 20–25 % of patients with diabetes. Immunizations against pneumococcal disease, influenza, and hepatitis B are recommended in addition to all other routine vaccinations. Patients should have annual fasting lipid profiles, assessments of kidney function (e.g., serum creatinine and urine microalbumin), monofilament foot exams, and dilated retinal exams [46].

Medication therapy, beginning with metformin, should be considered if patients are not attaining the recommended glycemic target goals. Whether targets are assessed using patient self-monitoring of blood glucose, plasma glucose, HbA1c, or other methods, treatment recommendations should acknowledge patient-specific goals, as well as risks and benefits of treatment. Contraindications to metformin are relatively rare and most side effects are manageable and abate over time. Although estimates suggest that over half of patients eligible for metformin have some conventionally regarded contraindication [48], the often-cited risk of lactic acidosis is reported to be only 6.3 per 100,000 patient years [49]. Gastrointestinal intolerance of any kind occurs in approximately 25 % of all patients who begin metformin [50], usually in the form of abdominal pain, flatulence, and diarrhea [51]. Most of these effects are transient and subside once the dose is reduced or when administered with meals. However, as much as 5 % of patients do not tolerate even the lowest dose of metformin [52].

If treatment goals are not achieved with metformin as monotherapy, then adding a second agent is indicated. A comparative effectiveness meta-analysis [53] suggests that overall each new class of non-insulin agents added to initial therapy lowers A1C approximately 0.9–1.1 %, regardless of what class of agents is chosen. Drug choice should be based on patient preferences as well as various patient, disease, and drug characteristics, with the goal of reducing blood glucose levels while minimizing side effects, especially hypoglycemia. Evidence in favor of one agent over another, however, is mixed. Initiating dual therapy for patients with HbA1c >9 % is recommended to achieve glycemic control more rapidly and early consideration of utilizing insulin for initiating dual therapy is reasonable when blood glucose is ≥300–350 mg/dL and/or A1C is ≥10–12 %. Long-acting insulin may be slightly more effective than oral antidiabetic agents as add-on therapy but may increase rate of hypoglycemic events. When initiating insulin, it is recommended that patients self-monitor blood glucose in order to anticipate and manage hypoglycemia [46].

Atrial Fibrillation

Atrial fibrillation is the most common dysrhythmia with a reported prevalence in the general population of 1–2 %. Men are slightly more predisposed to developing atrial fibrillation than women, due in large majority to the higher prevalence of risk factors among men (e.g., underlying coronary artery disease [CAD], HTN, valvular disease, obesity, and alcohol use). Diagnosis is made on the basis of electrocardiographic findings of rapid oscillatory ("fibrillatory") baseline waves varying in amplitude, shape, and timing, the absence of P waves, and an irregularly irregular ventricular response. Additional laboratory evaluation for underlying causes, especially thyroid disease, is recommended when first diagnosing atrial fibrillation. Serum levels of both B-type natriuretic peptide (BNP) (assessed by measuring BNP or N-terminal proBNP) and atrial natriuretic peptide are elevated in patients with paroxysmal or persistent atrial fibrillation but decrease rapidly after restoration of normal sinus rhythm [54].

Treatment for chronic atrial fibrillation consists primarily of rate control, as opposed to rhythm control, except for those patients whose symptoms persist despite rate control. Factors favoring rate control over rhythm control include advanced age, long-standing persistent atrial fibrillation, severe left atrial enlargement (and associated mitral valvular heart disease), several prior attempts to restore sinus rhythm minimal symptoms comorbidities with impact on quality of life [55]. Use of beta-blockers or non-dihydropyridine calcium channel blockers recommended as initial treatment, with a target resting heart rate below 110 beats per minute [56]. Ablation therapy by a catheter or surgery should be considered in the treatment of symptomatic patients with atrial fibrillation, especially if there is symptomatic paroxysmal AF without apparent structural heart disease [57].

Thromboembolism is a major complication of atrial fibrillation that can result in stroke or death. For this reason, the decision to offer prophylaxis against thromboembolism is a common clinical quandary for patients and clinicians alike. Antithrombotic therapy can reduce the risk of thromboembolism, but this benefit must be balanced against the risk of spontaneous or traumatic bleeding. Risk stratification scores (e.g., CHADS2 or CHA2DS2-VASc) can be helpful in this regard. The CHADS2 score gives 1 point for each of congestive heart failure, hypertension, age ≥75 years, diabetes mellitus; 2 points for prior stroke or transient ischemic attack. The CHA2DS2-VASc score assigns 1 point each for female sex, age 65–74 years, congestive heart failure or left ventricular dysfunction, hypertension, diabetes mellitus, history of myocardial infarction, or peripheral artery disease; 2 points for age ≥75 years; and 2 points for history of stroke, transient ischemic attack, or thromboembolism. There is strong evidence that antithrombotic therapy is indicated for most patients with atrial fibrillation or atrial flutter, along with anticoagulation for patients at high risk for stroke [58].

Dyslipidemia

Dyslipidemia, specifically increased LDL-C or decreased HDL-C, is one of the traditional risk factors for atherosclerotic cardiovascular disease. Evidence has shown that interventions to improve cholesterol levels decrease risk of cardiovascular events. The use of statin therapy decreases incidence of major cardiovascular events and all-cause mortality, with similar benefits shown in men as well as women [59–61]. As with other cardiovascular risk factors, healthy lifestyle modifications including increased physical activity and dietary modifications are also an important foundation in management.

The USPSTF guidelines recommend screening for dyslipidemia in adult men beginning at age 35 years or beginning at age 20 years for those who have cardiovascular risk factors, with a fasting serum lipid profile. An alternative screening modality would be non-fasting total cholesterol and high-density lipoprotein levels. Evidence has not shown an optimal screening frequency [31]. Previously, the indications of lipid-lowering treatment for primary prevention of cardiovascular disease had been based primarily on achievement of target cholesterol levels. However, updated ACC/AHA guidelines released in 2013 recommend a shift to lipid treatment for cardiovascular prevention based on 10-year risk and inclusion of cardiovascular risk factors, with less focus on initiation or goals of treatment based on specific cholesterol levels [62]. While these guidelines would notably increase the use of statins in the general population, studies using the presence of plaque and atherosclerosis on imaging as a surrogate marker for cardiovascular risk suggest that those with greater risk would more consistently be prescribed statin therapy when compared to prior treatment recommendations [63–65].

The ACC/AHA guidelines recommend initiation of statin therapy for primary prevention in individuals over 20 years of age with primary LDL-C greater than or equal to 190 mg/dL, individuals with diabetes aged 40–75 years, and individuals aged 40–75 years with 10-year risk for ASCVD greater than or equal to 7.5 %. The 10-year ASCVD risk is determined by use of the pooled cohort equations ASCVD risk calculator. Those with clinical atherosclerotic CVD (defined as prior myocardial infarction, acute coronary syndrome, angina, transient ischemic attack or stroke, arterial revascularization, or peripheral arterial disease) should also be treated with statin therapy for secondary prevention. Baseline serum liver transaminases should be measured prior to initiation of statin medication and followed yearly thereafter [62].

High-intensity statin therapy, if tolerated, is preferred for men with clinical ASCVD or LDL-C greater than or equal to 190 mg/dL, with moderate-intensity statin use being a secondary option. Individuals in the described benefit groups with diabetes or increased 10-year ASCVD risk should be treated with a moderate-intensity statin (see Table 8.1). For those with diabetes or increased risk, but outside of the specified age ranges or with LDL-C less than 70 mg/dL, initiation of statin therapy should be tailored to the individual with consideration of potential adverse effects versus benefits. Monitoring of lipid levels while on statin therapy should

Table 8.1 Intensity of statin therapy

Statin	High-intensity dose	Moderate-intensity dose	Low-intensity dose
Atorvastatin	80 mg daily (40 mg daily if not tolerated)	10–20 mg daily	–
Fluvastatin	–	80 mg daily or 40 mg BID	20–40 mg daily
Lovastatin	–	40 mg daily	20 mg daily
Pitavastatin	–	2–4 mg daily	1 mg daily
Pravastatin	–	40–80 mg daily	10–20 mg daily
Rosuvastatin	20–40 mg daily	5–10 mg daily	–
Simvastatin	–	20–40 mg daily	10 mg daily

occur within 4 months of dose adjustments and at least annually to assess for appropriate response to treatment. When indicated, addition of a non-statin lipid-lowering medication, such as fibric acid derivatives, niacin, bile acid-binding resins, or cholesterol absorption inhibitors, may be considered to further reduce ASCVD risk [62].

Atherosclerotic Vascular Disease

Dyslipidemia in particular is a risk factor that contributes to inflammation and atherosclerosis, thereby increasing the risk for ASCVD events. Atherosclerosis progresses with narrowing of vessels or causing thrombi, leading to clinical presentations including coronary heart disease, stroke, or peripheral vascular disease. With regard to gender, men have a higher risk of atherosclerosis as compared to women. Thus, promoting cardiovascular health in men is paramount in reducing risk of cardiovascular morbidity and mortality.

Stroke

Overall, women have a higher lifetime risk of stroke as compared to men, with lifetime risk from age 55 to 75 years being 1 in 5 for women and approximately 1 in 6 for men [66]. Coronary artery calcium (CAC) score, measured by CT imaging, provides assessment of coronary atherosclerosis and is an independent predictor of stroke. A lack of CAC is associated with reduced risk of cardiovascular events. Measurement of carotid intima media thickness (CIMT) by neck ultrasound is also a surrogate for early atherosclerosis and is associated with increased coronary disease risk. However, there is insufficient evidence to support routine screening with CAC or neck ultrasound in asymptomatic and low-risk individuals, and screening in higher risk populations have not been shown to clearly improve clinical outcomes [66, 67].

Modifiable risk factors of stroke are similar to those of other ASCVD, including hypertension, diabetes, dyslipidemia, atrial fibrillation, and carotid stenosis, as well as smoking status, obesity, physical inactivity, and diet. Reduction of elevated blood pressure is the most important risk factor modification in prevention of stroke, with less emphasis on the choice of specific antihypertensive medication. Statin therapy is indicated in those at risk given the associated benefits of decreased atherosclerosis, with evidence supporting greater beneficial effect with increasing intensity of statin treatment, as indicated by measured carotid intima media thickness. Carotid artery stenosis is associated with increased risk of stroke, though routine screening is not recommended as there is no evidence of reduction in population stroke risk. In certain instances for those with carotid artery stenosis, such as with 60 % or greater stenosis regardless of symptoms, prophylactic carotid endarterectomy (CEA) may be considered for reduction in stroke risk. Stroke risk assessment and management in individuals at risk for VTE is further addressed in the atrial fibrillation section [68].

Abdominal Aortic Aneurysm

The prevalence of abdominal aortic aneurysm (AAA) increases with age and is more predominant in men than in women. Typically, AAAs are asymptomatic prior to rupture. The larger the aneurysm size, the higher the risk of rupture, which is a life-threatening medical emergency that classically presents with hypotension, abdominal and/or back pain, and pulsatile mass of the abdomen. Dissected and ruptured AAAs are associated with high mortality rates [66]. Screening has been associated with decreased AAA rupture and AAA-related mortality. USPSTF guidelines recommend a one-time abdominal ultrasound screening in men aged 65–75 years of age with prior smoking history (at least 100 lifetime cigarettes) [69]. Additionally, ACC/AHA guidelines also recommend screening for men 60 years of age and older with family history of AAA [70].

Dilation of the abdominal aorta to size 3.0 cm or greater is diagnostic for AAA. Following diagnosis, management options include optimization of modifiable risk factors, ongoing ultrasound surveillance, and consideration of beta-blocker therapy, which has been shown to decrease perioperative mortality when undergoing repair and may slow AAA expansion. For aneurysms with high expansion rate or those greater than or equal to 5.5 cm, elective surgical repair is recommended [71, 72].

Peripheral Artery Disease

Peripheral artery disease (PAD) is defined by ankle-brachial index (ABI) less than or equal to 0.9 and represents a marker of atherosclerotic disease. Symptomatic lower extremity PAD may present with claudication. Following diagnosis, management should include optimization of modifiable risk factors, with consideration of antiplatelet therapy to decrease risk of cardiovascular events (including MI, stroke, and CV-related mortality). Aspirin is the preferred antiplatelet therapy, with clopidogrel also recommended as an alternative medication option. Further treatment with claudication medications and evaluation for possible revascularization may be considered for those with symptoms when clinically indicated [73].

Coronary Artery Disease

Coronary artery disease (CAD) is the leading cause of mortality in the USA, affecting approximately 1 in 7 deaths in 2011. It is accountable for over half of cardiovascular events occurring in those aged less than 75 years. The average age for first MI in men is younger compared to women, at 65.0 and 71.8 years, respectively. Additionally, men have a higher lifetime risk of coronary disease as compared to women, even when adjusted to assume optimal risk factors [66]. USPSTF guidelines recommend against routine screening for coronary artery disease with electrocardiogram in asymptomatic, low-risk individuals. There is insufficient evidence to provide recommendation regarding screening in those with higher CAD risk [74].

CAD is caused by atherosclerosis of the coronary arteries. Clinical presentation of disease may range from stable or unstable angina to symptoms of acute coronary syndrome and myocardial infarction. Management of CAD should include risk factor reduction with lifestyle modifications as well as pharmacotherapy to improve lipid levels and control blood pressure. Beta-blockers should be considered as initial antihypertensive therapy for individuals with comorbid CAD and should also be considered in those with CAD with normal blood pressure values when tolerated. Beta-blocker medications decrease myocardial oxygen demand, improving symptoms of angina, and further reduce risk of cardiovascular events following an MI as compared to other antihypertensive therapies. ACEIs should also be considered, which have been shown to decrease cardiovascular mortality following an MI. Calcium channel blockers would be a secondary or adjunctive option to beta-blockers if clinically indicated. Additional management for angina may include nitrate therapy, and antiplatelet therapy should be recommended in the absence of contraindications, as addressed elsewhere in this chapter [75]. For individuals with disease progression, surgical treatment options include revascularization by coronary artery bypass grafting (CABG) or percutaneous coronary intervention (PCI) [76].

Congestive Heart Failure

Congestive heart failure (CHF remains extremely common in the USA. About 2.7 million males alive today have CHF. Each year, about 350,000 new cases are diagnosed in males. In 2010, the overall prevalence for people age 20 and older is 2.1 %.

Table 8.2 NYHA functional classification of congestive heart failure

I	No limitation of physical activity. Ordinary physical activity does not cause symptoms of HF
II	Slight limitation of physical activity. Comfortable at rest, but ordinary physical activity results in symptoms of HF
III	Marked limitation of physical activity. Comfortable at rest, but less than ordinary activity causes symptoms of HF
IV	Unable to carry on any physical activity without symptoms of HF or symptoms of HF at rest

Among men, the following have heart failure: 2.2 % of non-Hispanic whites, 4.1 % of non-Hispanic blacks, and 1.9 % of Mexican Americans [38]. Gender-specific risk factors for CHF are related to the underlying causes, most commonly hypertension, coronary heart disease, history of MI, valvular heart disease, and cardiac dysrhythmias, among others. Regardless of the etiology, lifestyle modifications to reduce risk include smoking cessation, weight management, and regular exercise. In one large prospective cohort study, subjects rated as having diets in the highest quintile of quality (as measured by the modified Alternative Healthy Eating Index) had a 38 % lower risk of having heart failure [77]. Such diets were typically higher in vegetables, fruits, fish, nuts, and soy protein and low in deep-fried foods.

Although classic signs and symptoms can be suggestive of CHF [78], the diagnostic standard for HF is the transthoracic echocardiogram [79]. Clinical prediction rules incorporating novel biomarkers, such as NT-proBNP, along with other patient characteristics may be helpful in predicting CHF [80]. Once the diagnosis of HF is made, guideline-directed treatment should begin with risk factor modification in all individuals—smoking cessation and treatment of hypertension, ischemic heart disease, diabetes, and dyslipidemia. The assessment of CHF severity can be facilitated by the use of the NYHA classification of HF or the ACC/AHA classification.

Angiotensin-converting enzyme (ACE) inhibitors are indicated for all patients with reduced left ventricular ejection fraction, including asymptomatic patients, unless contraindicated or not tolerated. ACE inhibitors appear to reduce mortality and rates of myocardial infarction and hospital admission in patients with left ventricular dysfunction or symptomatic heart failure. Beta-blockers (e.g., bisoprolol, carvedilol, or sustained-release metoprolol succinate) reduce mortality in stable patients with New York Heart Association Class II and III heart failure [81] (Table 8.2). Calcium channel blocking drugs are not recommended as routine treatment for patients with systolic heart failure because there has been no documented clinical benefit for these agents in this setting [81]. Diuretics in patients with chronic heart failure may reduce risk of death and worsening systolic heart failure and improve exercise capacity. Aldosterone antagonists (e.g., spironolactone) are recommended for patients with symptomatic heart failure and moderate-to-severe symptoms. Once a mainstay of therapy in HF, digoxin should be considered only for patients with symptomatic HF because it may reduce hospitalization rate, but it has not been shown to reduce mortality in like other agents.

Summary

With the prevalence of cardiovascular disease, and the associated cost of care, projected to increase substantially [82], effective prevention strategies will be needed in order to reduce the overall burden of disease on the US population. We will need to expand capacity to address the complex needs of patients with cardiovascular disease, within primary care and subspecialty office settings, both inside and outside the hospital. We must simultaneously work to broaden our influence within traditionally marginalized communities and populations where often men bear a disproportionately higher burden of cardiovascular morbidity and mortality.

References

1. Holmes JS, Arise IE. Health, United States, 2013. With special feature on prescription drugs; 2013. http://www.cdc.gov/nchs/data/hus/hus13.pdf#024.
2. Heron M. Deaths: leading causes for 2008. Natl Vital Stat Rep. 2012;60(6):1–94.
3. Roger VL, Go AS, Lloyd-Jones DM, Benjamin EJ, Berry JD, Borden WB, et al. Heart disease and stroke statistics–2012 update: a report from the American Heart Association. Circulation. 2012;125(1):e2–e220.
4. Ritchey MD, Wall HK, Gillespie C, George MG, Jamal A, Division for Heart Disease and Stroke Prevention, CDC. Million hearts: prevalence of leading cardiovascular disease risk factors–United States, 2005–2012. MMWR Morb Mortal Wkly Rep. 2014;63(21):462–7.
5. Berry JD, Dyer A, Cai X, Garside DB, Ning H, Thomas A, et al. Lifetime risks of cardiovascular disease. N Engl J Med. 2012;366(4):321–9.
6. Goff Jr DC, Lloyd-Jones DM, Bennett G, Coady S, D'Agostino Sr RB, Gibbons R, et al. 2013 ACC/AHA guideline on the assessment of cardiovascular risk: a report of the American College of Cardiology/American Heart Association Task Force on Practice Guidelines. J Am Coll Cardiol. 2014;63(25 Pt B):2935–59.
7. de la Iglesia R, Lopez-Legarrea P, Abete I, Bondia-Pons I, Navas-Carretero S, Forga L, et al. A new dietary strategy for long-term treatment of the metabolic syndrome is compared with the American Heart Association (AHA) guidelines: the MEtabolic Syndrome REduction in NAvarra (RESMENA) project. Br J Nutr. 2014;111(4):643–52.
8. Rees K, Hartley L, Flowers N, Clarke A, Hooper L, Thorogood M, et al. 'Mediterranean' dietary pattern for the primary prevention of cardiovascular disease. Cochrane Database Syst Rev. 2013;8, CD009825.
9. Leblanc V, Begin C, Hudon AM, Royer MM, Corneau L, Dodin S, et al. Gender differences in the long-term effects of a nutritional intervention program promoting the Mediterranean diet: changes in dietary intakes, eating behaviors, anthropometric and metabolic variables. Nutr J. 2014;13:107.
10. Abete I, Romaguera D, Vieira AR, Lopez de Munain A, Norat T. Association between total, processed, red and white meat consumption and all-cause, CVD and IHD mortality: a meta-analysis of cohort studies. Br J Nutr. 2014;112(5):762–75.
11. Micha R, Wallace SK, Mozaffarian D. Red and processed meat consumption and risk of incident coronary heart disease, stroke, and diabetes mellitus: a systematic review and meta-analysis. Circulation. 2010;121(21):2271–83.
12. Micha R, Michas G, Mozaffarian D. Unprocessed red and processed meats and risk of coronary artery disease and type 2 diabetes–an updated review of the evidence. Curr Atheroscler Rep. 2012;14(6):515–24.

13. Mozaffarian D, Fahimi S, Singh GM, Micha R, Khatibzadeh S, Engell RE, et al. Global sodium consumption and death from cardiovascular causes. N Engl J Med. 2014;371(7): 624–34.
14. Moyer VA, U.S. Preventive Services Task Force. Vitamin, mineral, and multivitamin supplements for the primary prevention of cardiovascular disease and cancer: U.S. Preventive services Task Force recommendation statement. Ann Intern Med. 2014;160(8):558–64.
15. Schmidt M, Johannesdottir SA, Lemeshow S, Lash TL, Ulrichsen SP, Botker HE, et al. Obesity in young men, and individual and combined risks of type 2 diabetes, cardiovascular morbidity and death before 55 years of age: a Danish 33-year follow-up study. BMJ Open. 2013;3(4). doi: 10.1136/bmjopen-2013-002698. Print 2013.
16. Bogers RP, Bemelmans WJ, Hoogenveen RT, Boshuizen HC, Woodward M, Knekt P, et al. Association of overweight with increased risk of coronary heart disease partly independent of blood pressure and cholesterol levels: a meta-analysis of 21 cohort studies including more than 300 000 persons. Arch Intern Med. 2007;167(16):1720–8.
17. Kramer CK, Zinman B, Retnakaran R. Are metabolically healthy overweight and obesity benign conditions? a systematic review and meta-analysis. Ann Intern Med. 2013; 159(11):758–69.
18. Thomsen M, Nordestgaard BG. Myocardial infarction and ischemic heart disease in overweight and obesity with and without metabolic syndrome. JAMA Intern Med. 2014;174(1):15–22.
19. Jensen MD, Ryan DH, Apovian CM, Ard JD, Comuzzie AG, Donato KA, et al. 2013 AHA/ACC/TOS guideline for the management of overweight and obesity in adults: a report of the American College of Cardiology/American Heart Association Task Force on Practice Guidelines and The Obesity Society. J Am Coll Cardiol. 2014;63(25 Pt B):2985–3023.
20. Robertson C, Archibald D, Avenell A, Douglas F, Hoddinott P, van Teijlingen E, et al. Systematic reviews of and integrated report on the quantitative, qualitative and economic evidence base for the management of obesity in men. Health Technol Assess. 2014;18(35):v–vi, xxiii–xxix, 1–424.
21. Franco OH, de Laet C, Peeters A, Jonker J, Mackenbach J, Nusselder W. Effects of physical activity on life expectancy with cardiovascular disease. Arch Intern Med. 2005; 165(20):2355–60.
22. Leitzmann MF, Park Y, Blair A, Ballard-Barbash R, Mouw T, Hollenbeck AR, et al. Physical activity recommendations and decreased risk of mortality. Arch Intern Med. 2007;167(22):2453–60.
23. Peters SA, Huxley RR, Woodward M. Smoking as a risk factor for stroke in women compared with men: a systematic review and meta-analysis of 81 cohorts, including 3,980,359 individuals and 42,401 strokes. Stroke. 2013;44(10):2821–8.
24. Huxley RR, Woodward M. Cigarette smoking as a risk factor for coronary heart disease in women compared with men: a systematic review and meta-analysis of prospective cohort studies. Lancet. 2011;378(9799):1297–305.
25. Mons U, Muezzinler A, Gellert C, Schottker B, Abnet CC, Bobak M, et al. Impact of smoking and smoking cessation on cardiovascular events and mortality among older adults: meta-analysis of individual participant data from prospective cohort studies of the CHANCES consortium. BMJ. 2015;350:h1551.
26. Stead LF, Lancaster T. Combined pharmacotherapy and behavioural interventions for smoking cessation. Cochrane Database Syst Rev. 2012;10, CD008286.
27. Suls JM, Luger TM, Curry SJ, Mermelstein RJ, Sporer AK, An LC. Efficacy of smoking-cessation interventions for young adults: a meta-analysis. Am J Prev Med. 2012;42(6): 655–62.
28. US Preventive Services Task Force. Aspirin for the prevention of cardiovascular disease: U.S. Preventive Services Task Force recommendation statement. Ann Intern Med. 2009; 150(6):396–404.
29. Chobanian AV, Bakris GL, Black HR, Cushman WC, Green LA, Izzo Jr JL, et al. The Seventh Report of the Joint National Committee on Prevention, Detection, Evaluation, and Treatment of High Blood Pressure: the JNC 7 report. JAMA. 2003;289(19):2560–72.

30. Ogden LG, He J, Lydick E, Whelton PK. Long-term absolute benefit of lowering blood pressure in hypertensive patients according to the JNC VI risk stratification. Hypertension. 2000;35(2):539–43.
31. Heidelbaugh JJ, Tortorello M. The adult well male examination. Am Fam Physician. 2012;85(10):964–71.
32. Piper MA, Evans CV, Burda BU, Margolis KL, O'Connor E, Smith N, et al. Screening for high blood pressure in adults: a systematic evidence review for the U.S. Preventive Services Task Force; 2014 Dec.
33. U.S. Preventive Services Task Force. Screening for high blood pressure: U.S. Preventive Services Task Force reaffirmation recommendation statement. Ann Intern Med. 2007;147(11):783–6.
34. James PA, Oparil S, Carter BL, Cushman WC, Dennison-Himmelfarb C, Handler J, et al. 2014 Evidence-based guideline for the management of high blood pressure in adults: report from the panel members appointed to the Eighth Joint National Committee (JNC 8). JAMA. 2014;311(5):507–20.
35. National High Blood Pressure Education Program. The Seventh Report of the Joint National Committee on prevention, detection, evaluation, and treatment of high blood pressure; 2004 Aug.
36. Daugherty SL, Masoudi FA, Ellis JL, Ho PM, Schmittdiel JA, Tavel HM, et al. Age-dependent gender differences in hypertension management. J Hypertens. 2011;29(5):1005–11.
37. Wilkins K, Gee M, Campbell N. The difference in hypertension control between older men and women. Health Rep. 2012;23(4):33–40.
38. Go AS, Mozaffarian D, Roger VL, Benjamin EJ, Berry JD, Borden WB, et al. Heart disease and stroke statistics–2013 update: a report from the American Heart Association. Circulation. 2013;127(1):e6–e245.
39. DECODE Study Group. Age- and sex-specific prevalences of diabetes and impaired glucose regulation in 13 European cohorts. Diabetes Care. 2003;26(1):61–9.
40. King H, Aubert RE, Herman WH. Global burden of diabetes, 1995–2025: prevalence, numerical estimates, and projections. Diabetes Care. 1998;21(9):1414–31.
41. Schipf S, Werner A, Tamayo T, Holle R, Schunk M, Maier W, et al. Regional differences in the prevalence of known Type 2 diabetes mellitus in 45–74 years old individuals: results from six population-based studies in Germany (DIAB-CORE Consortium). Diabet Med. 2012;29(7):e88–95.
42. Pan C, Yang W, Jia W, Weng J, Tian H. Management of Chinese patients with type 2 diabetes, 1998–2006: the Diabcare-China surveys. Curr Med Res Opin. 2009;25(1):39–45.
43. Inoue M, Inoue K, Akimoto K. Effects of age and sex in the diagnosis of type 2 diabetes using glycated haemoglobin in Japan: the Yuport Medical Checkup Centre study. PLoS One. 2012;7(7), e40375.
44. Lin CC, Li CI, Hsiao CY, Liu CS, Yang SY, Lee CC, et al. Time trend analysis of the prevalence and incidence of diagnosed type 2 diabetes among adults in Taiwan from 2000 to 2007: a population-based study. BMC Public Health. 2013;13:318.
45. American Diabetes Association. (6) Glycemic targets. Diabetes Care. 2015;38(Suppl):S33–40.
46. Standards of medical care in diabetes–2015: summary of revisions. Diabetes Care. 2015;38(Suppl):S4–S003.
47. Haas L, Maryniuk M, Beck J, Cox CE, Duker P, Edwards L, et al. National standards for diabetes self-management education and support. Diabetes Care. 2014;37 Suppl 1:S144–53.
48. Sulkin TV, Bosman D, Krentz AJ. Contraindications to metformin therapy in patients with NIDDM. Diabetes Care. 1997;20(6):925–8.
49. Salpeter SR, Greyber E, Pasternak GA, Salpeter Posthumous EE. Risk of fatal and nonfatal lactic acidosis with metformin use in type 2 diabetes mellitus. Cochrane Database Syst Rev. 2010;(1):CD002967. doi(1):CD002967.
50. Blonde L, Dailey GE, Jabbour SA, Reasner CA, Mills DJ. Gastrointestinal tolerability of extended-release metformin tablets compared to immediate-release metformin tablets: results of a retrospective cohort study. Curr Med Res Opin. 2004;20(4):565–72.

51. Hermann LS. Metformin: a review of its pharmacological properties and therapeutic use. Diabete Metab. 1979;5(3):233–45.
52. Cusi K, DeFronzo RA. Metformin: a review of its metabolic effects. Diabetes Rev. 1998;6:89–131.
53. Bennett WL, Maruthur NM, Singh S, Segal JB, Wilson LM, Chatterjee R, et al. Comparative effectiveness and safety of medications for type 2 diabetes: an update including new drugs and 2-drug combinations. Ann Intern Med. 2011;154(9):602–13.
54. Fuster V, Ryden LE, Cannom DS, Crijns HJ, Curtis AB, Ellenbogen KA, et al. ACC/AHA/ ESC 2006 Guidelines for the Management of Patients with Atrial Fibrillation: a report of the American College of Cardiology/American Heart Association Task Force on Practice Guidelines and the European Society of Cardiology Committee for Practice Guidelines (Writing Committee to Revise the 2001 Guidelines for the Management of Patients With Atrial Fibrillation): developed in collaboration with the European Heart Rhythm Association and the Heart Rhythm Society. Circulation. 2006;114(7):e257–354.
55. Amerena JV, Walters TE, Mirzaee S, Kalman JM. Update on the management of atrial fibrillation. Med J Aust. 2013;199(9):592–7.
56. Wann LS, Curtis AB, January CT, Ellenbogen KA, Lowe JE, Estes NA, 3rd, et al. 2011 ACCF/ AHA/HRS focused update on the management of patients with atrial fibrillation (updating the 2006 guideline): a report of the American College of Cardiology Foundation/American Heart Association Task Force on Practice Guidelines. Circulation. 2011;123(1):104–23.
57. January CT, Wann LS, Alpert JS, Calkins H, Cigarroa JE, Cleveland Jr JC, et al. 2014 AHA/ ACC/HRS guideline for the management of patients with atrial fibrillation: a report of the American College of Cardiology/American Heart Association Task Force on Practice Guidelines and the Heart Rhythm Society. J Am Coll Cardiol. 2014;64(21):e1–76.
58. Ntaios G, Lip GY, Makaritsis K, Papavasileiou V, Vemmou A, Koroboki E, et al. CHADS(2), CHA(2)S(2)DS(2)-VASc, and long-term stroke outcome in patients without atrial fibrillation. Neurology. 2013;80(11):1009–17.
59. Cholesterol Treatment Trialists' (CTT) Collaboration, Fulcher J, O'Connell R, Voysey M, Emberson J, Blackwell L, et al. Efficacy and safety of LDL-lowering therapy among men and women: meta-analysis of individual data from 174,000 participants in 27 randomised trials. Lancet. 2015;385(9976):1397–405.
60. Taylor F, Huffman MD, Macedo AF, Moore TH, Burke M, Davey Smith G, et al. Statins for the primary prevention of cardiovascular disease. Cochrane Database Syst Rev. 2013;1, CD004816.
61. Kostis WJ, Cheng JQ, Dobrzynski JM, Cabrera J, Kostis JB. Meta-analysis of statin effects in women versus men. J Am Coll Cardiol. 2012;59(6):572–82.
62. Stone NJ, Robinson JG, Lichtenstein AH, Bairey Merz CN, Blum CB, Eckel RH, et al. 2013 ACC/AHA guideline on the treatment of blood cholesterol to reduce atherosclerotic cardiovascular risk in adults: a report of the American College of Cardiology/American Heart Association Task Force on Practice Guidelines. J Am Coll Cardiol. 2014;63(25 Pt B): 2889–934.
63. Johnson KM, Dowe DA. Accuracy of statin assignment using the 2013 AHA/ACC Cholesterol Guideline versus the 2001 NCEP ATP III guideline: correlation with atherosclerotic plaque imaging. J Am Coll Cardiol. 2014;64(9):910–9.
64. Pencina MJ, Navar-Boggan AM, D'Agostino Sr RB, Williams K, Neely B, Sniderman AD, et al. Application of new cholesterol guidelines to a population-based sample. N Engl J Med. 2014;370(15):1422–31.
65. Pursnani A, Mayrhofer T, Ferencik M, Hoffmann U. The 2013 ACC/AHA cardiovascular prevention guidelines improve alignment of statin therapy with coronary atherosclerosis as detected by coronary computed tomography angiography. Atherosclerosis. 2014;237(1): 314–8.
66. Mozaffarian D, Benjamin EJ, Go AS, Arnett DK, Blaha MJ, Cushman M, et al. Heart disease and stroke statistics–2015 update: a report from the American Heart Association. Circulation. 2015;131(4):e29–322.

67. Muhlestein JB, Lappe DL, Lima JA, Rosen BD, May HT, Knight S, et al. Effect of screening for coronary artery disease using CT angiography on mortality and cardiac events in high-risk patients with diabetes: the FACTOR-64 randomized clinical trial. JAMA. 2014;312(21):2234–43.
68. Goldstein LB, Bushnell CD, Adams RJ, Appel LJ, Braun LT, Chaturvedi S, et al. Guidelines for the primary prevention of stroke: a guideline for healthcare professionals from the American Heart Association/American Stroke Association. Stroke. 2011;42(2):517–84.
69. Guirguis-Blake JM, Beil TL, Senger CA, Whitlock EP. Ultrasonography screening for abdominal aortic aneurysms: a systematic evidence review for the U.S. Preventive Services Task Force. Ann Intern Med. 2014;160(5):321–9.
70. Rooke TW, Hirsch AT, Misra S, Sidawy AN, Beckman JA, Findeiss L, et al. Management of patients with peripheral artery disease (compilation of 2005 and 2011 ACCF/AHA Guideline Recommendations): a report of the American College of Cardiology Foundation/American Heart Association Task Force on Practice Guidelines. J Am Coll Cardiol. 2013;61(14): 1555–70.
71. Aggarwal S, Qamar A, Sharma V, Sharma A. Abdominal aortic aneurysm: a comprehensive review. Exp Clin Cardiol. 2011;16(1):11–5. Spring.
72. Keisler B, Carter C. Abdominal aortic aneurysm. Am Fam Physician. 2015;91(8):538–43.
73. Hirsch AT, Haskal ZJ, Hertzer NR, Bakal CW, Creager MA, Halperin JL, et al. ACC/AHA 2005 guidelines for the management of patients with peripheral arterial disease (lower extremity, renal, mesenteric, and abdominal aortic): executive summary a collaborative report from the American Association for Vascular Surgery/Society for Vascular Surgery, Society for Cardiovascular Angiography and Interventions, Society for Vascular Medicine and Biology, Society of Interventional Radiology, and the ACC/AHA Task Force on Practice Guidelines (Writing Committee to Develop Guidelines for the Management of Patients With Peripheral Arterial Disease) endorsed by the American Association of Cardiovascular and Pulmonary Rehabilitation; National Heart, Lung, and Blood Institute; Society for Vascular Nursing; TransAtlantic Inter-Society Consensus; and Vascular Disease Foundation. J Am Coll Cardiol. 2006;47(6):1239–312.
74. Moyer VA, U.S. Preventive Services Task Force. Screening for coronary heart disease with electrocardiography: U.S. Preventive Services Task Force recommendation statement. Ann Intern Med. 2012;157(7):512–8.
75. Pflieger M, Winslow BT, Mills K, Dauber IM. Medical management of stable coronary artery disease. Am Fam Physician. 2011;83(7):819–26.
76. Hall SL, Lorenc T. Secondary prevention of coronary artery disease. Am Fam Physician. 2010;81(3):289–96.
77. Dehghan M, Mente A, Teo KK, Gao P, Sleight P, Dagenais G, et al. Relationship between healthy diet and risk of cardiovascular disease among patients on drug therapies for secondary prevention: a prospective cohort study of 31 546 high-risk individuals from 40 countries. Circulation. 2012;126(23):2705–12.
78. Davie AP, Francis CM, Caruana L, Sutherland GR, McMurray JJ. Assessing diagnosis in heart failure: which features are any use? QJM. 1997;90(5):335–9.
79. Dosh SA. Diagnosis of heart failure in adults. Am Fam Physician. 2004;70(11):2145–52.
80. Kelder JC, Cramer MJ, van Wijngaarden J, van Tooren R, Mosterd A, Moons KG, et al. The diagnostic value of physical examination and additional testing in primary care patients with suspected heart failure. Circulation. 2011;124(25):2865–73.
81. Yancy CW, Jessup M, Bozkurt B, Butler J, Casey Jr DE, et al. 2013 ACCF/AHA guideline for the management of heart failure: a report of the American College of Cardiology Foundation/American Heart Association Task Force on practice guidelines. Circulation. 2013;128(16):e240–327. Writing Committee Members.
82. Heidenreich PA, Trogdon JG, Khavjou OA, Butler J, Dracup K, Ezekowitz MD, et al. Forecasting the future of cardiovascular disease in the United States: a policy statement from the American Heart Association. Circulation. 2011;123(8):933–44.

Chapter 9
Male Sexual Health

Harland Holman and Mark Armstrong

Introduction

This chapter starts with a discussion of the sexual history, which is used to screen for sexual dysfunction and the risk for sexually transmitted infections in men. However, this is often omitted in the primary care setting for several reasons including inadequate time and provider and patient discomfort. Tips are discussed to help providers overcome these barriers. Several sexual dysfunctions are reviewed in this chapter. Erectile dysfunction is highlighted due to its high prevalence and association with multiple other conditions including cardiovascular, psychiatric, and endocrine disorders. Treatment for erectile dysfunction can be costly but is often very effective with multiple options. Various treatments for erectile dysfunction with risks and benefits are discussed. Premature ejaculation is also very common, and pharmacologic and behavioral treatments are discussed in detail. Other less common sexual dysfunctions briefly discussed are hematospermia and painful ejaculation. Over-the-counter treatments to enhance sexual dysfunction are becoming increasingly prevalent, yet efficacy and risks of common ingredients may pose some risk to men who take them. Finally, men play a factor in many cases of infertility. Terminology, etiology, diagnostics, and treatments of male infertility will be reviewed.

H. Holman, MD (✉)
Spectrum Family Medicine, Family Medicine Residency Clinic, Grand Rapids, MI, USA
e-mail: htholman@gmail.com

M. Armstrong, DO
Department of Family Medicine, Spectrum Health, Grand Rapids, MI, USA

© Springer International Publishing Switzerland 2016
J.J. Heidelbaugh (ed.), *Men's Health in Primary Care*, Current Clinical Practice,
DOI 10.1007/978-3-319-26091-4_9

Obtaining a Male Sexual History

Introduction

Many primary care physicians fail to obtain a male sexual history during health maintenance examinations despite their patients being at risk for sexual dysfunction and sexual transmitted infections (STIs) [1]. Approximately 15 % of primary care providers routinely ask their patients about sexual dysfunction; longer medical appointments and patients who take medications with known sexual side effects increase this statistic [2]. While some men prefer starting the conversation about sexual concerns with their provider, most have reported that they are agreeable with their provider starting this discussion. Other reasons for medical providers not obtaining an appropriate sexual history include time restraints, provider character- istics (including gender discordance), and provider knowledge [2]. Most patients want their medical provider to give information (74 %) and be asked (69 %) about sexual dysfunction [3]. Providers should normalize the sexual history by including it in the overall history, explaining that these questions are asked of all patients, and ensuring confidentiality (see Fig. 9.1).

History/Counseling

The United States Preventive Services Task Force (USPSTF) recommends high- intensity counseling to sexually active adolescent and adult men at high risk for STIs (Grade B, there is high certainty that the benefit is moderate, or moderate certainty the benefit is moderate to high) [5]. High-risk sexual activity includes improper or inconsistent use of barrier contraceptives, multiple sexual partners, having a sexual partner with a history of or current STI, or having sexual interac- tions under the influence of a mind-altering substances [5]. The other component of a sexual history is to assess for sexual dysfunction. Individual sexual dysfunctions will be discussed in further detail including erectile dysfunction, premature ejacula- tion, hematospermia, and painful ejaculation.

Onset and timing of the sexual dysfunction is important to obtain, as it may be a clue to the etiology of the dysfunction. For example, while antidepressants have been associated with sexual side effects, it has been shown that there is a high rate of sexual dysfunction prior to starting antidepressant therapy [6]. Several standard- ized forms have been developed to help obtain and monitor male sexual health. These have been used in both the clinical and research setting [7]. The international index of erectile function (IIEF) is a frequently used screening tool that addresses the severity of erectile dysfunction and sexual satisfaction within a short form (5 questions) or longer version (15 questions). Questions on the IIEF include topics about the ability to obtain or maintain an erection and satisfaction with sexual intercourse.

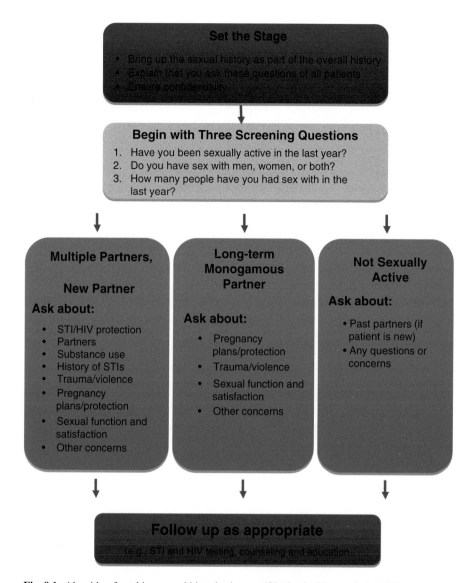

Set the Stage
- Bring up the sexual history as part of the overall history
- Explain that you ask these questions of all patients
- Ensure confidentiality

Begin with Three Screening Questions
1. Have you been sexually active in the last year?
2. Do you have sex with men, women, or both?
3. How many people have you had sex with in the last year?

Multiple Partners,

New Partner

Ask about:
- STI/HIV protection
- Partners
- Substance use
- History of STIs
- Trauma/violence
- Pregnancy plans/protection
- Sexual function and satisfaction
- Other concerns

Long-term Monogamous Partner

Ask about:
- Pregnancy plans/protection
- Trauma/violence
- Sexual function and satisfaction
- Other concerns

Not Sexually Active

Ask about:
- Past partners (if patient is new)
- Any questions or concerns

Follow up as appropriate
(e.g., STI and HIV testing, counseling and education

Fig. 9.1 Algorithm for taking sexual histories in men (Obtained with permission) [4]

Men may have myths or perceptions they would like to discuss when sexual health is approached. Briefly, several common myths will be investigated:

1. Male circumcision has no effect on sexual function or satisfaction based on a systematic review [8].
2. While vigorous sexual activity may increase the cardiac demand (about the equivalent of walking 2 flights of stairs), the addition of a PDE5i has not been shown to cause any additional harm, and PDE5is may actually reduce the risk of MI [9, 10].

3. More frequent pornographic use in men was associated with decreased enjoyment with intimate sexual partners [11].
4. Adolescents should be reminded that all different types of sexual contact: oral, anal, or vaginal can lead to sexual transmitted infections.

Special Populations

Adolescents may legally discuss sexual concerns with their medical provider confidentially, without parental consent, in the USA per the Health Insurance Portability and Accountability Act (HIPAA) law passed in 2002. Two validated screening surveys that assess sexual history in adolescents include the RAAPS (Rapid Assessment for Adolescent Preventive Services, www.raaps.org) and the HEADDSSS (Home, Education/Employment, Activities, Drugs, Sexuality, Suicide, Sleep, https://depts.washington.edu/dbpeds/Screening%20Tools/HEADSS.pdf) [12, 13]. The HEADDSSS has two versions of sexual questions: a short and long form. The short form asks about sexual attraction, activity, and prevention against STIs. The longer form asks multiple other questions including prior STIs, number of sexual partners, and unwilling sexual contact. The RAAPS survey has identified in a large population that 38 % of adolescents were sexually active and 32 % of this population failed to use barrier protection [14].

Older men may have several chronic diseases which affect their sexual performance. There is a natural decline in men's sexual frequency often as a result of poor physical health [15]. Chronic pain, respiratory, cardiac, and mental health diseases may all play a factor. Likewise, sexual dysfunction may be an early precursor to depression [16] and negatively impact overall quality of life. Figure 9.2 demonstrates this decline in sexual frequency in men compared to women.

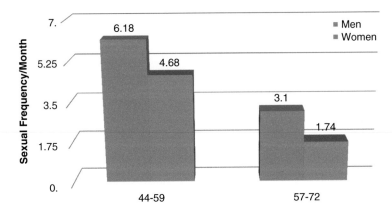

Fig. 9.2 Gender difference in sexual decline (Adapted from data from Karraker A, Delamater J, Schwartz CR. Sexual frequency decline from midlife to later life. J Gerontol B Psychol Sci Soc Sci)

Sexual orientation should be addressed in a nonjudgmental, factual manner. However, a physician's knowledge about how to comfortably obtain information about a patient's sexual preference and/or gender identity is a barrier [17]. Cultural differences may affect how sexual history is approached, and asking permission to discuss a sexual history is recommended [18]. One study has shown that migrant population's sexual practices adapt to their host country [19]. Men are less frequently sexually abused than women. However, male sexual abuse may affect a man's masculine identity and may lead to multiple other psychiatric comorbidities [20, 21]; thus, intensive counseling is highly recommended in this situation.

Erectile Dysfunction

Epidemiology/Etiology/Evaluation

The frequency of erectile dysfunction (ED) increases with age, with a prevalence of less than 10 % in men younger than 40-year-olds and up to 75 % in 75-year-old or older men [22]. The cost of treatment with sildenafil, tadalafil, and vardenafil to treat ED exceeds $1 billion dollars worldwide per year [23]. Erectile dysfunction has also shown to inversely impact the quality of life of men [24]. The diagnosis of ED is based on a patient's self-report of difficulties forming or maintaining an erection. A careful history might help determine the major causes of ED such as hormonal, neurologic, vascular, or psychogenic. Diseases such as diabetes mellitus and renal disease may cause ED through all of the above mechanisms [25]. A careful medication and substance history should be obtained, as many medications including opioids and alcohol are implicated in erectile dysfunction [26].

A history of penile and spinal cord trauma and urologic procedures such as radical prostatectomy history should be determined. Multiple other medical problems have been shown to be risk factors for ED including chronic kidney disease, with an estimate of 80 % of patients having ED [25]. A limited physical exam is recommended including evaluation for neurologic deficits, prostate disease, penile deformities, cardiovascular disease, and signs of hypogonadism [27]. Laboratory evaluation may include screening for diabetes, hyperlipidemia, and low testosterone [27] (Fig. 9.3).

One expert guideline includes an algorithm with routine screening of thyroid-stimulating hormone and a behavioral therapy referral if there isn't a definable medical etiology [28]. Imaging studies for difficult-to-treat ED can be ordered usually by a urologist in a few unique situations. This testing includes (1) dynamic penile Doppler to evaluate blood flow in high-risk vascular patients who would benefit from curative vascular surgery and (2) RigiScan or nocturnal penile tumescence to evaluate neurologic function in patients with complex psychologic disease [28, 29]. However, recent expert opinion recommends avoiding the term psychogenic ED, since all ED likely has some psychological component [30].

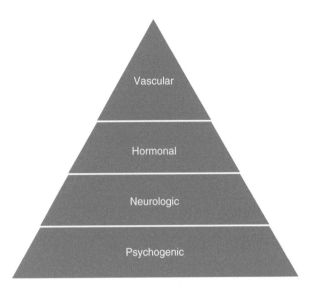

Fig. 9.3 Overlap of multiple etiologies of ED with psychogenic ED central to all causes

Erectile Dysfunction: Associations and Risks

Since detecting ED at an early age has helped patients find out about silent CAD, diagnosing ED has been described as lifesaving [31]. Microvascular damage causing endothelial dysfunction is the etiology of both coronary disease and vascular ED. However, it appears that this damage leads to ED symptoms often before cardiac symptoms. It is recommended that men with ED be risk stratified with the Framingham risk calculator, with low-risk (<5 %, 10 year CVD) factors be addressed, medium risk (5–20 %) be evaluated with a stress test, and high risk (>20 %) be referred to a cardiologist [32]. Men in between the ages of 40 and 50 with erectile dysfunction are at a 50-fold higher risk for CAD [33] (Fig. 9.4). The third Princeton Consensus guidelines on ED recommend obtaining a resting EKG on patients with ED who also have risks such as diabetes and hypertension, and the guidelines base further testing depending on exercise tolerance [34].

Depression and anxiety are also associated with erectile dysfunction. Both can be a result or a cause of ED. Newly diagnosed men with ED had a twofold greater risk of developing depression in next 5 years [35]. While surgical abdominal aneurysm repair has been shown to cause ED, a preoperative screening found 82 % had ED prior to surgery [36]. Men with hypertension have been found to have a twofold increase in ED, and hypertension medications may also contribute to ED [37]. Therefore, a careful sexual history and counseling in hypertensive patients may help with management.

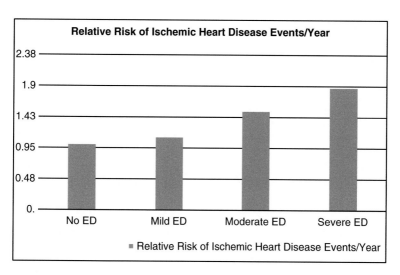

Fig. 9.4 Association of erectile dysfunction severity and ischemic heart disease (Adapted from Banks E, Joshy G, Abhayaratna WP, et al. Erectile dysfunction severity as a risk marker for cardio-vascular disease hospitalization and all-cause mortality: a prospective cohort study)

ED Treatment

Many men with ED are not treated [38]. The rates of treatment tend to be based on patient income level, with the wealthy far more likely to receive treatment, due to the current high cost and limited access to care [39]. Current guidelines recommend lifestyle change as a first-line treatment for men with ED [27]. While smoking doubles the risk of ED, smoking cessation rapidly decreases that risk back to baseline [40]. Diet and exercise have also shown to be helpful with improving ED [41]. Treatment options and approach should involve shared decision making. A recent study demonstrated that Hispanic men prefer to discuss lifestyle changes versus becoming "viagraed" [42]. In a randomized control trial, about one-third of obese patients had improved ED based on IIEF scores over a 2-year diet and exercise program [43]. Diets high in soy may have beneficial cardiovascular effects, and they may negatively affect testosterone levels leading to ED [44].

After discussing lifestyle modifications, treatment of other possible etiologies should be the next step in treating patient with ED. Common medications implicated with ED will be discussed below and include antidepressants, antihypertensive medications, and opioids. In depression treatment, bupropion may be a better option for depressed patients with ED than SSRIs [45]. In the hypertension class, experts advise avoiding beta blockers and diuretics and recommend the use of ARBs in hypertensive patients with ED [37]. Opioid dose and duration have also been found to be associated with ED [46]. Discussing with patients other pain control options might be useful. Testosterone replacement in men with hypogonadism has shown to improve ED; however, this is not an additive effect to phosphodiesterase type-5 inhibitors (PDE5is) [47]. It is also not useful to treat ED with testosterone in men with baseline normal testosterone levels [48]. A Cochrane review has shown that psychotherapy is effective for treatment of ED and adds to the effectiveness of pharmacologic therapy [49].

The mainstay of pharmacologic treatment for ED is the PDE5i class of medications which include sildenafil, tadalafil, and vardenafil. In 2012, a fourth medication, avanafil, was approved by the US Food and Drug Administration (FDA). Studies have shown similar efficacy and side effects between all four medications, with improved erections in 50–80 % of men and a number needed to treat of two patients [27]. Treatment also has been shown to improve the sexual satisfaction of the man's sexual partner [50]. Time of onset (30–60 min) is similar with these medications, except oral disintegrating vardenafil, and avanafil's onset is 15 min.

Each of these drugs has some potential benefits: sildenafil has been studied the longest, tadalafil has longest duration of action, and vardenafil has shown promise in difficult-to-treat patients. Cost is the most common cause for discontinuation of PDE5is [39]. Several online resources cite the typical patient's cost ranging from $10 to $40 per pill (goodrx.com). The starting doses are as follows: sildenafil (50 mg), tadalafil (10 mg), avanafil (100 mg), and vardenafil (10 mg). These doses then can be adjusted based on tolerance and/or efficacy. Daily tadalafil (5 mg) is an option for patients that prefer spontaneity in their sexual life and has been shown to have positive effects on lower urinary tract symptoms in patients with benign prostatic hyperplasia (BPH). Many insurance programs currently do not cover PDE5i therapy.

Side effects and risks of these medications should be discussed prior to prescribing them. Phosphodiesterase receptors are present in several other areas of the body, and this leads to a variety of adverse effects. Headache and flushing are the most common side effects noted in the PDE5is with a low rate of 6 % in avanafil and high rate of 14 % in sildenafil [51]. There are PDE6 receptors in the eye, and therefore visual changes can occur like blue vision (self-limited) or, more seriously, optic neuropathy [52]. While PDE5is have been associated with sudden hearing loss, sudden hearing loss has also been shown to be a risk factor for ED [53]. A 2014 study showed sildenafil use increased the risk of melanoma (HR: 2.2), and while the mechanism isn't clear, it is felt to be a class effect [54]. Other unique individual side effects include tadalafil's association with back pain and vardenafil's potential to increase the QT interval [55].

PDE5is and alpha-blockers have efficacy in treating both BPH and ED. However, this combination should be used with caution as it can lead to severe hypotension. Likewise, nitrates and PDE5is also can cause severe hypotension and syncope due to a synergistic effect, and this combination is an absolute contraindication. Apomorphine is a sublingual dopamine agonist and is not as effective as PDE5is but is safe to take with nitrates when indicated for treatment of ED. Other drug interactions to be aware of with PDE5is include rifampin and human immunodeficiency (HIV) protease inhibitors [52].

Alprostadil has been available in the past only in an injectable formulation, but now recently a topical intraurethral version is available. Intraurethral alprostadil may be an option if oral treatments are not warranted, and efficacy has been reported over 80 % [56]. Injectable alprostadil is also effective, but side effects including urethral pain, UTI, priapism, fibrosis, and permanent erectile dysfunction have been noted, so intensive patient education is recommended [27]. Unlike PDE5i, alprostadil avoids the nitrous oxide pathway and therefore doesn't require erectogenic stimulus to form an erection. This may be an advantage to patients with difficulties in the initiation phase of erectile dysfunction.

Proper patient education mainly about PDE5i timing is recommended to increase the effectiveness of PDE5is. PDE5is are not erotogenic and so patients should be advised they require sexual arousal to work properly. One study determined that in a primary care office, when patients who did not respond to PDE5is were reeducated, improvement in ED was seen in 40 % of cases [57].

When patients fail to respond to PDE5i treatment, and other lifestyle changes and underlying disease management have failed, alternative options exist. These include vacuum constriction devices (Fig. 9.5), alprostadil intracavernous injections, or penile prostheses. Advantages of the vacuum device include rapid action (30 s to 7 min), few contraindications (which are anticoagulation, bleeding diatheses, and sickle cell), and one-time cost [58]. Disadvantages include bluish erection, pain, and petechia (25–39 % of cases) [58]. Penile implants for refractory ED have shown to be effective with low risks of infection [59]. Penile prosthesis is a good option for patients who have failed other treatments or want a permanent treatment. Their success rate and patient satisfaction rates are 70–80 % [60].

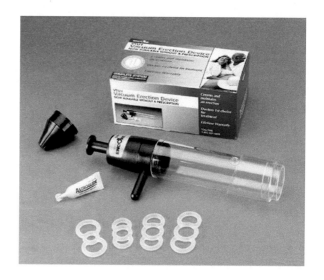

Fig. 9.5 Encore Standard Manual Vacuum Erection Device produced by Encore Medical (Obtained with permission from Hector Pimentel, MD)

Premature Ejaculation

Definitions/Epidemiology/Etiology

Normal intravaginal ejaculatory latency time has been found to be between half a minute and 5 min. The definition of premature ejaculation (PE) has changed over the last 20 years to be more specific. In order to treat and study men who suffer from this condition, the International Society on Sexual Medicine formed a committee who published a paper defining premature ejaculation as [61]:

1. Ejaculation that occurs prior or within 1 min of vaginal penetration (lifelong PE) or a clinically significant or bothersome reduction in latency time to about 3 min or less (acquired PE)
2. The inability to delay ejaculation in all or nearly all vaginal penetrations
3. Negative personal consequences such as distress, bother, frustration, and/or avoidance of sexual intimacy

The panel acknowledged this definition does not include the same gender sexual intercourse, or oral or anal penetration, citing lack of evidence to define problematic early ejaculation in these situations [61]. The *Diagnostic and Statistical Manual of Mental Disorders*, 5th edition (DSM-5), uses a similar definition for PE with the addition of a fourth criteria that the condition is not related to another nonsexual mental disorder or a severe relationship or other significant stressor or medication use. Given the prior history of vague definitions and men's reluctance to discuss this condition, the exact number of men suffering from PE is not well known. A recent survey over 2000 men in China found that 25 % of men had some PE symptoms, and of those with symptoms, 18 % fit the criteria for acquired PE and 12 % fit the criteria for lifelong PE [62].

Premature ejaculation, like ED, can be caused by both physiological and psychological factors. There have not been as many medical comorbidities associated with PE as there is with ED. The exact etiology is often unknown. There is association with PE and other sexual disorders such as ED and infertility [63]. Many studies use a stopwatch to measure intravaginal ejaculatory latency time (IELT), but the use in clinical practice has been discouraged as it can disrupt spontaneity and pleasure. Studies have found that self-report is often as accurate as a stopwatch in defining measurable time. A physical exam for lifelong PE is usually not as helpful as for acquired PE, when the thyroid and prostate function and glands should be examined. PE can be very disruptive to a relationship causing significant emotional distress for the patient and their partner [64].

Treatment

Both pharmacologic and behavioral therapies have been found to be effective for PE. Combining behavioral and pharmacologic treatment increases effectiveness. Despite studies showing the effectiveness of SSRIs, currently no FDA-approved medications are available for PE. Treatments can be divided into either daily dosing or on-demand treatment. Daily dosing medications that have shown to be effective include paroxetine, citalopram, fluoxetine, and clomipramine. On-demand medications include paroxetine, clomipramine, dapoxetine (not available in the USA), and topical lidocaine or prilocaine.

Topical EMLA (eutectic mixture of local anesthetics) cream has been shown to be effective when applied 15 min before sexual activity [65]. The authors encourage a trial of condom use for patients with PE. Although studies with condom use alone were not found to demonstrate effectiveness, most studies evaluating topical anesthetic used condoms to avoid diffusion into the vaginal wall and numbing of the partner. The most effective daily dosing SSRI appears to be paroxetine with over an eightfold delay in ejaculation [66]. The on-demand medications usually take 3–6 h to be effective and are not as effective as daily dosing. However, men often are reluctant to take any medications for PE, and despite effectiveness of treatment, one study found that 90 % of men stopped after a year [67]. Other potential treatments for PE which have limited evidence include acupuncture and caffeine 100 mg orally, 2 h prior to sexual intercourse [68].

Non-Ejaculation Ejaculatory Disorders

Hematospermia

Hematospermia, or hemospermia, is a rare condition where blood is found in the ejaculate. While it is often distressing for men, it is rarely a sign of a more significant disease. A single episode in men less than 40 without other systemic or urinary symptoms like hematuria does not require an extensive evaluation [68]. For men greater than 40, or those whom have recurrent symptoms, an evaluation for urologic disorders such as genitourinary infections or cancers or systemic diseases like uncontrolled hypertension or bleeding disorders is recommended [69]. This evaluation depends upon the history and physical examination but may include a serum prostate-specific antigen (PSA) assay, prostate ultrasound, testicular ultrasound, prostate biopsy, or serologic evaluation for coagulation disorders. Treatment is directed based on any etiology discovered.

Painful Ejaculation

Painful ejaculation has been described to be prevalent in about 1 % of the male population over 50 years of age [70]. Painful ejaculation is a known complication of a radical prostatectomy and has been implicated in other prostate disorders such as benign prostate hypertrophy and chronic prostatitis [71]. While the frequency of painful ejaculation in patients with BPH is low (15 %), the frequency in men with interstitial cystitis is quite high (60 %) [71]. Other causes include hernia repair, intra-abdominal cancer or abscesses, or urethral stricture, but often the etiology is unknown. A review of the literature did not find a valid treatment for this condition, but a small randomized controlled clinical trial (RCT) showed no effect with tamsulosin versus placebo [72]. Treatment should be focused at the underlining condition, and referral to a urologist may be appropriate.

Supplements and Over-the-Counter (OTC) Treatments to Enhance Male Sexuality

In many societies throughout history, treatments to improve or enhance sexual function have been highly sought after. This has resulted in "quackery" where charismatic salesman flourishes, such as John Brinkley who, in the 1950s, promoted transplanting goat glands into humans to improve erections [73]. Currently, it has been found that the main ingredients in web-based sexual enhancement products are yohimbine, maca, gingko biloba, and horny goat weed [74]; please see Table 9.1 for further details on these. Also, many over-the-counter supplements have been found

Table 9.1 Common sexual enhancement products found online [74]

Key ingredient	Source	Active ingredient	Efficacy	Safety
Maca	Peruvian plant grown in the Andes at high elevations	Benzyl glucosinolates and polyphenols	Inconclusive data on elderly and sexual desire in men, small positive study on ED	Potential mutagenic, induces craving behavior, moodiness, insomnia, gastritis
Horny goat weed	Chinese herb found by goat farmer, who noticed increased sexual activity of his goats	Icariin, which works on nitric oxide synthesis, and PDE5	Some animal trials with positive effects but no human trials in literature	No long-term data but case reports of tachyarrhythmia and hypomanic symptoms
Gingko biloba	Tall, living fossil trees in China	Common extract is EGb761, flavonoid glycosides	Randomized controlled trials have found no benefit	MAO inhibitor, animal studies have shown increased thyroid cancer, increases bleeding risks
Yohimbine	Extracted from the bark of African and Asian plants	Yohimbine binds to alpha 2-adrenergic receptors, low affinity to serotonin and dopamine	Meta-analysis showed positive effect on ED, but AUA recommends against routine use for ED	Central adrenergic effects such has increased pulse, blood pressure, and mania

to have detectable PDE5i elements like sildenafil [75]. There is evidence from a small single-blinded study for supplementation with L-carnitine, L-arginine, and niacin combination to improve ED [76].

Male Infertility

Definitions/Epidemiology/Etiology

Infertility is defined as the inability for a couple to become pregnant after 12 months of unprotected intercourse [77]. Prior studies have looked at prevalence based upon referrals to infertility clinics, but a 2014 study looking at a wide male population found rates of infertility at 12 %, confirming data from older studies [78]. Factors associated with longer time to pregnancy in this study included male age (35–45 years vs. 17–24 years), biologic childlessness, and no health insurance [78]. Of the total infertility cases in one population study, men were found to be the cause 20 % of the time, women 33 % of the time, a combination of male and female factors 39 % of the time, and 8 % were unexplained [79]. The cost of diagnosing and treating infertility is often substantial, and many insurances do not cover this cost. Therefore, there is a socioeconomic disparity in the diagnosis and treatment of infertility [80].

The diagnosis of male infertility is based on having an abnormal semen analysis (SA). Azoospermia is defined as undetectable sperm in an SA; oligospermia is a diminished sperm count in an SA; asthenospermia is abnormal sperm motility; teratospermia is abnormal sperm morphology. The etiology of an abnormal SA is often unknown but could be due to pre-testicular, testicular, or post-testicular causes [81]. Environment, trauma, prior infections, and pharmaceuticals such as exogenous testosterone, spironolactone, carbamazepine, and calcium channel blockers may affect spermatogenesis [81].

Evaluation and Treatment

Key points to determine in a man who is concerned about infertility include if he has had prior biologic children, his partner's history of biologic children, testicular trauma, mumps, bicycling, hot tub use, smoking, dairy intake, sugar substitute intake, urologic procedures, medications (including over-the-counter), sexual activity, and illicit drug use. A 2014 cohort study of over 10,000 men found a significant decrease in semen volume and sperm concentration in men with obesity [82]. Physical examination should be conducted to evaluate for signs of hypogonadism or abnormalities in the genitourinary exam. Varicocele repair has been shown to improve sperm measurements and fertility, but the improvement may decrease over time [83]. Other physical findings that can affect male fertility are cryptorchidism, hernia or hernia repair, prostate disease, penile deformities (e.g., hypospadias), and the lack of a vas deferens.

The recommended initial laboratory testing for male infertility is the SA. Updated SA parameters by the World Health Organization (WHO) in 2010 include lower normal limits for sperm count (15 million/ml), total motility, and normal morphology [84]. This may result in a lower number of men diagnosed with male infertility. There is frequent day-to-day variability within a man's SA, and any abnormal SA should be repeated to confirm a diagnosis of suspected male infertility [80]. Studies have obtained SA by masturbation at a clinic site after men had been asked to abstain from ejaculation for 48 h [85]. Home testing is available that reliably tests for sperm counts but not motility or morphology [86].

It is estimated that approximately 30 % of male infertility may be missed on SA, and so other special testing should include anti-sperm antibody tests and sperm penetration assays [84]. Routine endocrine testing (e.g., diabetes, thyroid disease) prior to obtaining SA has been found to be of low yield [87]. However, if there are significant abnormalities on the SA, then serum testosterone and follicle-stimulating hormone (FSH) levels are recommended to evaluate for hypogonadotropic hypogonadism. A testicular long axis less than 4.6 cm and an FSH level greater than 7.6 indicate nonobstructive azoopermia with high certainty, limiting the need for testicular biopsy [88].

Treatment for infertility depends on the etiology. Specific treatments based on etiology include alpha-adrenergic agonists for retrograde ejaculation, gonadotropin replacement for hypogonadotropic hypogonadism, and surgical varicocele repair. Treatments should also focus on lifestyle modification of factors mentioned above such as smoking cessation, weight loss, and dietary modifications to promote weight loss. Empiric treatment has been evaluated, and antioxidants, gonadotropins, and antiestrogens may be effective at improving sperm parameters and fertility rates [89]. Treatment for severe oligospermia or azoospermia often involves testicular sperm extraction (TESE) with intracytoplasmic injection (ICSI). There is a high rate of Y chromosome microdeletions in this population which would be passed on to offspring, so this testing is recommended prior to treatment [90].

Conclusion

While medical providers and male patients may be reluctant to discuss sexual health, this conversation can reveal many other underlying health concerns. Physiologic and psychologic conditions overlap in male sexual dysfunction, and often evaluation and treatment need to be focused on addressing both. Hopefully, after this review, strategies mentioned above can be used to improve knowledge, comfort, and efficiency when addressing men's sexual health. While there are many treatments that are effective in conditions including ED, premature ejaculation, and male infertility, costs can be prohibitive for some patients. Likewise, some insurance companies choose not to cover costs of infertility treatments. With improved insurance coverage by the Affordable Care Act, more men will be able to gain access and seek treatment for sexual concerns in the future. At the same time, insurance coverage should treat reproductive health as an integral part of a male's overall health.

Best Practice Recommendations

1. Patients with high-risk sexual behavior should receive high-intensity counseling [5].
2. Men with erectile dysfunction should be screened for cardiovascular disease [32, 33].
3. Lifestyle changes such as increased exercise, weight loss, and smoking cessation can improve erectile dysfunction [40, 41].
4. Phosphodiesterase inhibitors are first-line medical treatment for erectile dysfunction [27].
5. Premature ejaculation (less than 3 min latency) can cause significant psychological distress to the patient and his partner [64].
6. Hematospermia in men less than 40 is rarely associated with any significant disease [68].
7. Over-the-counter supplements to enhance sexuality should be discouraged given limited efficacy and potential toxicity [74].

References

1. Dubois-Arber F, Meystre-Agustoni G, André J, De Heller K, Alain P, Bodenmann P. Sexual behaviour of men that consulted in medical outpatient clinics in Western Switzerland from 2005–2006: risk levels unknown to doctors? BMC Public Health. 2010;10:528. Available from: http://www.pubmedcentral.nih.gov/articlerender.fcgi?artid=2939648&tool=pmcentrez&rendertype=abstract.
2. Ribeiro S, Alarcão V, Simões R, Miranda FL, Carreira M, Galvão-Teles A. General practitioners' procedures for sexual history taking and treating sexual dysfunction in primary care. J Sex Med. 2014;11(2):386–93. Available from: http://www.ncbi.nlm.nih.gov/pubmed/24261826.
3. Clark RD, Williams AA. Patient preferences in discussing sexual dysfunctions in primary care. Fam Med. 2014;46(2):124–8. Available from: http://www.ncbi.nlm.nih.gov/pubmed/24573520.
4. Publications|National LGBT Health Education Center. Available from: http://www.lgbthealtheducation.org/publications/top/.
5. Recommendation Summary – US Preventive Services Task Force. Available from: http://www.uspreventiveservicestaskforce.org/Page/Topic/recommendation-summary/sexually-transmitted-infections-behavioral-counseling1.
6. Ishak WW, Christensen S, Sayer G, Ha K, Li N, Miller J, et al. Sexual satisfaction and quality of life in major depressive disorder before and after treatment with citalopram in the STAR*D study. J Clin Psychiatry. 2013;74(3):256–61. Available from: http://www.ncbi.nlm.nih.gov/pubmed/23561231.
7. Cappelleri JC, Stecher VJ. An assessment of patient-reported outcomes for men with erectile dysfunction: Pfizer's perspective. Int J Impot Res. 2008;20(4):343–57. Available from: http://dx.doi.org/10.1038/ijir.2008.8.
8. Morris BJ, Krieger JN. Does male circumcision affect sexual function, sensitivity, or satisfaction? – A systematic review. J Sex Med. 2013;10(11):2644–57. Available from: http://www.ncbi.nlm.nih.gov/pubmed/23937309.
9. Kontaras K, Varnavas V, Kyriakides ZS. Does sildenafil cause myocardial infarction or sudden cardiac death? Am J Cardiovasc Drugs. 2008;8(1):1–7. Available from: http://www.ncbi.nlm.nih.gov/pubmed/18303932.
10. Cheitlin MD. Sexual activity and cardiac risk. Am J Cardiol. 2005;96(12B):24M–8M. Available from: http://www.ncbi.nlm.nih.gov/pubmed/16387562.

11. Sun C, Bridges A, Johnason J, Ezzell M. Pornography and the male sexual script: an analysis of consumption and sexual relations. Arch Sex Behav. 2014 Dec 3. Available from: http://www.ncbi.nlm.nih.gov/pubmed/25466233.

12. Klein DA, Goldenring JM, Adelman WP. HEEADSSS 3.0: The psychosocial interview for adolescents updated for a new century fueled by media. 2014. Available from: http://contemporarypediatrics.modernmedicine.com/contemporary-pediatrics/content/tags/adolescent-medicine/heeadsss-30-psychosocial-interview-adolesce?page=full.

13. Yi CH, Martyn K, Salerno J, Darling-Fisher CS. Development and clinical use of Rapid Assessment for Adolescent Preventive Services (RAAPS) questionnaire in school-based health centers. J Pediatr Health Care. 2009;23(1):2–9. Available from: http://www.pubmedcentral.nih.gov/articlerender.fcgi?artid=2696801&tool=pmcentrez&rendertype=abstract.

14. Case Studies|Rapid Assessment for Adolescent Preventive Services. Available from: https://www.raaps.org/caseStudies.php.

15. Karraker A, Delamater J, Schwartz CR. Sexual frequency decline from midlife to later life. J Gerontol B Psychol Sci Soc Sci. 2011;66(4):502–12. Available from: http://www.pubmedcentral.nih.gov/articlerender.fcgi?artid=3132270&tool=pmcentrez&rendertype=abstract.

16. Bahouq H, Allali F, Rkain H, Hajjaj-Hassouni N. Discussing sexual concerns with chronic low back pain patients: barriers and patients' expectations. Clin Rheumatol. 2013;32(10):1487–92. Available from: http://www.ncbi.nlm.nih.gov/pubmed/23743660.

17. Kitts RL. Barriers to optimal care between physicians and lesbian, gay, bisexual, transgender, and questioning adolescent patients. J Homosex. 2010;57(6):730–47. Available from: http://www.tandfonline.com/doi/abs/10.1080/00918369.2010.485872?url_ver=Z39.88-2003&rfr_id=ori:rid:crossref.org&rfr_dat=cr_pub%3dpubmed#.VOjI5Lk5DmQ.

18. The Proactive Sexual Health History: Key to Effective Sexual Health Care – American Family Physician. Available from: http://www.aafp.org/afp/2002/1101/p1705.html.

19. Kramer MA, van Veen MG, Op de Coul ELM, Coutinho RA, Prins M. Do sexual risk behaviour, risk perception and testing behaviour differ across generations of migrants? Eur J Public Health. 2014;24(1):134–8. Available from: http://eurpub.oxfordjournals.org/content/24/1/134.long.

20. Breiding MJ, Smith SG, Basile KC, Walters ML, Chen J, Merrick MT. Prevalence and characteristics of sexual violence, stalking, and intimate partner violence victimization–national intimate partner and sexual violence survey, United States, 2011. MMWR Surveill Summ. 2014;63(8):1–18. Available from: http://www.ncbi.nlm.nih.gov/pubmed/25188037.

21. Andersen TH. Speaking about the unspeakable: sexually abused men striving toward language. Am J Mens Health. 2008;2(1):25–36. Available from: http://www.ncbi.nlm.nih.gov/pubmed/19477767.

22. Miller DC, Saigal CS, Litwin MS. The demographic burden of urologic diseases in America. Urol Clin North Am. 2009;36(1):11–27. v. Available from: http://www.pubmedcentral.nih.gov/articlerender.fcgi?artid=2614213&tool=pmcentrez&rendertype=abstract.

23. Polinski JM, Kesselheim AS. Where cost, medical necessity, and morality meet: should US government insurance programs pay for erectile dysfunction drugs? Clin Pharmacol Ther. 2011;89(1):17–9. Available from: http://www.ncbi.nlm.nih.gov/pubmed/21170064.

24. Claes HIM, Andrianne R, Opsomer R, Albert A, Patel S, Commers K. The HelpED study: agreement and impact of the erection hardness score on sexual function and psychosocial outcomes in men with erectile dysfunction and their partners. J Sex Med. 2012;9(10):2652–63. Available from: http://www.ncbi.nlm.nih.gov/pubmed/22906210.

25. Suzuki E, Nishimatsu H, Oba S, Takahashi M, Homma Y. Chronic kidney disease and erectile dysfunction. World J Nephrol. 2014;3(4):220–9. Available from: http://www.pubmedcentral.nih.gov/articlerender.fcgi?artid=4220354&tool=pmcentrez&rendertype=abstract.

26. Grover S, Mattoo SK, Pendharkar S, Kandappan V. Sexual dysfunction in patients with alcohol and opioid dependence. Indian J Psychol Med. 2014;36(4):355–65. Available from: http://www.pubmedcentral.nih.gov/articlerender.fcgi?artid=4201785&tool=pmcentrez&rendertype=abstract.

27. Hatzimouratidis K, Amar E, Eardley I, Giuliano F, Hatzichristou D, Montorsi F, et al. Guidelines on male sexual dysfunction: erectile dysfunction and premature ejaculation. Eur Urol. 2010;57(5):804–14. Available from: http://www.sciencedirect.com/science/article/pii/S0302283810001338.

28. Aversa A, Sarteschi LM. The role of penile color-duplex ultrasound for the evaluation of erectile dysfunction. J Sex Med. 2007;4(5):1437–47. Available from: http://www.ncbi.nlm.nih.gov/pubmed/17645448.

29. Jannini EA, Granata AM, Hatzimouratidis K, Goldstein I. Use and abuse of Rigiscan in the diagnosis of erectile dysfunction. J Sex Med. 2009;6(7):1820–9. Available from: http://www.ncbi.nlm.nih.gov/pubmed/19575775.

30. Jannini EA, McCabe MP, Salonia A, Montorsi F, Sachs BD. Organic vs. psychogenic? The Manichean diagnosis in sexual medicine. J Sex Med. 2010;7(5):1726–33. Available from: http://www.ncbi.nlm.nih.gov/pubmed/20537061.

31. Brock G. Diagnosing erectile dysfunction could save your patient's life. Can Urol Assoc J. 2014;8((7–8 Suppl 5)):S151–2. Available from: http://journals.sfu.ca/cuaj/index.php/journal/article/view/2311.

32. Miner M, Nehra A, Jackson G, Bhasin S, Billups K, Burnett AL, et al. All men with vasculogenic erectile dysfunction require a cardiovascular workup. Am J Med. 2014;127(3):174–82. Available from: http://www.amjmed.com/article/S0002934313009273/fulltext.

33. Gades NM, Jacobson DJ, McGree ME, St Sauver JL, Lieber MM, Nehra A, et al. Longitudinal evaluation of sexual function in a male cohort: the Olmsted county study of urinary symptoms and health status among men. J Sex Med. 2009;6(9):2455–66. Available from: http://www.pubmedcentral.nih.gov/articlerender.fcgi?artid=2862565&tool=pmcentrez&rendertype=abstract.

34. Nehra A, Jackson G, Miner M, et al. The Princeton III Consensus recommendations for the management of erectile dysfunction and cardiovascular disease. Mayo Clin Proc. 2012;87(8):766–78. doi:10.1016/j.mayocp.2012.06.015.

35. Chou P-S, Chou W-P, Chen M-C, Lai C-L, Wen Y-C, Yeh K-C, et al. Newly diagnosed erectile dysfunction and risk of depression: a population-based 5-year follow-up study in Taiwan. J Sex Med. 2014;12(3):804–12. Available from: http://www.ncbi.nlm.nih.gov/pubmed/25475605.

36. Falkensammer J, Hakaim AG, Falkensammer CE, Broderick GA, Crook JE, Heckman MG, et al. Prevalence of erectile dysfunction in vascular surgery patients. Vasc Med. 2007;12(1):17–22. Available from: http://vmj.sagepub.com/cgi/doi/10.1177/1358863X06076043.

37. Viigimaa M, Vlachopoulos C, Lazaridis A, Doumas M. Management of erectile dysfunction in hypertension: tips and tricks. World J Cardiol. 2014;6(9):908–15. Available from: http://www.pubmedcentral.nih.gov/articlerender.fcgi?artid=4176800&tool=pmcentrez&rendertype=abstract.

38. Frederick LR, Cakir OO, Arora H, Helfand BT, McVary KT. Undertreatment of erectile dysfunction: claims analysis of 6.2 million patients. J Sex Med. 2014;11(10):2546–53. Available from: http://www.ncbi.nlm.nih.gov/pubmed/25059314.

39. Ströberg P, Hedelin H, Bergström A. Is sex only for the healthy and wealthy? J Sex Med. 2007;4(1):176–82. Available from: http://www.ncbi.nlm.nih.gov/pubmed/17233783.

40. McVary KT, Carrier S, Wessells H. Smoking and erectile dysfunction: evidence based analysis. J Urol. 2001;166(5):1624–32. Available from: http://www.ncbi.nlm.nih.gov/pubmed/11586190.

41. Moyad MA, Park K. What do most erectile dysfunction guidelines have in common? No evidence-based discussion or recommendation of heart-healthy lifestyle changes and/or Panax ginseng. Asian J Androl. 2012;14(6):830–41. Available from: http://www.pubmedcentral.nih.gov/articlerender.fcgi?artid=3720104&tool=pmcentrez&rendertype=abstract.

42. Wentzell E, Salmerón J. You'll get viagraed:" Mexican men's preference for alternative erectile dysfunction treatment. Soc Sci Med. 2009;68(10):1759–65. Available from: http://www.ncbi.nlm.nih.gov/pubmed/19362402.

43. Esposito K, Giugliano F, Di Palo C, Giugliano G, Marfella R, D'Andrea F, et al. Effect of lifestyle changes on erectile dysfunction in obese men: a randomized controlled trial. JAMA.

2004;291(24):2978–84. Available from: http://jama.jamanetwork.com/article.aspx?articleid=198993.

44. Siepmann T, Roofeh J, Kiefer FW, Edelson DG. Hypogonadism and erectile dysfunction associated with soy product consumption. Nutrition. 2015;27(7–8):859–62. Available from: http://www.ncbi.nlm.nih.gov/pubmed/21353476.

45. Clayton AH, Croft HA, Handiwala L. Antidepressants and sexual dysfunction: mechanisms and clinical implications. Postgrad Med. 2014;126(2):91–9. Available from: http://www.ncbi.nlm.nih.gov/24685972.

46. Deyo RA, Smith DHM, Johnson ES, Tillotson CJ, Donovan M, Yang X, et al. Prescription opioids for back pain and use of medications for erectile dysfunction. Spine (Phila Pa 1976). 2013;38(11):909–15. Available from: http://www.pubmedcentral.nih.gov/articlerender.fcgi?artid=3651746&tool=pmcentrez&rendertype=abstract.

47. Ramasamy R, Scovell JM, Wilken NA, Kovac JR, Lipshultz LI. Management of erectile dysfunction in the hypogonadal man: a case-based review. Rev Urol. 2014;16(3):105–9. Available from: http://www.pubmedcentral.nih.gov/articlerender.fcgi?artid=4191629&tool=pmcentrez&rendertype=abstract.

48. Corona G, Isidori AM, Buvat J, Aversa A, Rastrelli G, Hackett G, et al. Testosterone supplementation and sexual function: a meta-analysis study. J Sex Med. 2014;11(6):1577–92. Available from: http://www.ncbi.nlm.nih.gov/pubmed/24697970.

49. Melnik T, Soares BGO, Nasselo AG. Psychosocial interventions for erectile dysfunction. Cochrane Database Syst Rev. 2007;3:CD004825.

50. Chevret-Méasson M, Lavallée E, Troy S, Arnould B, Oudin S, Cuzin B. Improvement in quality of sexual life in female partners of men with erectile dysfunction treated with sildenafil citrate: findings of the Index of Sexual Life (ISL) in a couple study. J Sex Med. 2009;6(3):761–9. Available from: http://www.ncbi.nlm.nih.gov/pubmed/19143916.

51. Cui Y-S, Li N, Zong H-T, Yan H-L, Zhang Y. Avanafil for male erectile dysfunction: a systematic review and meta-analysis. Asian J Androl. 2014;16(3):472–7. Available from: http://www.pubmedcentral.nih.gov/articlerender.fcgi?artid=4023381&tool=pmcentrez&rendertype=abstract.

52. Sadovsky R, Brock GB, Gutkin SW, Sorsaburu S. Toward a new "EPOCH": optimising treatment outcomes with phosphodiesterase type 5 inhibitors for erectile dysfunction. Int J Clin Pract. 2009;63(8):1214–30. Available from: http://www.pubmedcentral.nih.gov/articlerender.fcgi?artid=2779984&tool=pmcentrez&rendertype=abstract.

53. Hsu H-T, Chen J-Y, Weng S-F, Huang K-H, Lin Y-S. Increased risk of erectile dysfunction in patients with sudden sensorineural hearing loss: a nationwide, population-based cohort study. Otol Neurotol. 2013;34(5):862–7. Available from: http://www.ncbi.nlm.nih.gov/pubmed/23739556.

54. Li W-Q, Qureshi AA, Robinson KC, Han J. Sildenafil use and increased risk of incident melanoma in US men: a prospective cohort study. JAMA Intern Med. 2014;174(6):964–70. Available from: http://www.pubmedcentral.nih.gov/articlerender.fcgi?artid=4178948&tool=pmcentrez&rendertype=abstract.

55. Smith WB, McCaslin IR, Gokce A, Mandava SH, Trost L, Hellstrom WJ. PDE5 inhibitors: considerations for preference and long-term adherence. Int J Clin Pract. 2013;67(8):768–80. Available from: http://www.ncbi.nlm.nih.gov/pubmed/23869678.

56. Moncada I, Cuzin B. Clinical efficacy and safety of Vitaros©/Virirec© (Alprostadil cream) for the treatment of erectile dysfunction. Urologia. 2015;82(2):84–92. Available from: http://www.ncbi.nlm.nih.gov/pubmed/25744707.

57. Atiemo HO, Szostak MJ, Sklar GN. Salvage of sildenafil failures referred from primary care physicians. J Urol. 2003;170(6 Pt 1):2356–8. Available from: http://www.ncbi.nlm.nih.gov/pubmed/14634415.

58. Hoyland K, Vasdev N, Adshead J. The use of vacuum erection devices in erectile dysfunction after radical prostatectomy. Rev Urol. 2013;15(2):67–71. Available from: http://www.pubmedcentral.nih.gov/articlerender.fcgi?artid=3784970&tool=pmcentrez&rendertype=abstract.

59. Trost LW, McCaslin R, Linder B, Hellstrom WJG. Long-term outcomes of penile prostheses for the treatment of erectile dysfunction. Expert Rev Med Devices. 2013;10(3):353–66. Available from: http://www.ncbi.nlm.nih.gov/pubmed/23668707.

60. Albersen M, Orabi H, Lue TF. Evaluation and treatment of erectile dysfunction in the aging male: a mini-review. Gerontology. 2012;58(1):3–14. Available from: http://www.karger.com/Article/FullText/329598.
61. Serefoglu EC, McMahon CG, Waldinger MD, Althof SE, Shindel A, Adaikan G, et al. An evidence-based unified definition of lifelong and acquired premature ejaculation: report of the second international society for sexual medicine ad hoc committee for the definition of premature ejaculation. J Sex Med. 2014;2(2):41–59. Available from: http://www.pubmedcentral.nih.gov/articlerender.fcgi?artid=4184676&tool=pmcentrez&rendertype=abstract.
62. Gao J, Zhang X, Su P, Liu J, Xia L, Yang J, et al. Prevalence and factors associated with the complaint of premature ejaculation and the four premature ejaculation syndromes: a large observational study in China. J Sex Med. 2013;10(7):1874–81. Available from: http://www.ncbi.nlm.nih.gov/pubmed/23651451.
63. Shindel AW, Nelson CJ, Naughton CK, Mulhall JP. Premature ejaculation in infertile couples: prevalence and correlates. J Sex Med. 2008;5(2):485–91. Available from: http://www.ncbi.nlm.nih.gov/pubmed/18086172.
64. Revicki D, Howard K, Hanlon J, Mannix S, Greene A, Rothman M. Characterizing the burden of premature ejaculation from a patient and partner perspective: a multi-country qualitative analysis. Health Qual Life Outcomes. 2008;6:33. Available from: http://www.pubmedcentral.nih.gov/articlerender.fcgi?artid=2390524&tool=pmcentrez&rendertype=abstract.
65. Atan A, Basar MM, Tuncel A, Ferhat M, Agras K, Tekdogan U. Comparison of efficacy of sildenafil-only, sildenafil plus topical EMLA cream, and topical EMLA-cream-only in treatment of premature ejaculation. Urology. 2006;67(2):388–91. Available from: http://www.ncbi.nlm.nih.gov/pubmed/16461091.
66. International Journal of Impotence Research – Figure 1 for article: relevance of methodological design for the interpretation of efficacy of drug treatment of premature ejaculation: a systematic review and meta-analysis. Available from: http://www.nature.com/ijir/journal/v16/n4/fig_tab/3901172f1.html#figure-title.
67. Mondaini N, Fusco F, Cai T, Benemei S, Mirone V, Bartoletti R. Dapoxetine treatment in patients with lifelong premature ejaculation: the reasons of a "Waterloo". Urology. 2013;82(3):620–4. Available from: http://www.ncbi.nlm.nih.gov/pubmed/23987156.
68. Akhter W, Khan F, Chinegwundoh F. Should every patient with hematospermia be investigated? A critical review. Cent Eur J Urol. 2013;66(1):79–82. Available from: http://www.pubmedcentral.nih.gov/articlerender.fcgi?artid=3921834&tool=pmcentrez&rendertype=abstract.
69. Stefanovic KB, Gregg PC, Soung M. Evaluation and treatment of hematospermia. Am Fam Physician. 2009;80(12):1421–7. Available from: http://www.ncbi.nlm.nih.gov/pubmed/20000304.
70. Blanker MH, Bosch JLHR, Groeneveld FPM, Bohnen AM, Prins A, Thomas S, et al. Erectile and ejaculatory dysfunction in a community-based sample of men 50 to 78 years old: prevalence, concern, and relation to sexual activity. Urology. 2001;57(4):763–8. Available from: http://www.goldjournal.net/article/S0090429500010918/fulltext.
71. Matsushita K, Tal R, Mulhall JP. The evolution of orgasmic pain (dysorgasmia) following radical prostatectomy. J Sex Med. 2012;9(5):1454–8. Available from: http://www.ncbi.nlm.nih.gov/pubmed/22458302.
72. Safarinejad MR. Safety and efficacy of tamsulosin in the treatment of painful ejaculation: a randomized, double-blind, placebo-controlled study. Int J Impot Res. 2006;18(6):527–33. Available from: http://dx.doi.org/10.1038/sj.ijir.3901466.
73. McMahon CG. Get a better erection!–Hope for sale–use sexual snake oil. J Sex Med. 2010;7(5):1699–702. Available from: http://doi.wiley.com/10.1111/j.1743-6109.2010.01821.x.
74. Corazza O, Martinotti G, Santacroce R, Chillemi E, Di Giannantonio M, Schifano F, et al. Sexual enhancement products for sale online: raising awareness of the psychoactive effects of yohimbine, maca, horny goat weed, and Ginkgo biloba. Biomed Res Int. 2014;841798. Available from: http://www.pubmedcentral.nih.gov/articlerender.fcgi?artid=4082836&tool=pmcentrez&rendertype=abstract.
75. Cohen PA, Venhuis BJ. Adulterated sexual enhancement supplements: more than mojo. JAMA Intern Med. 2013;173(13):1169–70. Available from: http://archinte.jamanetwork.com/article.aspx?articleid=1710101.

76. Gianfrilli D, Lauretta R, Di Dato C, Graziadio C, Pozza C, De Larichaudy J, et al. Propionyl-L-carnitine, L-arginine and niacin in sexual medicine: a nutraceutical approach to erectile dysfunction. Andrologia. 2012;44 Suppl 1:600–4. Available from: http://www.ncbi.nlm.nih.gov/pubmed/21966881.
77. Definitions of infertility and recurrent pregnancy loss: a committee opinion. Fertil Steril. 2013;99(1):63. Available from: http://www.ncbi.nlm.nih.gov/pubmed/23095139.
78. Louis JF, Thoma ME, Sørensen DN, McLain AC, King RB, Sundaram R, et al. The prevalence of couple infertility in the United States from a male perspective: evidence from a nationally representative sample. Andrology. 2013;1(5):741–8. Available from: http://www.pubmedcentral.nih.gov/articlerender.fcgi?artid=3752331&tool=pmcentrez&rendertype=abstract.
79. Thonneau P, Marchand S, Tallec A, Ferial ML, Ducot B, Lansac J, et al. Incidence and main causes of infertility in a resident population (1,850,000) of three French regions (1988–1989). Hum Reprod. 1991;6(6):811–6. Available from: http://www.ncbi.nlm.nih.gov/pubmed/1757519.
80. Keel BA. Within- and between-subject variation in semen parameters in infertile men and normal semen donors. Fertil Steril. 2006;85(1):128–34. Available from: http://www.ncbi.nlm.nih.gov/pubmed/16412742.
81. Brezina PR, Yunus FN, Zhao Y. Effects of pharmaceutical medications on male fertility. J Reprod Infertil. 2012;13(1):3–11. Available from: http://www.pubmedcentral.nih.gov/articlerender.fcgi?artid=3719368&tool=pmcentrez&rendertype=abstract.
82. Belloc S, Cohen-Bacrie M, Amar E, Izard V, Benkhalifa M, Dalléac A, et al. High body mass index has a deleterious effect on semen parameters except morphology: results from a large cohort study. Fertil Steril. 2014;102(5):1268–73. Available from: http://www.ncbi.nlm.nih.gov/pubmed/25225071.
83. Cavallini G, Beretta G, Biagiotti G, Mallus R, Maretti C, Pescatori E, et al. Subsequent impaired fertility (with or without sperm worsening) in men who had fathered children after a left varicocelectomy: a novel population? Urol Ann. 2015;7(1):79–85. Available from: http://www.pubmedcentral.nih.gov/articlerender.fcgi?artid=4310124&tool=pmcentrez&rendertype=abstract.
84. Esteves SC. Clinical relevance of routine semen analysis and controversies surrounding the 2010 world health organization criteria for semen examination. Int Braz J Urol. 2014;40:443–53. Available from: http://brazjurol.com.br/july_august_2014/Esteves_443_453.htm.
85. Sperm Morphology, Motility, and Concentration in Fertile and Infertile Men—NEJM. Available from: http://www.nejm.org/doi/full/10.1056/NEJMoa003005.
86. Coppola MA, Klotz KL, Kim K, Cho HY, Kang J, Shetty J, et al. SpermCheck Fertility, an immunodiagnostic home test that detects normozoospermia and severe oligozoospermia. Hum Reprod. 2010;25(4):853–61. Available from: http://www.pubmedcentral.nih.gov/articlerender.fcgi?artid=2839906&tool=pmcentrez&rendertype=abstract.
87. Sigman M, Jarow JP. Endocrine evaluation of infertile men. Urology. 1997;50(5):659–64. Available from: http://www.ncbi.nlm.nih.gov/pubmed/9372871.
88. Schoor RA, Elhanbly S, Niederberger CS, Ross LS. The role of testicular biopsy in the modern management of male infertility. J Urol. 2002;167(1):197–200. Available from: http://www.ncbi.nlm.nih.gov/pubmed/11743304.
89. Jung JH, Seo JT. Empirical medical therapy in idiopathic male infertility: promise or panacea? Clin Exp Reprod Med. 2014;41(3):108–14. Available from: http://www.pubmedcentral.nih.gov/articlerender.fcgi?artid=4192450&tool=pmcentrez&rendertype=abstract.
90. Stahl PJ, Masson P, Mielnik A, Marean MB, Schlegel PN, Paduch DA. A decade of experience emphasizes that testing for Y microdeletions is essential in American men with azoospermia and severe oligozoospermia. Fertil Steril. 2010;94(5):1753–6. Available from: http://www.ncbi.nlm.nih.gov/pubmed/19896650.

Chapter 10
Sexually Transmitted Infections in Men

Charles Kodner

Overview

Sexually transmitted infections (STIs) are among the most common clinical conditions encountered in primary care and urgent care settings. The prevention, early detection, and effective treatment of STIs represent a significant clinical and public health burden, with a critical role for patient behavioral counseling as an important part of an overall prevention strategy. The majority of clinical care recommendations regarding STIs focus on the care of women, in whom STIs can result in sequelae such as pelvic inflammatory disease (PID), infertility, increased morbidity and mortality during pregnancy, chronic pelvic pain syndromes, neonatal transmission and complications, and others. STIs in women are more frequently evident clinically due to presentation with vaginal discharge or other related symptoms, and they are diagnosed incidentally or during STI screening during routine pelvic examinations as part of an established preventive health program for women.

Most STIs in men are more often asymptomatic, and men are less likely to present for routine health maintenance visits, especially as young adults. There is no male equivalent of the routine Pap smear test to drive an opportunity for reproductive-age male patients to have a regular discussion of general health issues including sexual health and STI risk and prevention. A recent set of guidelines for male sexual and reproductive health [1] emphasizes the relative lack of training and clear recommendations regarding men's sexual health issues.

The public health considerations regarding STIs in men are considerable, particularly in terms of the risk of transmission of asymptomatic STIs to female partners, with attendant health risks as above. Men who are homosexual or bisexual

C. Kodner, MD (✉)
Department of Family and Geriatric Medicine, University of Louisville School of Medicine,
Med Center One Building, Louisville, KY 40202, USA
e-mail: charles.kodner@louisville.edu

© Springer International Publishing Switzerland 2016
J.J. Heidelbaugh (ed.), *Men's Health in Primary Care*, Current Clinical Practice,
DOI 10.1007/978-3-319-26091-4_10

(men who have sex with men [MSM]) are at an increased risk of STIs including human immunodeficiency virus (HIV), and multiple other STIs are seen as statistical risk factors and biological cofactors for acquiring HIV infection.

There are important clinical, biological, and behavioral differences in the presentation, diagnosis, management, and prevention of STIs in men compared to women. This chapter will review these aspects in the management of STIs, including current epidemiology of STIs, current clinical treatment and screening guidelines, and evolving recommendations for STI prevention in men, including vaccination against preventable STIs. This chapter will also address societal issues including different sexual health-related behaviors and beliefs more common among men, and how these translate into physician communication and counseling skills when caring for male patients with STIs or STI risk factors.

This chapter will focus on the care of adult and adolescent ("reproductive age") male patients in the United States (USA) and will emphasize the detection, prevention, and management of STIs other than HIV. HIV care, STIs in developing countries, and the management of STIs in children are beyond the scope of this chapter. The focus of the chapter will be on chlamydia, gonorrhea, syphilis, viral hepatitis C (HCV), human papillomavirus (HPV), and herpes simplex type 2 (HSV2); chancroid and other STIs are significantly less common or even rare in the USA.

Assessing a patient's overall sexual health involves discussions of sexual symptoms or dysfunction, relationship issues, reproductive plans and pregnancy prevention, and other areas; these topics are as important for men as for women [1], but this chapter will focus solely on issues related to STIs.

Before addressing screening, counseling, or treatment recommendations regarding STIs in men, it is important to review the following factors on which such recommendations are based for an individual patient; these topics will be addressed in the following sections:

- An understanding of the epidemiology of STIs in men
- The biological and clinical differences in STI presentation in men versus women
- Risk factors for STIs in men
- Obtaining a comprehensive sexual health history in male patients
- An understanding of cultural or perceptual beliefs common among men regarding STIs

Epidemiology of STIs in Men

The US Centers for Disease Control and Prevention (CDC) collects and publishes extensive data on the frequency of STIs in multiple populations (see http://www.cdc.gov/std/stats/ for additional information). Table 10.1 summarizes key epidemiologic statistics for chlamydia and gonorrhea, the most common STIs, according to CDC data (CDC); the table shows data from 2000, 2009, and 2013 (the most recent year with full data) to briefly represent trends in these statistics; the table shows the number of cases and the case rate per 100,000 for the total US population and for men and women.

Table 10.1 Epidemiology of selected sexually transmitted diseases in the USA for selected years

Infection	Year	2000	2009	2013
Chlamydia	Total cases	702,039	1,244,180	1,401,906
	Rate	257.5	405.3	446.6
	Cases in women	563,206	912,718	993,348
	Rate	404.0	586.7	623.1
	Cases in men	137,049	328,783	405,652
	Rate	102.8	217.1	262.6
Gonorrhea	Total cases	358,995	301,174	333,004
	Rate	131.6	98.1	106.1
	Cases in women	178,854	162,568	163,208
	Rate	128.3	104.5	102.4
	Cases in men	179,375	137,819	169,130
	Rate	134.6	91.0	109.5

Drawn from references [2] and [3]

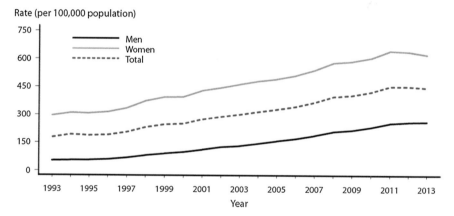

Fig. 10.1 Rates of reported cases of chlamydia in the USA by year [3]

Chlamydia

The total case rate for *Chlamydia trachomatis* infection in 2013 decreased by 1.5 % compared to the rate in 2012; this is the first time since nationwide reporting for chlamydia began that the overall rate of reported cases of chlamydia has decreased. The rate in women decreased 2.4 %, while the rate in men increased 0.8 %. During 2009–2013, the chlamydia rate in men increased 21 %, compared with a 6.2 % increase in women during this period [3]. In 2013, 949,270 cases of chlamydial infection were reported among persons aged 15–24 years of age, representing 68 % of all reported chlamydia cases.

Figure 10.1 shows the rates of reported cases of chlamydia in the USA by year, and Fig. 10.2 shows the rates of chlamydia infection by state in 2013. Figure 10.3 shows the rates of chlamydia by age and gender in 2013.

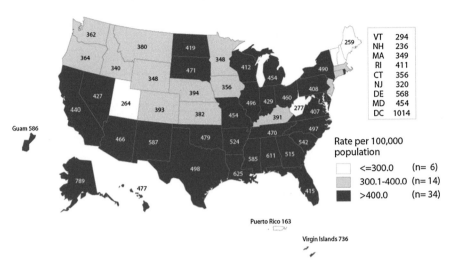

Fig. 10.2 Rates of reported cases of chlamydia in the USA by State, 2013 [3]

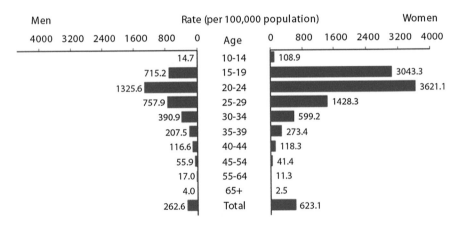

Fig. 10.3 Rates of reported cases of chlamydia in the USA by age and gender, 2013 [3]

The larger number of chlamydia cases in women reflects the impact of screening for this infection; however, the increased use and availability of urine testing helps to explain the increased infection rate in men. The lower rate among men also suggests that many of the sex partners of women with chlamydia are not receiving a diagnosis of chlamydia or being reported as having chlamydia [3].

Gonorrhea

Following a 74 % decline in the rate of reported *Neisseria gonorrhea* during 1975–1997, overall gonorrhea rates in the USA plateaued for 10 years. After the decline halted for several years, gonorrhea rates decreased further to 98.1 cases per 100,000 population in 2009, the lowest rate since recording of gonorrhea rates began. Since then, the rate of gonorrhea has fluctuated from year to year with an overall trend toward a slight increase. In 2013, the rate of reported gonorrhea was higher in men than in women for the first time since 2000 [3]. This increase may be due to increased disease transmission or may be due to increased detection of cases due to screening high-risk patient populations or to the ease of urine-based diagnostic testing compared to urethral swab testing.

The highest rates of gonorrhea tend to be in the southern and southeastern USA; in 2013, the rate of reported gonorrhea was higher in men than in women for the first time since 2000, corresponding to the similar trend with reported chlamydia. In 2013, as in previous years, men aged 20–24 years had the highest rate of gonorrhea (459.4 cases per 100,000 males) compared with males across other age groups.

Syphilis

After declining throughout the 1990s, the rate of primary and secondary (P&S) syphilis reported in the USA increased each year from 2001 through 2009 and has continued a slower increase from 2010 through 2013 [3]. The increased rates are due almost solely to an increased rate in men; in 2013, men accounted for 91 % of all P&S syphilis cases, and 75 % of these cases are in MSM. In this population, about one-half of MSM patients with syphilis also were infected with HIV, whereas the coinfection rate during the same time was approximately 10 % in men who have sex with women (MSW) and 5 % in women. During 2000–2013, the rate of P&S syphilis among men 20–24 years old increased from 4.3 to 27.7 cases per 100,000, representing the highest rate of P&S syphilis among any age group in men. From the standpoint of STI and sexual health care in men, syphilis has once more become an important disease to consider when assessing patients' STI risk factors. Figure 10.4 shows the reported cases of syphilis by gender and sexual behavior from 2007 to 2013.

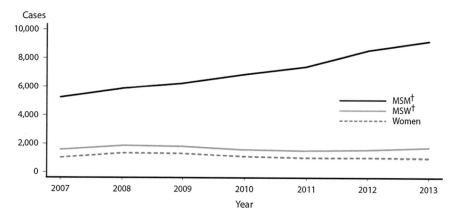

Fig. 10.4 Reported cases of syphilis by gender and sexual behavior, 2007–2013 [3]

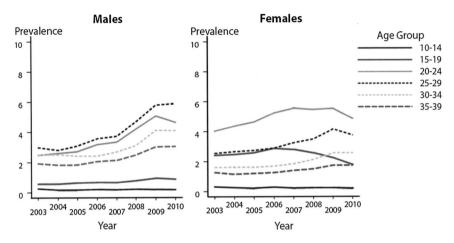

Fig. 10.5 Rates of genital warts in the USA by age and gender [3]

HPV

Prevalence data on genital warts due to human papillomavirus (HPV) were compiled by information via provider diagnosis or by documentation from the physical examination. Gay, bisexual, and other MSM and men who have sex with women only (MSW) were defined by self-report or by reported sex partners. Between 2010 and 2013, among patients in STI clinics who were diagnosed with genital warts, 17.0 % were women, 20.5 % were MSM, and 62.5 % were MSW.

In 2013, the prevalence of diagnosed genital warts among MSM was 3.0 times that of women, and the prevalence among MSW was 4.0 times that of women [3]. During 2010–2013, prevalence of genital warts among MSW increased (6.8–7.4 %), while prevalence among MSM decreased (6.3–5.5 %). The proportion of women diagnosed with genital warts decreased slightly over time, from 1.9 % in 2010 to 1.6 % in 2013. Figure 10.5 shows the rates of genital warts by age and gender.

HSV

Herpes simplex virus 2 (HSV2) is essentially ubiquitous in the US population and throughout the world and is an important cause of genital ulcer disease and genital herpes. Genital ulcer disease is associated with an increased risk of acquiring HIV disease, presumably due to exposure of mucosal surfaces that allow increased transmission of infection. Since genital herpes is not a reportable illness, it is impossible to create similarly detailed epidemiologic data and assessments compared to other STIs; the CDC reports only HSV-related physician visits rather than complete case data which is unavailable. Approximately 90 % of patients who are HSV seropositive are unaware of this [3]. Serology for HSV2 is not generally useful in

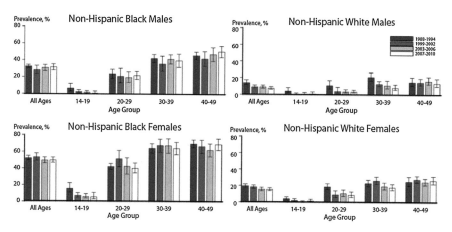

Fig. 10.6 Seroprevalence of HSV2 by age group, ethnicity, and year [3]

predicting clinical symptoms or transmission, but is often used as a surrogate in place of more specific epidemiologic data. In general, while HSV-2 seroprevalence is increasing, HSV-related physician visits are increasing, possibly due to increased recognition and awareness of infection [3]. Figure 10.6 shows the seroprevalence of HSV2 by age group, ethnicity, and year.

Clinical Features of STIs in Men

The common STIs produce generally predictable clinical syndromes; the presenting features and symptoms of these infections differ from men to women, and a review of the key clinical features of these disorders specific to men can help physicians maintain an appropriate index of suspicion for STIs in patients with various presenting complaints.

During sexual intercourse or other contact, STIs are typically transmitted at the site of breaks in mucosal surfaces that are exposed to STI-causing organisms [4]. Women have a greater exposed mucosal surface than do men, and these surfaces are subjected to greater trauma, which in part explains the increased risk women have for STIs.

Men's physical examination to evaluate for evidence of STIs is easier and less invasive than in women, in whom the vagina and cervix must be visualized. Despite this, the ready availability of urine-based STI testing may limit the actual physical examination of men for STIs, particularly in "express treatment" STI clinics that rely heavily on urine-based testing and forego the clinical examination. One study found an increased rate of missed STI diagnoses in men presenting to an STI clinic with symptoms (10.4 %) compared to the group of asymptomatic patients (2.6 %) and the group of patients presenting after identification of an STI in a sexual contact (4.5 %) [5]. This suggests that even when a diagnosis of urethritis seems evident based on history and can be confirmed on urine testing, a physical examination is still important to identify other or unsuspected STIs or genital infections, such as balanitis, scabies, epididymitis, penile warts, or genital herpes, as well as a disseminated gonococcal infection and the small proportion of primary syphilis cases [5].

Clinical Syndromes

The clinical syndromes for STIs in men include the following: urethritis, presenting with urethral discharge or irritation; genital ulcer disease; HPV causing genital warts; and disorders presenting with irritative voiding. Table 10.2 lists the most common clinical syndromes and causative organisms for STIs in men.

Urethritis

Chlamydia trachomatis infection in men is often asymptomatic but is more often symptomatic than in women. Chlamydia in men typically presents with urethral pain and dysuria rather than urethral discharge. These symptoms of urethritis are the most common presentation for STIs in men. Gonorrheal infections behave similarly in terms of clinical presentation in men, although they are more commonly

Table 10.2 Clinical syndromes and causative organisms for male STIs

Syndrome	Agent
Urethritis	*N. gonorrhoeae*, *C. trachomatis*, herpes simplex virus (HSV), *T. vaginalis*, *M. genitalium*
Epididymitis	*C. trachomatis*, *N. gonorrhoeae*
Genital ulceration	HSV, *T. pallidum*, *H. ducreyi*, *Klebsiella granulomatis*, *C. trachomatis* (LGV strains)
Nonulcerative genital skin lesions	*T. pallidum*, *C. albicans*, HSV
Genital warts	Human papillomavirus (HPV) types 6 and 11
Molluscum contagiosum	Pox virus
Ectoparasite infestations	*Sarcoptes scabiei*, *Phthirus pubis*
Cervical intraepithelial neoplasia, carcinoma	HPV types 16 and 18 and other oncogenic HPV types
Anal carcinoma	HPV types 16 and 18 and other oncogenic types
Hepatocellular carcinoma	Hepatitis B
Kaposi's sarcoma	HIV, HHV-8
Hepatitis	Hepatitis A, B and C viruses, cytomegalovirus, *T. pallidum*
Acquired immune deficiency syndrome (AIDS)	HIV-1, HIV-2
Acute arthritis with urogenital or intestinal infection	*N. gonorrhoeae*, *C. trachomatis*, *Shigella* sp., *Campylobacter* sp.

Information drawn from reference [6]

symptomatic. Post-gonococcal urethritis is a syndrome of recurrent urethral discharge and/or dysuria following single-dose treatment for gonococcal urethritis and likely represents untreated chlamydia infection [7, 8].

Epididymitis/Orchitis

Ascending infection with chlamydia or gonorrhea can cause clinical syndromes of epididymitis or orchitis; these syndromes are more commonly due to STI-causing organisms in men younger than 35 years of age, while in men older than 35 years they are most often due to *E. coli* or other gastrointestinal organisms. An infection with a systemic inflammatory response, for example, due to *N. gonorrhea*, can cause reactive arthritis. Some serovars of chlamydia can cause proctitis in MSM, resulting in rectal pain or discharge [9].

Extragenital manifestations of chlamydia and gonorrhea include pharyngitis, which usually presents as an exudative pharyngitis; laboratory testing is required since the physical exam cannot confirm the causative organism. Chlamydia, gonococcal, and trichomonas infections have in the past been thought to be causative factors in the development of chronic prostatitis, but subsequent research has not found a clear association between STIs and prostatitis syndromes. Some authors proposed that most chronic prostatitis syndromes are inflammatory and not bacterial/infectious in nature and antibiotic therapy is often unsatisfying in symptom resolution [2].

Genital Warts

In men, genital warts present as flesh-colored lesions on the skin of the penis, perianal region, or urethral mucous membrane. They can appear as flat, verrucous, or pedunculated lesions and may range in size from 1 mm to 10 cm or more. Associated symptoms may include discomfort, pain, bleeding, or difficulty with sexual intercourse, although these symptoms are more common with larger, cauliflower-like lesions that may develop. Urethral lesions may impair the passage of urine or semen and lead to obstructive symptoms in severe cases [2].

Genital Herpes

The primary infection with herpes simplex virus (HSV) is often accompanied by prodromal viral symptoms of headache, fever, malaise, and myalgias, with subsequent outbreak of painful vesicles on the external genitalia that may then ulcerate or erode. Infection is transmitted by direct contact with infected mucosa or secretions, and the incubation period ranges between 2 and 20 days. New outbreaks may occur in the second week after the primary infection and is commonly associated with tender regional lymphadenopathy. In men, lesions occur on the penile shaft, glans, and prepuce. Men who engage in receptive anal intercourse can develop HSV proctitis with pain, tenesmus, and rectal discharge/fecal incontinence [2].

Assessing STI Risk

Interventions to prevent STIs depend upon an accurate assessment of a man's STI risks as well as on epidemiologic and clinical understanding of the disorders involved. Clinical recommendations regarding behavioral counseling, screening, and other preventive health measures are often recommended for men considered to be at "high risk" for STIs, and it is critical to effectively assess these risk factors in men in primary care practices, urgent or emergency care, or STI clinic settings. As with women, STI risk factors include modifiable risks (e.g., sexual behavior) and non-modifiable risk factors (e.g., ethnicity, demographics); STI risk assessment for men should also address the patient's social context including work and/or living arrangements as possible risk factors that can guide preventive health interventions. Table 10.3 lists modifiable and non-modifiable as well as contextual STI risk factors for men; many of these are the same risk factors as for women.

Additional behavioral and contextual risk factors have been investigated; for example, in one study, first leaving the parental home, poor self-regulation or planning skills, emotional distress and hostility, poor attitudes toward condom use, and

Table 10.3 STI risk factors in men

Modifiable risk factors
Sexually active adolescents
Current or recent (1 year) STI
Multiple sexual partners
No consistent condom use
Men who have sex with men (MSM)
Exchanging sex for money or drugs
Current or former intravenous drug use
Demographic risk factors
African Americans
Native Americans, Latinos
History of sexual abuse
Situational risk factors
Low income living in urban setting
Current or former inmate
Military recruits
Mental illness or disability
Patients seen at STI clinics
Information from reference [10]

alcohol binge drinking predicted unprotected sexual contact in rural African American men, but not in women [11]. These factors suggest that obtaining a detailed and patient-centered social history, including an understanding of patient beliefs regarding sexual behavior and STI risks, represents an important area for determining a patient's overall STI risk profile.

A number of scoring systems and risk calculators (including online scoring systems or cell phone "apps" such as http://www.stdriskcalculator.com/ or http://www.medindia.net/patients/calculators/hiv-risk-calculator.asp) have been developed in an attempt for providers or patients themselves to quantify their degree of STI risk [12]. However, the studies on which such scoring systems have been conducted vary widely in their patient population, baseline STI risk, methods and outcomes assessment, and other factors. As such it is nearly impossible to determine a useful quantitative risk profile for various STI risk factors, and attempts to calculate or quantify such risks have not performed well outside very limited settings.

Physicians and other health-care providers should, instead of attempting to quantify STI risk, simply be aware of the multiple possible risk factors that patients might have for STIs and should try to elicit these details in their history-taking. Assessing an individual patient's overall STI risk becomes more of a subjective global risk assessment based on the patient's unique social and medical history, rather than a more quantifiable or scientific risk estimate.

Male Circumcision

Male circumcision has long been felt to have a protective effect against acquiring STIs, particularly HIV and particularly in MSM. Different studies have had variable results, largely as a result of varying patient populations and varying sexual practices. A meta-analysis of 15 studies of over 500,000 MSM [13] found that the odds of being HIV positive were lower in circumcised than in non-circumcised MSM, but the difference was not statistically significant; this study also found that there was no evidence of a protective effect against other STIs.

This study noted that earlier trials showing a protective effect from circumcision were conducted before the advent of highly active antiretroviral therapy (HAART) for chronic HIV disease and that changes in sexual behavior and/or disease transmission may limit the actual current protective effect of circumcision. Also, it is possible that male circumcision can still provide an aggregate protective effect in areas where STI prevalence is high and circumcision prevalence is low (<50 %).

Obtaining the Sexual Health History

Applying a knowledge of STI epidemiology, clinical features, and risk factors depends on eliciting a medical and sexual health history from the patient. Obtaining the sexual history requires the physician to take extra time to ensure that the environment and the physician communication are optimal to protect patient privacy and confidentiality, so that the most effective history and counseling can be conducted. Effective history-taking and communication can be thought of in the following steps:

1. Ensuring an appropriate setting
2. Obtaining basic information
3. Obtaining more detailed information
4. Using appropriate communication methods
5. Attending to specific patient circumstances (e.g., MSM, gay, cultural concerns, gender difference, etc.)

Appropriate Setting

Ensuring an environment and setting conducive to an effective discussion of sexual health and STI risks or treatment is vital for obtaining the necessary information from patients as well as increasing the likelihood of behavioral change or adherence to treatment. Arranging such a setting typically entails limiting external interruptions such as nursing questions and personal phone use (by physician or patient) and ensuring that physician and patient have sufficient time for the discussion. Providers should also pay attention to nonverbal communication issues. Taking active steps to sit down, setting the physical chart or electronic record aside, and actively demonstrating an active interest in the patient are critical to convey to the patient that their health needs are the focus of the discussion. Having the patient seated in an exam room chair, rather than on the end of the exam table, can also help ensure that the discussion is a productive one among equal partners, rather than a more formalized physician advice which may not be followed.

Other aspects of ensuring an appropriate setting include assessing patient's competency to make decisions (or have a suitable surrogate decision-maker present) and discussing in advance an agreed-upon method of giving results of diagnostic testing, particularly for HIV testing.

Basic Information

Once a suitable conversation setting is ensured, providers should obtain basic health history information; clearly this includes fundamental information such as the patient's symptoms, agenda of questions or concerns, and/or reason for presentation for medical attention, as well as their general medical history, current medications and allergies, and full social history. The history data to be obtained regarding STI risks or treatment should also include any previous history of STIs and any previous immunizations against STIs such as vaccination against HBV or HPV. The focused sexual health and STI discussion however will address additional information pertinent to these areas.

This history can be triggered or initiated based on a number of different factors:

- Men presenting with sexual health symptoms or symptoms suggesting an STI
- Men presenting to an STI clinic
- As part of a routine health maintenance visit that includes questions specifically to assess sexual health or as part of a "review of systems"
- When prompted by factors in the social history (e.g., new partner, multiple partners, history of previous STI, etc.)
- A medical encounter conducted while the patient is in the military, in prison, or in institutionalized settings that represent a situational risk factor for STIs

A number of guidelines [1, 14] describe the content for a basic sexual health history and STI risk assessment when evaluating male patients. The content of the basic STI/sexual health history includes the following data elements or questions:

- Last sexual contact, partner's gender, anatomic sites of exposure, and sexual practices used
- Previous sexual partners and sexual practices used, if in the last 3 months, and a note of total number of partners in the last 3 months if more than two
- Any suspected infection, infection risk, or symptoms in recent partners
- Previous STIs
- Methods used to prevent STIs and methods used to prevent female partner from becoming pregnant, if any (including condom use)
- Blood-borne virus risk assessment and vaccination history for those at risk
- Reproductive history, including history of previous fathered children, and any plans for future children

When obtaining the sexual health history, physicians should allow sufficient time to obtain all of the above information and should inform patients that this will be used to help address the patient's concerns and improve their overall health.

Detailed Information

Either as part of a routine sexual health history or when prompted by patient-specific concerns or known medical history, it is often necessary to ask more in-depth questions pertaining to a patient's sexual health and STI risks. While the above basic data pertains to most or all patients, the following data will likely be obtained only when prompted by various patient factors:

- History of domestic or intimate partner violence
- History of alcohol and/or drug use or abuse
- Mental health history including history of mental health disorders
- Any history of trading sex for money or drugs
- History of sex while under the influence of drugs or alcohol

Arguably, these questions could also constitute "screening" information that should be obtained for all patients, and some physicians may find it more suitable to ask all of these questions routinely so that the questions do not seem judgmental to some patients and would not be omitted for others. These decisions ultimately depend critically on the setting, the physician, and the patient. It is reasonable to have a low threshold for asking these questions and to ask them whenever triggered by patient circumstances or concerns.

Communication Methods

Once the patient history is obtained, it can be used along with the clinician's risk assessment to guide patient treatment recommendations and counseling. There are however a number of other communication issues that should be addressed.

First, it is vital to check with patients whether they have any other concerns that have not yet been discussed. Patients may have questions about psychosocial concerns, issues related to "coming out" or disclosing their sexual orientation, relationship safety, questions about STI transmission, or others.

The question about other possible concerns should be asked as an open-ended question, and physicians should make every effort to let the question truly invite further discussion and not appear to be the close of the conversation. Eliciting the patient's full spectrum of concerns early in the interview can both ensure thorough patient-centered care and can also prevent unwanted "By the way, doc" questions as the physician is leaving the exam room.

When the patient history is concluded, prior to performing any relevant physical examination steps, physicians should explain the need for testing, the nature of any tests or exam steps that will be performed, and how this information will be used to improve their care. Finally, men should be offered the opportunity to have a chaperone present for the examination. This may be particularly relevant for gay or transgender patients or for those who are uncertain about their sexual orientation or gender identity.

Table 10.4 summarizes the key information to obtain and lists a reasonable set of intake history question for men regarding STIs and STI risk.

Physical Examination

In light of the potential importance for physical examination in male patients with suspected STIs, the physical examination for men with a suspected STD should include the following [15]:

1. Inspection of the skin of the genitals, inguinal areas, thighs, lower abdomen, hands, palms, soles, and forearms
2. Inspection of the pubic hair for lice and nits
3. Inspection of the penis, including the urethral meatus, with retraction of the foreskin, if present, and milking of the urethra
4. Palpation of the scrotal contents
5. Palpation for inguinal and femoral lymphadenopathy

Table 10.4 Suggested history for men with suspected STIs

1.	What brings you in today?
2.	Do you have specific symptoms and, if so, which is your main symptom?
3.	Do you have a urethral discharge and, if so, for how long? How would you describe it, for example, clear and thin? White and thick? Yellow and thick?
4.	Do you have any burning when you pass urine and, if so, for how long have you noticed it?
5.	Have you noticed any skin lesions on your penis, scrotum, or groin and, if so, for how long?
6.	Have you noted any skin rash in your genital area or anywhere else on your body?
7.	Have you had any rectal symptoms, diarrhea, or constipation?
8.	Have you had sex with more than one partner in the last 2 months and, if so, how many? Have you had sex with any new partners in the last 2 months? How many partners have you had in the last year? As far as you know, do any of your sex partners have signs of infection? Are any of your partners infected with HIV?
9.	Do you have sex with men, women, or both?
10.	When was your last sexual encounter?
11.	In the last 2 months, have you had vaginal sex? Given or received oral sex? Given or received anal sex?
12.	Have you taken any antibiotics in the last month?
13.	Have you had allergic reactions to any medications?
14.	Have you had any sexually transmitted disease diagnosed previously and, if so, which one(s) and when? Have you had an HIV test? If so, what was the date and result of your last HIV test? Are you concerned that you may have been exposed to a partner with HIV or at risk for HIV?
15.	Do you regularly use alcohol or drugs, injection or others? If you use injection drugs, do you share needles? Have you used or are you using methamphetamine?
16.	(If with a female partner) Is your partner trying to get pregnant? If not, what are you doing to prevent pregnancy? What has your experience with using condoms been? Are there any partners you tend to use condoms with more often?
17.	(If with a male partner) What has your experience been using condoms with men? Have you been vaccinated against hepatitis A and hepatitis B?
18.	Do you regularly use alcohol or drugs? If you use injection drugs, do you share needles? How do you feel that drugs or alcohol impacts your sex life?
19.	Have you been vaccinated against hepatitis B? HPV?

From reference [15]

For MSM, additional physical examination steps should include:

6. Palpation for cervical, supraclavicular, and axillary lymphadenopathy
7. Inspection of the mouth, throat/pharynx, perineum, and anus
8. Consideration of anoscopy for MSM complaining of rectal symptoms

Counseling Men for STI Risk Reduction

The USPSTF recommends intensive behavioral counseling for all sexually active adolescents and for adults who are at increased risk for STIs [10]. Behavioral counseling interventions can reduce a person's likelihood of acquiring an STI, typically measured over the course of 12 months. In general, the content of these interventions includes training in pertinent skills, such as condom use; communication about safe sexual practices; problem solving; and goal setting [10]. Many successful interventions used a targeted approach to the age, sex, and ethnicity of the participants and also aimed to increase motivation or commitment to safe sex practices. A wide variety of counseling approaches and formats have been used, and the CDC provides information about various methods and studies regarding counseling to prevent STIs (http://www.cdc.gov/hiv/prevention/research/compendium/rr/index.html).

If physicians or other providers are working in a dedicated adolescent or STI clinic or have access to trained behavioral counselors, resources will likely be available to provide longer, more in-depth behavioral counseling. Studies of behavioral interventions have consistently shown that the intensity of counseling is the strongest predictor of subsequent STI risk reductions; interventions ranging in intensity from 30 min to more than 2 h of contact time are the most beneficial. Some physicians may not work in such a setting but will have the capacity to refer patients at increased risk to a decided STI clinic or other resource which can provide in-depth counseling services. Such approaches incorporate videos, interactive computer programs, face-to-face counseling, telephone follow-up, and other modalities.

There is a wide range of efficacy for counseling interventions using different modalities in different groups. Most studies of counseling directed toward adolescents showed at least a 50 % decrease in the odds of acquiring an STI after behavioral counseling, though most studies have been conducted with female patients. There is no evidence of any increased risk of subsequent sexual activity or STI as a result of counseling [10].

The USPSTF did not find enough evidence to determine whether factors such as the degree of cultural tailoring, group versus individual format, condom negotiation or other communication as an intervention component, counselor characteristics, setting, or type of control group influenced the effectiveness of behavioral counseling [10]. A good portion of STI risk-reduction counseling, however, will continue to take place in typical primary care or urgent care settings, between the physician and patient in a more time-constrained setting. In such settings, a number of effective strategies for STI risk-reduction counseling can still be employed; these are similar to most other motivational interviewing methods.

First, physicians should determine the patient behavior that they would like the patient to change. Typical sexual behavioral changes may include any of the following [16]:

- Increasing condom use with the "main" partner or other partners
- Reducing the number of sexual partners
- Enhancing partner communication about sexual activities
- Practicing monogamy or abstinence
- Partner testing for STIs
- Use of noncoital sexual activities or other means to reduce STI risk
- Reducing use of alcohol and/or drugs in relation to sexual activity
- Understanding and acceptance of personal or partner STI risks
- Awareness or consideration of any of the above factors at the time of the sexual encounter

Once the desired behavioral change is identified, physicians should counsel patients regarding this change. In general, physicians should only aim to have patients change one important sexual behavior at a time. Changing individual behavior is generally challenging, and the same barriers that limit behavioral change for smoking, substance use, physical activity, and others also affect patients' ability to change sexual behaviors. It is often helpful to ask patients themselves to indicate one behavioral change that they could make; such changes that are patient-initiated are more likely to be followed.

When engaging in risk-reduction counseling for behavioral change, physicians should keep in mind some general principles regarding such counseling [16]:

- Knowledge alone is insufficient to produce behavioral change.
- Self-efficacy (belief in one's ability to carry out a behavioral change) may be limited, and patients may need counseling on this topic specifically.
- Social norms and/or societal sources of information may work against the planned behavioral change, and this may need to be addressed also.
- Risk-reduction activities should be acceptable to the patient and should be realistically achievable in his situation.

Counseling adolescents regarding sexual behavior represents a special challenge, given the inherent risk-taking behaviors, lack of future-oriented planning, and extensive social media exposure prevalent in this age group. Lack of health insurance, lack of a usual provider or source of health care, and lack of a need for regular physician contact (such as for contraceptives in young women) all represent additional barriers to reducing STI risk in adolescent men; black and Hispanic young men, particularly MSM, are at further increased risk [17].

When counseling adolescent men, the same principles described above still apply; it is even more important than in adult men to focus on correcting misinformation obtained through public media, focusing on achievable and realistic behavioral change, and emphasizing present-time benefits rather than future benefits. As above, a wide variety of creative measures for counseling adolescents have been studied and implemented, including use of multiple communication media and community engagement. In settings where it is possible, intensive or longer-duration counseling may be more beneficial than brief or focused counseling.

Regular, consistent, and correct use of condoms remains both an important clinical STI prevention step and an important focus for behavioral counseling. The CDC has a brief fact sheet regarding correct condom use; Fig. 10.7 shows some of this information.

Cultural and Belief Issues in Counseling

As above, in all areas of health behavior counseling, the provision of information alone is insufficient to change behavior; patients may be very familiar with the clinical consequences of STIs and the preventive role of consistent condom use, but may have other beliefs that overcome their desire to obtain these benefits. Physicians and other providers should not simply counsel men about the role and use of

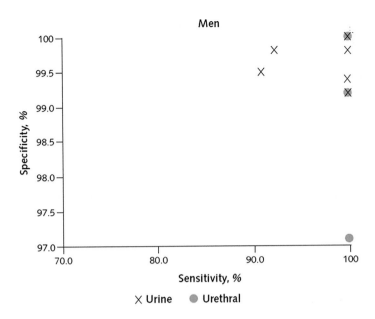

Fig. 10.7 Gonorrhea Testing Accuracy

condoms, and other topics as above, but should strive to explore patients' beliefs and knowledge regarding STIs and STI prevention. Some of these beliefs are mediated by culture or social context, which may require a careful social history to elicit. Assessing a few key items can be done swiftly in the context of an outpatient or urgent care visit, and the brief amount of time spent on this discussion may translate into significant patient benefits and a higher likelihood of adherence.

One study showed that male survey participants in areas with high STI rates had appropriate knowledge and beliefs about the benefits of male or female condom use, monogamy, or abstinence as suitable methods of preventing STI or unwanted pregnancy [18]. However, they also had other beliefs that may have limited the effectiveness of any of these methods. For example, men who otherwise recognized the benefits of sexual abstinence also felt that abstinence would be sexually frustrating and interfere with the development of a close relationship; likewise, men who acknowledged the benefits of condom use also felt that this would interfere with sex or would limit the enjoyment of either partner. These beliefs were not strongly correlated with educational or socioeconomic status, but did appear to be consistent with actual behavior. Assessing these beliefs may be an important part of overall patient assessment for risk or treatment for STIs.

Often, these beliefs stem from typical or perceived male gender roles; men often perceive themselves as authority figured, decision-makers, or providers; these are clearly not universal, and many men have different gender or social roles based on their own ethnic or cultural background [19]. While not all men adopt or represent these "power" roles, recognition of these factors can represent a potentially useful approach to break down barriers to effective behavioral counseling. As barriers to behavioral change, socially constructed expectations about men's sexual behavior can result in men engaging in risky behaviors, such as having unprotected sex and sex with multiple partners. This behavior can contribute to men transmitting STIs to their female partners. Likewise, many men have concerns about how to tell their wives that they have an STI. Men may fear that their wives will ask them where the STI came from, which may put the men in an uncomfortable situation if they have other partners that they have not mentioned to their wives. While physicians may see such situations as at least partially the patient's "fault" and may wish to avoid contributing to the man's perception of his status, the end goal of patient-centered communication is the health and well-being of the patient and potentially his partner.

Men are not accustomed to seeking reproductive health care and are often uncomfortable accessing reproductive health services. This may be because they view the services as being for women only or because they have been socially conditioned to believe that an important part of being a man is to be "strong" and not ask for assistance.

Some potential ways to use perceived male gender roles or beliefs to improve acceptance of, or adherence to, behavioral change include the following [19]:

- Emphasize the man's role as a protector figure by describing the role of STI prevention in reducing the clinical impact and disease burden in women.
- Emphasize the appropriate decision-making role of the male patient in presenting for clinical attention.
- Focus on behavioral change as a challenge to be confronted or a problem to be solved.
- Rather than emphasizing lack of condom use as a disease risk, focus on past successful condom use and discuss "what worked" in those situations.
- Rather than asking if the patient has questions, emphasize what he "already knows" and use the opportunity to fill in gaps or details as patient education.
- Universalize or normalize the patient's experience, e.g., indicate "a lot of men are initially uncomfortable asking about that,"

Screening Men for STIs

Screening men for STIs represents a challenging issue. There is not sufficient evidence that screening for STIs in men, with subsequent effective treatment, changes subsequent sexual behavior or reduces STI incidence or sequelae in women. Screening asymptomatic men who are at low behavioral or statistical risk for STI has not been shown to be clinically effective or cost-effective, and the possibility of a large number of false-positive tests in a low-risk population may lead to increased costs, medical visits, anxiety, and further testing, with potentially limited benefit. Different organizations often promote different recommendations for screening, and all such recommendations are limited by insufficient evidence for the health impact of STI screening at the patient and population levels.

As with other disease prevention efforts, physicians and other providers should focus on assessing individual patient factors and determining an individualized and appropriate screening plan to address patient's health risks. As a broad summary recommendation, universal screening is currently recommended for particular age groups for HIV and hepatitis C, while in general STI screening in male patients is limited to those at higher risk.

Screening Tests for Chlamydia and Gonorrhea

While all STI tests have similar issues regarding diagnostic accuracy, appropriate testing assay, and possible confirmatory testing, the nature of screening and diagnostic test for chlamydia and gonorrhea, the most common STIs in men, has changed the most in recent years. It is helpful to review current testing recommendations for these infections before addressing screening recommendations specifically.

Nucleic Acid Amplification Tests

Multiple culture and non-culture diagnosis and detection methods are available for chlamydia and gonorrhea, including culture, antigen detection, nucleic acid hybridization, and nucleic acid amplification tests (NAATs), which are approved by the Food and Drug Administration (FDA) for detection of genital tract infections caused by *Chlamydia trachomatis* and *Neisseria gonorrhoeae* infections in men and women with and without symptoms [20]. Optimal specimens in men are "first-catch" urine samples.

Current practice supports the nearly exclusive use of NAAT testing, due to the high degree of diagnostic accuracy and patient acceptance of these tests. Older tests such as serologic tests and other non-culture- or culture-based tests have inferior sensitivity and specificity and are no longer recommended for diagnosis or screening [21, 22]. However, chlamydia and gonorrhea culture testing is still clinically appropriate when evaluating suspected cases of treatment failure (i.e., persistent symptoms after otherwise appropriate treatment), monitoring antimicrobial susceptibility, or when evaluating possible child sexual assault in boys and extragenital infections in girls.

The accuracy of NAATs for detection of rectal and oropharyngeal infections caused by *C. trachomatis* and *N. gonorrhoeae* is likely to be high, and the CDC is recommending NAATs to test for these extragenital infections based on increased sensitivity and ease of specimen transport and processing. However, these tests are not currently FDA-approved for these scenarios, and providers should be aware of possible false-positive tests as well as Clinical Laboratory Improvement Amendments (CLIA) and/or local or state regulatory requirements if they use NAATs to test for rectal or oropharyngeal infections.

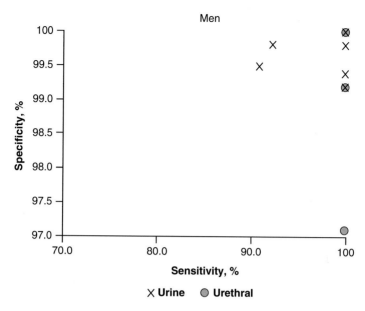

Fig. 10.8 Sensitivity and specificity of nucleic acid amplification tests for gonorrhea screening in men (across various studies) (from reference [20])

The improved diagnostic accuracy of NAATs raises the question of what constitutes a "gold standard" for STI testing, since other diagnostic methods are thought to have lower sensitivity and specificity and significantly lower predictive value in a lower-risk population. While routine repeat testing of NAAT-positive genital tract specimens is not recommended because this does not improve the positive predictive value of the test [20], it is possible that the best confirmatory strategy is to use a different NAAT assay product that has improved accuracy. One (corporate-sponsored) study [21] suggests using the APTIMA COMBO 2 assay (AC2) test for initial screening and the APTIMA CT assay (ACT) for confirmation, since 98 % of AC2 positive results were confirmed by ACT.

The high acceptability and ease of use and transportation of NAAT testing have raised the possibility of patient self-testing as well as home-based, mail-in, or Internet-based screening [20]. This would undoubtedly increase the rate of detection of asymptomatic infection but would introduce logistic, follow-up, and potentially false-positive testing issues that need to be addressed before patient self-testing becomes broadly implemented.

Figures 10.8 and 10.9 show the ranges of diagnostic accuracy for NAAT testing of urine and urethral swab samples from men in various studies, for gonorrhea and chlamydia, respectively. NAAT testing is now considered the standard for screening and diagnosis of chlamydia and gonorrhea, due to their high sensitivity and specificity [22]. Urine testing with NAATs is at least as sensitive as testing with endocervical specimens, clinician or self-collected vaginal specimens, or urethral specimens that are self-collected in clinical settings. The same specimen can be used to test for chlamydia and gonorrhea.

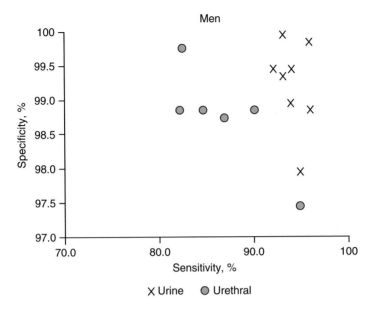

Fig. 10.9 Sensitivity and specificity of nucleic acid amplification tests for chlamydia screening in men (across various studies) (from reference [20])

Screening Recommendations

The USPSTF does not recommend STI screening for asymptomatic men who are not at increased risk. The USPSTF recommends HIV and syphilis screening for men engaging in high-risk sexual behavior [23]. Syphilis screening should be offered if the geographic or community risk or prevalence of syphilis is high enough to justify population-based testing, although there are not specific cutoffs for these parameters to indicate a need for screening. The following sections will summarize STI screening recommendations in men; however, as above, it is important that physicians take a thorough sexual history to assess if the patient engages in high-risk sexual behavior. In MSM, it is important to focus on high-risk sexual behavior and not on sexual orientation in making decisions about which screening tests to offer.

Chlamydia and Gonorrhea

Screening strategies for *C. trachomatis* and *N. gonorrhoeae* in men differ from those in women. While chlamydial or gonorrheal infections may cause urethritis or epididymitis in men, these infections typically do not cause PID or other serious complications as they do in women. Screening and treating young men at increased risk may reduce the incidence of chlamydial infections; however, the USPSTF found no published prospective trials of the effect of routine screening in men in comparison with the strategy of screening women and treating their male partners [24, 25].

The USPSTF concludes that the current evidence is insufficient to assess the balance of benefits and harms of screening for chlamydia and gonorrhea in heterosexual men at increased risk of infection (I recommendation). It is not recommended to screen for gonorrhea infection in men at low risk for infection. Although there are no recommendations to screen heterosexual men in the general population, the USPSTF suggests testing sexually active heterosexual men in clinical settings with a high prevalence of *C. trachomatis* (e.g., STD clinics, adolescent clinics, and detention and correctional facilities) as well as men entering the Armed Forces or the National Job Training Program [22].

As above, physicians should be guided by clinical judgment and by their assessment of individual patient STI risk factors, including the likelihood of seeking care for either symptoms or for routine health maintenance visits. In the absence of studies on screening intervals, a reasonable approach would be to screen patients at higher STI risk, particularly those whose sexual history reveals new or persistent risk factors since the last negative test result.

Hepatitis C

The USPSTF recommends screening for HCV infection in persons at high risk for infection [26]. The USPSTF also recommends offering 1-time screening for HCV infection to adults born between 1945 and 1965 (B recommendation). The most important risk factor for HCV infection is past or current injection drug use. Additional risk factors include receiving a blood transfusion before 1992, having sex with an injection drug user, long-term hemodialysis, being born to an HCV-infected mother, incarceration, intranasal drug use, getting an unregulated tattoo, and other percutaneous exposures. Patients born in the year range listed need only be screened once; patients with ongoing injection drug use or other risks may be rescreened, but there are no guidelines on screening interval or frequency. HCV is transmitted inefficiently through sexual contact, so patients with high-risk sexual behaviors as above are at increased risk, but the magnitude of the risk is probably low, and it is difficult to determine if this is an independent risk factor or a confounding variable that is also associated with other risky behaviors.

HPV

There is currently no approved test for HPV in men, and there is no recommendation to screen men for asymptomatic HPV or HPV-related diseases. While subclinical HPV can lead to anal, penile, or throat cancers in men, the population-based risk of these cancers is relatively low and universal screening is not recommended [27].

However, some physicians do offer Pap screening tests to men who might be at increased risk for anal cancer, for example, due to receptive anal intercourse with multiple partners, particularly men with these behaviors who have HIV. There are no clear guidelines or recommendations for such screening.

HIV

The USPSTF recommends universal screening of all adolescents and adults aged 15–65 years for HIV infection, with a strong (grade A) recommendation [28]. The recommended testing strategy is rapid serum immunoassay, followed by confirmatory Western blot or immunofluorescent assay. The rationale for this recommendation is based on the relatively high prevalence of HIV, the ease and acceptability of rapid testing, and the substantial benefit of early initiation of antiretroviral therapy. Screening at younger or older ages is recommended for higher-risk patients. The available evidence does not suggest a specific testing interval; an expert recommendation for a testing strategy is a 1-time HIV screen for low-risk patients, presumably during a routine health maintenance visit when such testing is convenient and can be discussed with patients. Patients at higher risk can be rescreened on a semi-regular basis (every 3–5 years for patients at moderately increased risk up to annually for patients at very high risk). The screening intensity or interval might be increased in areas with a particularly high prevalence of HIV infection, defined as >1 % [1, 28].

Syphilis

The USPSTF strongly recommends that physicians screen patients at increased risk for syphilis (A recommendation) but recommends against routinely screening asymptomatic patients who are not at increased risk (D recommendation) [23]. Despite the accuracy of screening for diagnosing syphilis and the availability of effective treatment, there is no direct evidence that screening at-risk patients for syphilis leads to improved outcomes. Though there are potential harms such as antibiotic exposure, patient anxiety, and false-positive testing, the USPSTF concludes that the benefits of screening at-risk patients outweigh the harms.

Populations at increased risk for syphilis include MSM, men who engage in high-risk sexual behavior, commercial sex workers, persons who exchange sex for drugs, and those in adult correctional facilities. There is no evidence to recommend a specific screening strategy or screening frequency in these at-risk groups. Patients diagnosed with other STIs may be more likely than others to engage in high-risk behavior, thus increasing their risk for acquiring syphilis, but there is no evidence that supports the routine screening of individuals diagnosed with other STIs for syphilis infection. Physicians should use clinical judgment to individualize screening for syphilis infection based on local infection rates and unique patient risk factors [23].

Table 10.5 summarizes STI screening recommendations for men.

Table 10.5 STI screening recommendations for men

Group	Screening recommendations			
	Ch/GC	Syphilis	HIV	HCV
Adolescent males at average STI risk			√[a]	
Adolescent males at increased STI risk	√	√	√	
Adult men at average STI risk			√	√
Adult men at increased STI risk	√	√	√	
MSM	√	√	√	

Information from references [1, 23–26, 28]

[a]The USPSTF recommends screening all patients age 13–64 and subsequently retesting patients at high risk or who develop new risk factors; the optimal screening interval is known, but annual screening is recommended

Other STI Prevention Measures

A population-based program for STI prevention includes not only direct provider-to-patient counseling with appropriate laboratory testing but other population-based prevention measures. Prevention methods include vaccinations where appropriate, behavioral changes to reinforce monogamy or abstinence, and ongoing public education efforts. The CDC and other organizations are engaged in multiple different educational campaigns to encourage individuals to "take control" of their health by knowing their sexual health risks, taking steps to prevent infection, and obtain accurate information regarding STIs and other topics. In an era of tremendous information overload, particularly for adolescents, it is challenging for the right "message" to take precedence. While there are no clear guidelines for this aspect of counseling, physicians may well wish to talk to their patients about their sources of information regarding STIs and to help guide patients toward reliable resources. This may be most relevant for adolescent patients.

HPV vaccination recommendations have recently been updated, and vaccination is now recommended for males age 11–26 years [6]. Catch-up vaccination is recommended for males age 13–21 who have not been vaccinated previously or have not completed the 3-dose series by age 21. Routine vaccination is recommended for at-risk males including MSM and immune-compromised males through age 26. There are at present no published studies showing that vaccination of male patients reduces rates of female cervical cancer, though vaccination does seem to reduce the burden of symptomatic HPV infection and disease.

Hepatitis B vaccination series is recommended for all unvaccinated and uninfected patients being treated or evaluated for STIs [6].

Preexposure prophylaxis for prevention of HIV in high-risk populations is a relatively new method to prevent STIs. For patients at substantially increased risk for acquiring HIV (including patients with an HIV-positive sexual partner, a recent bacterial STI, a high number of sex partners, a history of inconsistent or no condom use, and commercial sex workers), a daily regimen of a fixed-dose combination of tenofovir disoproxil fumarate 300 mg and emtricitabine 200 mg has been shown to be safe and effective in reducing the risk of sexual HIV acquisition in adults but not in adolescents [29].

Treatment Considerations

Urethritis

There are multiple treatment regimens available for men diagnosed with urethritis. It is typical to treat for both chlamydia and gonorrhea concurrently given the likelihood of coinfection and the imperfection of diagnostic testing. Guidelines for treatment of uncomplicated gonococcal urethritis have been updated recently, with oral cephalosporins no longer recommended [6].

Recommended treatment options for gonococcal urethritis include any one of the following:

- Ceftriaxone 250 mg in a single intramuscular dose plus azithromycin 1 g orally in a single dose
- Doxycycline 100 mg orally twice daily for 7 days

Alternative regimens if ceftriaxone is not available include:

- Cefixime 400 mg in a single oral dose plus azithromycin 1 g orally in a single dose or doxycycline 100 mg orally twice daily for 7 days plus test-of-cure in 1 week if the patient has severe cephalosporin allergy
- Azithromycin 2 g in a single oral dose plus test-of-cure in 1 week

Recommended treatment options for chlamydial urethritis include:

- Azithromycin 1 g orally in a single dose
- Doxycycline 100 mg orally twice a day for 7 days

Alternative treatment recommendations for chlamydia include:

- Erythromycin base 500 mg orally four times a day for 7 days
- Erythromycin ethylsuccinate 800 mg orally four times a day for 7 days
- Levofloxacin 500 mg orally once daily for 7 days
- Ofloxacin 300 mg orally twice a day for 7 days

Among sexually active men aged <35 years, acute epididymitis is most frequently caused by *C. trachomatis* or *N. gonorrhoeae*, and the same treatment regimens can be used to treat this infection that are used to treat urethritis [6]. Specific treatment recommendations for epididymitis due to sexually transmitted chlamydia and gonorrhea include:

- Ceftriaxone 250 mg IM in a single dose plus doxycycline 100 mg orally twice a day for 10 days

For acute epididymitis most likely caused by sexually transmitted chlamydia and gonorrhea and enteric organisms (men who practice insertive anal sex), treatment options include:

- Ceftriaxone 250 mg IM in a single dose plus levofloxacin 500 mg orally once a day for 10 days
- Ofloxacin 300 mg orally twice a day for 10 days

HSV

Most patients with symptomatic genital herpes should be offered antiviral treatment based on the efficacy and safety of the available agents [6]. Available treatment regimens include any one of the following:

- Acyclovir 400 mg orally three times a day for 7–10 days
- Acyclovir 200 mg orally five times a day for 7–10 days
- Famciclovir 250 mg orally three times a day for 7–10 days
- Valacyclovir 1 g orally twice a day for 7–10 days

Patients with recurrent herpes outbreaks can be treated on an episodic basis, though many patients with frequent recurrences prefer a daily preventive treatment regimen. The following are typical options for preventive HSV treatment:

- Acyclovir 400 mg orally twice a day
- Famciclovir 250 mg orally twice a day
- Valacyclovir 500 mg orally once a day
- Valacyclovir 1 g orally once a day

Treatment recommendations for newly diagnosed HIV, syphilis, and more unusual STIs are described in recent CDC/MMWR treatment guidelines, available at http://www.cdc.gov/std/tg2015/.

HPV

Treatment of HPV in men is directed at clinically evident symptomatic lesions, i.e., genital or perianal warts. Subclinical, asymptomatic HPV infections generally have a higher spontaneous clearance rate in men than in women [27], though in HIV-infected men, anal HPV infection does not clear as quickly. Therefore, there is no recommendation to specifically treat asymptomatic HPV infections in men with the goal of eradicating the infection.

Treatment of genital warts should be guided by the preference of the patient, available resources, and the experience of the health-care provider. No definitive evidence suggests that any of the available treatments are superior to any other, and no single treatment is ideal for all patients or all warts [6]. Available treatment options include cryotherapy, patient-applied podofilox solution or gel, imiquimod cream, or provider-applied podophyllin resin or trichloroacetic acid. Surgical removal by various methods is an option for larger warts. Complete treatment recommendations are available in CDC/MMWR guidelines.

Partner Management

One aspect of the public health management of diagnosed STIs is identification and treatment of potentially infected sexual partners of the index patient. For some STIs, particularly trichomonas, syphilis, gonorrhea, and chlamydia, this depends on reporting to local public health departments with subsequent tracking sexual contacts or on physicians advising patients to urge their partners to seek assessment and treatment. Both of these options are limited in their effectiveness by a number of barriers, including overburdened public health departments, patient failure to notify their partners, partners failing to seek medical care, or lack of insurance coverage or provider access [30].

One means of overcoming these barriers is the option of patient-delivered partner therapy (PDPT) which is one method for expedited partner therapy (EPT) [31]. Though the evidence for completed partner therapy and reduced incidence or duration of partner STIs is limited, a small number of randomized trials that have been completed show a trend toward efficacy of the PDPT approach. Rates of partner notification and treatment were increased in some trials but were equal to patient referral without PDPT in others. No studies have been published evaluating the benefit of PDPT for STIs among MSM.

In PDPT, when patients diagnosed with an STI seem unwilling or unlikely to advise their partners to see testing and treatment, providers can offer treatment for the partners of infected patients, often by prescribing enough antibiotics to treat both partners. PDPT is generally limited to the most recent sexual partner, and it is atypical to treat multiple partners in this way.

Partners treated via PDPT do not undergo medical testing or counseling, and in this context PDPT is considered a suboptimal approach to partner therapy, but in cases when partners are not likely to receive notification or treatment otherwise, PDPT may still offer a significant benefit. PDPT may be prohibited in some states but is supported by legislation and guidelines in others, and physicians and other providers should review their states' laws regarding this practice.

Implementation of PDPT involves a number of potential barriers, including [31]:

- Undiagnosed PID in female partners treated via PDPT
- Limitations on insurance coverage for increased quantities of antibiotics to treat both partners
- Missed opportunities to counsel partners regarding sexual behavior and STIs
- Risk of allergic reactions or adverse effects to antibiotics
- Partner/patient privacy issues
- Potential ethical or professional beliefs of providers regarding treatment of people not directly evaluated

PDPT clearly represents suboptimal management and should not be used as a first-line option for partner management; but in some cases, for some providers, PDPT is an attractive option to achieve some benefit in terms of STI reduction rather than potentially no benefit at all.

Current CDC STI guidelines [6] strengthen this recommendation and recommend EPT to heterosexual patients with chlamydia or gonorrhea infection, when the provider cannot confidently ensure that all of a patient's sexual partners in the previous 60 days will be treated and when this practice is not prohibited by law or other regulations.

Test for Cure

Patients diagnosed with urethritis due to chlamydia or gonorrhea who have received appropriate antibiotic treatment generally do not require a test of cure, i.e., repeat STI testing 3–4 weeks after completing treatment.

However, if patients remain symptomatic, then repeat testing should be performed to confirm the diagnosis, with possible retreatment or treatment with a different regimen. Likewise, if patients remain symptomatic and nonadherence to their medication regimen is suspected, repeat diagnostic testing is generally appropriate to confirm their infection as the cause of persistent symptoms.

Because men have a high rate of reinfection within 6 months after treatment, current CDC STI guidelines do recommend repeat testing of all men diagnosed with urethritis, within 6 months after treatment, regardless of whether partners were treated or not [6].

Management of Men Who Have Sex with Men

Compared to women and men who have sex with women only, MSM (which may include gay or bisexual men and others) are at increased risk for STIs including infection with antibiotic-resistant organisms. This increased STI risk confers an increased risk of HIV infection due to behavioral and biologic factors as above. MSM who have lower economic status, or who are members of ethnic minorities, are particularly vulnerable to poorer health outcomes, in part due to cultural and societal risk factors as described above [32].

After a decrease in reported rates of STIs and incident HIV infection in MSM through the 1980s and 1990s, increased rates of early syphilis, gonorrhea, chlamydia, and unsafe sexual behaviors have been observed among MSM. While data are not conclusive, this increase is thought to be due to a number of possible factors [6]: advances in HIV care and quality of life for patients with chronic HIV disease, changes in patterns of substance abuse, and changes in sex partner networks due to new methods for acquiring partners, primarily via the Internet. Thus far a clear increase in HIV infection due to these factors has not been observed [6, 32].

Because of these increased risks, physicians should devote extra attention to assessing STI-related health risks for all MSM patients. This includes obtaining a nonjudgmental history as outlined above, including routinely asking sexually active MSM about potential STI-related symptoms including urethral discharge, dysuria, genital and perianal ulcers, regional lymphadenopathy, skin rash, and anorectal symptoms consistent with proctitis or discharge and pain on defecation or during anal intercourse.

Also in light of these known risks and risk factors, physicians should offer current STI screening tests to MSM patients; current CDC recommendations state that the following screening tests should be performed at least annually for sexually active MSM, including those with HIV infection [6]:

- HIV serology, if HIV status is unknown or negative and the patient himself or his sex partner(s) has had more than one sex partner since most recent HIV test.
- Syphilis serology to establish whether persons with reactive tests have untreated syphilis, have partially treated syphilis, or have a slow response to appropriate treatment.
- Urine NAAT (preferred) or other testing for urethritis due to chlamydia or gonorrhea, in men who have had insertive intercourse during the preceding year.
- Rectal specimen NAAT (preferred) to test for rectal infection with chlamydia or gonorrhea, in men who have had receptive anal intercourse during the preceding year.
- Pharyngeal specimen NAAT (preferred) to test for gonococcal pharyngitis in men who have had receptive oral intercourse during the preceding year; testing for *C. trachomatis* pharyngeal infection is not recommended.
- Data are insufficient to recommend routine anal cancer screening with anal cytology.
- All MSM should be tested for HBsAg to detect chronic HBV infection.
- Serologic screening for HCV is recommended at initial evaluation of MSM with newly diagnosed HIV infection.

Conclusions

While the presenting symptoms, risk factors, clinical features, diagnosis, and management of STIs in men are very similar to those in women, there are important differences. Men may have greater risks of asymptomatic infection from a number of STI-causing organisms, and they may have significant delays in accessing care. Men do not have an equivalent of the routine Pap test, and many younger adult men may have little or no reason to present for routine health maintenance visits.

Counseling men regarding sexual behaviors to reduce STI risks may need to be conducted differently than in women to account for important differences in culture, perceived societal roles, expectations for sexual behavior, the role of popular media, and other factors. Communication methods that focus on preserving men's decision-making authority or other societal roles may be more effective in gaining their active participation and adherence to treatment.

Treatment recommendations for STIs in men are the same as those for women, but screening recommendations are significantly different, with less emphasis on testing asymptomatic men and a stronger emphasis on screening based on high-risk sexual behaviors. MSM have different recommendations for STI screening based on a higher statistical likelihood of such behaviors.

While female patients have appropriately been the focus of most clinical attention on identification and treatment of STIs, male patients represent an important and sometimes neglected population where the public and individual health benefits of STI recognition and treatment are considerable.

References

1. Marcell AV. Preventive male sexual and reproductive health care: recommendations for clinical practice. Philadelphia, PA: Male Training Center for Family Planning and Reproductive Health and Rockville, MD: Office of Population Affairs; 2014.
2. Kodner C. Sexually transmitted infections in men. Prim Care Clinics. 2003;30(1):173–91.
3. Sexually Transmitted Disease Surveillance 2013. US DHHS Centers for Disease Control and Prevention National Center for HIV/AIDS, Viral Hepatitis, STD, and TB Prevention Division of STD Prevention Atlanta, Georgia; December 2014.
4. Madkan VK. Sex differences in the transmission, prevention, and disease manifestations of sexually transmitted diseases. Arch Dermatol. 2006;142:365–70.
5. Tuddenham S. Toward enhancing sexually transmitted infection clinic efficiency in an era of molecular diagnostics: the role of physical examination and risk stratification in men. Sex Trans Dis. 2013;40(11):886–93.
6. Workowski KA. Sexually Transmitted Diseases Treatment Guidelines, 2015. MMWR Recomm Rep. 2015;64(3):1–137.
7. Augenbraun LH. Urethritis. In: Bennett JE, Dolin R, Blaser MJ, editors. Mandell, Douglas, and Bennett's principles and practice of infectious diseases. 8th ed. Philadelphia, PA: Elsevier Churchill Livingstone; 2014 (Chapter 109).
8. Karnath BM. Manifestations of gonorrhea and chlamydial infection. Hospital Physician 2009; 44–48.
9. McGowan CC. Prostatitis, epididymitis, and orchitis. In: Bennett JE, Dolin R, Blaser MJ, editors. Mandell, Douglas, and Bennett's principles and practice of infectious diseases. 8th ed. Philadelphia, PA: Elsevier Churchill Livingstone; 2014 (Chapter 112).
10. LeFevre ML. Behavioral counseling interventions to prevent sexually transmitted infections: U.S. preventive services task force recommendation statement. Ann Intern Med. 2014;161(12): 894–901.
11. Kogan SM. Risk and protective factors for unprotected intercourse among rural African American young adults. Public Health Rep. 2010;125:709–17.
12. Guimaraes EMB. Lack of utility of risk score and gynecological examination for screening for sexually transmitted infections in sexually active adolescents. BMC Med. 2009;7:8.
13. Millet GA. Circumcision status and risk of HIV and sexually transmitted infections among men who have sex with men: a meta-analysis. JAMA. 2008;300(14):1674–84.
14. Brook G, Clinical Effectiveness Group. 2013 UK national guideline for consultations requiring sexual history taking. London (UK): British Association for Sexual Health and HIV (BASHH); 2013.
15. Celum CL. The Practitioner's handbook for the management of sexually transmitted diseases, 3rd ed. Seattle, WA: Seattle STD/HIV Prevention Training Center, University of Washington; 2002.
16. Creegan L. Brief, individual behavioral counseling for STD/HIV risk reduction. National Network of STD/HIV Prevention Training Centers Curriculum Committee 2011. http://nnptc.

org/wp-content/uploads/Behavioral-Counseling-Risk-Reduction-Curriculum-Module-2011. pdf. Accessed 8/31/2015.

17. Lanier Y. Reframing the context of preventive health care services and prevention of HIV and other sexually transmitted infections for young men: new opportunities to reduce racial/ethnic sexual health disparities. Am J Public Health. 2013;103:262–9.

18. Gillmore MR. Heterosexually active men's beliefs about methods for preventing sexually transmitted diseases. Perspect Sex Reprod Health. 2003;35(3):121–9.

19. Counseling and Communicating with Men. In: Men's Reproductive Health Curriculum, EngenderHealth; 2003. https://www.engenderhealth.org/pubs/gender/mens-rh-curriculum.php

20. Zakher B. Screening for Gonorrhea and Chlamydia: a systematic review for the U.S. preventive services task force. Ann Intern Med. 2014;161:884–93. doi:10.7326/M14-1022.

21. Schachter J. Confirming positive results of nucleic acid amplification tests (NAATs) for Chlamydia trachomatis: all NAATs are not created equal. J Clin Microbiol. 2005;43(3): 1372–3.

22. Papp JR. Recommendations for the Laboratory-Based Detection of Chlamydia trachomatis and Neisseria gonorrhoeae – 2014. MMWR. 2014;63(2):1–19.

23. U.S. Preventive Services Task Force. Screening for syphilis: recommendation statement. Ann Fam Med. 2004;2(4):362–5.

24. U.S. Preventive Services Task Force. Screening for chlamydial infection: U.S. Preventive Services Task Force recommendation statement. Ann Intern Med. 2007;147(2):128–34.

25. U.S. Preventive Services Task Force. Screening for Gonorrhea: recommendation statement. Ann Fam Med. 2005;3(3):263–7.

26. Moyer VA. Screening for hepatitis C virus infection in adults: U.S. Preventive services task force recommendation statement. Ann Intern Med. 2013;159:349–57.

27. Moscicki AB. HPV in men: an update. J Low Genit Tract Dis. 2011;15(3):231–4.

28. Moyer VA. Screening for HIV: U.S. preventive services task force recommendation statement. Ann Intern Med. 2013;159(1):51–60.

29. U.S. Public Health Service: Preexposure prophylaxis for the prevention of HIV infection in the United States – 2014 – A Clinical Practice Guideline. CDC 2014. http://www.cdc.gov/hiv/pdf/ prepguidelines2014.pdf. Accessed 2 Sep 2015.

30. California Department of Public Health Sexually Transmitted Diseases (STD) Control Branch. Patient-Delivered Partner Therapy (PDPT) for Chlamydia, Gonorrhea, and Trichomoniasis: Guidance for Medical Providers in California; 2012. https://www.cdph.ca.gov/pubsforms/ Guidelines/Documents/CA-STD-PDPT-Guidelines.pdf. Accessed 9/2/2015.

31. Centers for Disease Control and Prevention. Expedited partner therapy in the management of sexually transmitted diseases. Atlanta, GA: US Department of Health and Human Services, 2006.

32. Centers for Disease Control and Prevention. Sexually Transmitted Disease Surveillance 2013. Atlanta: U.S. Department of Health and Human Services; 2014. http://www.cdc.gov/std/stats.

Chapter 11
Benign Prostatic Hyperplasia and Lower Urinary Tract Symptoms

Abdul Waheed

Background and Introduction

The lower urinary tract refers to the urogenital organs anatomically located in the pelvis and perineum that have direct bearing on the content, storage, and flow of urine beyond the ureterovesical junction and from the urinary bladder through the external urethral meatus. These structures include the urinary bladder, bladder neck and internal and external sphincters, and the urethra in both males and females. There are multiple adjacent organs differing in males and females which are significantly important parts of the lower urinary tract both structurally and functionally.

In males, the prostate gland is the most prominent organ located at the level of the bladder neck anatomically. This has a large bearing on the urogenital structure and the function of urinary outflow as described in the coming sections. Other adjacent organs that are not directly related structurally to the lower urinary tract but have significant bearing on a sense of normalcy and disease states involving the lower urinary tract include the testicles, epididymis, vas deferens, and the spermatic cord.

Urine flow through the lower urinary tract involves a complex interplay of these anatomic structures of lower urinary tract, autonomic nervous system, and an input from higher neurologic centers including voluntary cerebral control. This interplay results in desired storage of urine, addition of urine over time, and periodic and

A. Waheed, MD (✉)
Department of Family and Community Medicine, Penn State University College of Medicine,
Milton S. Hershey Medical Center, Hershey, PA, USA
e-mail: awaheed1@hmc.psu.edu

© Springer International Publishing Switzerland 2016
J.J. Heidelbaugh (ed.), *Men's Health in Primary Care*, Current Clinical Practice,
DOI 10.1007/978-3-319-26091-4_11

Table 11.1 Summary of lower urinary tract symptoms [1, 2, 5]

Frequency	Refers to need to urinate more than usual, commonly taken as need to go back to urinate within 2 h
Urgency	Refers to inability to postpone the urge to urinate
Intermittency	Refers to interrupted stream because patient has to stop and start again several times to finish a single act of urination
Weak urinary stream	May manifest as less amount of urine passage as a function of time or dribbling
Hesitancy and straining	Refers to inability to initiate urine stream despite the urge and patient ends up straining to initiate urination
Nocturia	Refers to waking up from sleep with an urge to urinate
Incomplete bladder emptying	Refers to residual urge after finishing an act of urination or feeling/sensation of not having the bladder completely emptied after finishing urination

voluntary voiding in normal physiologic states. Many structurally and functionally pathologic states can alter the sense of normalcy giving rise to a host of symptoms, collectively referred to as lower urinary tract symptoms (LUTS).

Historically, a compendium of terminologies existed for long period of time to describe these symptoms and related disease states. After a heated debate in Paul Abrams' articles [1, 2], all urologic societies favored uniform use of terminologies to avoid confusion and to provide safe patient care and meaningful research in these thematic areas. Since then, new terms have been proposed [3]. There is still considerable variation and some controversy that exists to date in this area [4]. Some consensus that we have in this area universally favors the use of the term "lower urinary tract symptoms" or "LUTS." These symptoms refer to both storage and dynamic voiding function or immediately post micturition [5]. Table 11.1 summarizes commonly described LUTS with their acceptable definitions.

LUTS related to different pathologic disease states affect both men and women and are common presenting complaints in both primary care and urologic outpatient offices. The present working theories, however, are focused on the presence of LUTS in men. Bothersome LUTS are highly prevalent in elderly men and require careful clinical attention to minimize potential complications that would impair urologic tract functioning [5]. Multiple population-based studies have shown that the prevalence of LUTS increases with age and that moderate to severe LUTS occur in 25 % of men over the age of 50 years [6, 7]. The pathophysiology of LUTS is often multifactorial. In most cases, obstructive as well as nonobstructive or dynamic factors may contribute to the development of LUTS [5].

One of the major causes of LUTS in middle-aged to elderly men is bladder outflow obstruction (BOO) related to prostate enlargement. It may be caused by a static component which is related to the size of prostate and a dynamic component which is due to the increased alpha-adrenergic smooth muscle tone within the prostate. The prostatic enlargement is most commonly due to benign prostatic hyperplasia (BPH) but may also be from prostatic intraepithelial neoplasia and prostate cancer. LUTS suggestive of BPH are very common in older men, occurring commonly in

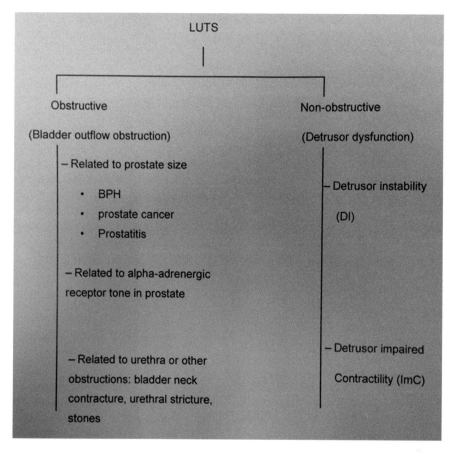

Fig. 11.1 A schematic flowchart summarizing LUTS and common etiology [2, 5]. *BPH* benign prostatic hyperplasia, *ImC* impaired detrusor contractility

over one-half of men aged 50 years or older. Patients with LUTS/BPH may present with storage symptoms (e.g., increased daytime frequency, nocturia, urgency) and/ or voiding symptoms (e.g., weak force and caliber of stream, hesitancy, terminal dribble) [2]. Figure 11.1 is a schematic flow that summarizes broad etiologic categories of LUTS.

Benign Prostatic Hyperplasia

Benign prostatic hyperplasia (BPH) refers to benign enlargement of the prostate gland. In a normal healthy male adult, the prostate gland weighs approximately 20 g. Leissner and colleagues described the average prostate to be 11 g with two standard deviations being 7 and 16 g in one case series of autopsies in healthy young males [8]. Some data suggests that average prostate size increases considerably above 50 years of age. This trend coincides with, and is likely resultant from, an increasing prevalence of BPH and resultant LUTS [9, 10]. Chute and colleagues reported the prevalence BPH and LUTS to range from 26 % to 46 % as men age from the fifth to the eighth decade of life [10]. Another study reported the prevalence to be 19 % when diagnosed using a cutoff of 30 g prostate size and the presence of significant clinical symptoms [11]. In summary, BPH causing clinically significant symptoms is very commonly encountered in primary care practices.

BPH is a histologic diagnosis whereby a glandular hyperplasia is demonstrated along with gross enlargement of the gland as opposed to benign prostate enlargement (BPE), which refers to a clinical diagnosis of an enlarged prostate with clinically assessed benign disease. Paul Abrams emphasizes the use of bladder outlet obstruction (BOO) until a final dynamic obstructive component can be demonstrated by flow/urodynamic studies along with demonstrated structural enlargement secondary to benign hyperplasia [4]. However, in routine primary care practices, BPH is often diagnosed with significant LUTS in men if prostate-specific antigen (PSA) levels are normal and prostate gland size is enlarged on digital rectal exam (DRE) with benign features.

Evaluation for Suspected BPH

Typically, a man with suspected BPH presents with LUTS (Table 11.1); however, microscopic hematuria, urinary retention, or chronic renal failure can be additional presentations of BPH. LUTS usually have a gradual and progressive course with a vague point of symptom onset. Patients commonly present due to either worsening in the intensity of symptoms leading to lifestyle disturbance or newly associated symptoms including hematuria or urinary retention. More rarely, BPH could be discovered when evaluating someone with chronic kidney disease. Patients with hematuria should be evaluated thoroughly for a full range of etiologies including infection, urologic neoplasm (e.g., bladder, kidney, urothelial), and nephritic syndrome to avoid anchoring diagnostic error in cases where man has a known diagnosis of BPH.

The evaluation of a man for BPH centers on a detailed history and thorough physical examination.

History

The history should focus on the presence or absence of LUTS, the extent of compromise on quality of lifestyle, and the presence of absence of "red flag symptoms" (Table 11.2). Red flag symptoms require prompt evaluation to rule out more serious disorders. A comprehensive review of systems is also very important in deriving a

Table 11.2 Red flag symptoms indicating additional broad-based evaluation [12–16]

Hematuria	Evaluate for urolithiasis, urethral stricture, glomerulonephritis, cancers of urinary tract including renal cell cancer, transitional cell cancer, bladder cancer
Chronic perennial pain	Evaluate for chronic prostatitis, proctalgia because of disorders of lower gastrointestinal tract, neuralgia
Neurologic symptoms/deficits of lower extremity	Evaluate for neurogenic bladder, back and spine disorders, or other causes of peripheral nerve issues
Fever, fatigue, dysuria	Evaluate for urinary tract infection, bacterial prostatitis, orchitis, epididymitis, orchid-epididymitis, or other infection elsewhere as suggested by review of systems
Urinary retention	Evaluate for neurogenic bladder, urethral stricture, detrusor-sphincter dyssynergia, and urethral stone. Should also lead to prompt decompression of bladder with Foley's catheter or suprapubic catheter

cogent differential diagnosis. Standardized symptom score tools like the American Urological Association Symptom Index (AUA-SI) [17] shown in Table 11.3 or the International Prostate Symptom Score (IPSS) [18] should be used to estimate the severity of symptoms and the impact of these symptoms on quality of life. These symptom scores are based upon symptoms shown in Table 11.1, along with questions specifically aimed at assessing quality of life parameters.

The standardized tools like AUA-SI and IPSS can provide a method of quantification to be followed longitudinally to guide clinicians in the initiation and monitoring of symptomatic therapy. The AUA-SI is shown in Fig. 11.2 and IPSS in Table 11.3, respectively. Voiding diaries can also be helpful in charting symptom progress.

Physical Examination

The physical examination should be complete, including evaluations of the head and neck and pulmonary, cardiac, abdominal, and pelvic systems and a detailed assessment to evaluate for lymphadenopathy. The genital (penile and scrotal) examination should detect any gross abnormalities or lesions, and the digital rectal examination (DRE) should be conducted thoroughly as detailed below.

Digital rectal examination (DRE) is one of the most important, readily available, cost-effective tools for prostate evaluation. The prostate gland is walnut-shaped structure located at the base of the urinary bladder; the apex is caudal and the base cranial as shown above. Normally, it weighs approximately 20 g and measures approximately 4 cm in transverse diameter, 3 cm in vertical, and 2 cm in anteroposterior diameter. It has an anterior surface, a posterior surface, and two inferolateral surfaces.

Table 11.3 International Prostate Symptom Score (IPSS) [18]

In the past month	Not at all	Less than 1 in 5 times	Less than half of the times	About half the time	More than half the time	Almost always	Your score
1. Incomplete emptying How often have you had the sensation of not emptying your bladder?	0	1	2	3	4	5	
2. Frequency How often have you had to urinate less than every 2 h?	0	1	2	3	4	5	
3. Intermittency How often have you found you stopped and started again several times when you urinated?	0	1	2	3	4	5	
4. Urgency How often have you found it difficult to postpone urination?	0	1	2	3	4	5	
5. Weak stream How often have you had a weak urinary stream?	0	1	2	3	4	5	
6. Straining How often have you had to strain to start urination?	0	1	2	3	4	5	
7. Nocturia How many times did you typically get up at night to urinate?	0	1	2	3	4	5	

Add up your scores for total AUA scores: ------
Quality of life due to urinary symptoms: If you were to spend the rest of your life with your urinary condition just the way it is now, how would you feel about that? (bold, highlight, or underline)
Delighted   Pleased   Mostly satisfied   Mixed   Mostly dissatisfied   Unhappy   Terrible
Score: mild 1–7, moderate 8–19, severe 20–35

AUA SYMPTOM SCORE

Last Name		First Name	Date

Highlight or bold or change font color of the response correct for you and type in your score in the far right box for all SEVEN questions.

1. **Incomplete emptying:** Over the past month, how often have you had a sensation of not emptying your bladder completely after you finished urinating?

Not at all	Less than 1 time in 5	Less than half the time	About half the time	More than half the time	Almost always	Your Score
0	1	2	3	4	5	

2. **Frequency:** Over the past month, how often have you had to urinate again less than 2 hours after you finished urinating?

Not at all	Less than 1 time in 5	Less than half the time	About half the time	More than half the time	Almost always	Your Score
0	1	2	3	4	5	

3. **Intermittency:** Over the past month, how often have you found that you stopped and started again several times when you urinated?

Not at all	Less than 1 time in 5	Less than half the time	About half the time	More than half the time	Almost always	Your Score
0	1	2	3	4	5	

4. **Urgency:** Over the past month, how often have you found it difficult to postpone urination?

Not at all	Less than 1 time in 5	Less than half the time	About half the time	More than half the time	Almost always	Your Score
0	1	2	3	4	5	

5. **Weak-stream:** Over the past month, how often have you had a weak stream?

Not at all	Less than 1 time in 5	Less than half the time	About half the time	More than half the time	Almost always	Your Score
0	1	2	3	4	5	

6. **Straining:** Over the past month, how often have you had to push or strain to begin urination?

Not at all	Less than 1 time in 5	Less than half the time	About half the time	More than half the time	Almost always	Your Score
0	1	2	3	4	5	

7. **Nocturia:** Over the past month or so, how many times did you get up to urinate from the time you went to bed until the time you got up in the morning?

None	1 time	2 times	3 times	4 times	5 or more times	Your Score
0	1	2	3	4	5	

Add up your scores for total AUA score = _____

Quality of Life Due to Urinary Symptoms: If you were to spend the rest of your life with your urinary condition just the way it is now, how would you feel about that? (Bold, Highlight or Underline)

Delighted   Pleased   Mostly satisfied   Mixed   Mostly dissatisfied   Unhappy   Terrible

Fig. 11.2 American Urological Association Symptom Index (AUA-SI) [17]

Table 11.4 DRE prostate features concerning of disease processes other than benign prostate disease [12–14]

Prostatitis	Boggy, moderately to severely tender, may or may not be enlarged
Prostate cancer	Indurations, nodules, hard consistency, mass, asymmetry, distortion of median sulcus, commonly non-tender

The DRE can be performed in several different positions, most commonly the left lateral decubitus and the knee-elbow positions. In one example, the patient may lie on the examination table in the left lateral decubitus position when the finger of the examiner is inserted in the rectum to palpate the prostate. The knee-elbow position allows the patient to lean over the examination table using elbows and bends his knees to allow for the examiner to insert the finger into rectum. The examiner should palpate for appropriate anal sphincter tone, generalized characteristics of the anal wall mucosa, and anteriorly the prostate including size, consistency, symmetry of the lobes, median sulcus, frank masses, indurations, nodules, and tenderness/bogginess. Understanding these characteristics while performing a "blind" examination can assist in differentiating among normal findings, benign enlargement, prostatitis, and prostate cancer (Table 11.4).

The size of the prostate can be estimated by using the "finger pad sweep" technique. Essentially, one finger pad sweep (the estimated surface area of the palmar surface of the index finger) over the prostate gland measures to be approximately 15–20 g (the normal weight of the prostate). Additional finger pad sweeps in both lateral and vertical directions should be added to estimate the total prostate size.

Another method of estimating and documenting prostate gland volume is to define one finger pad sweep as being a normal-sized gland; two finger pad sweeps would be estimated as double the normal size or "+2"; three finger pad sweeps estimated as triple the normal size or "+3"; etc. Another schematic used by primary care clinicians is estimating if the examiner can reach and feel both upper and lateral limits of the prostate with a finger sweep, then it is less than 30 g (+1 to +2 size), whereas if the examiner can reach the lateral limits only and not the vertical limits, then it is between 30 and 50 g (+2 to +3), while if both lateral and vertical limits are not reachable, then prostate volume is likely more than 50 g (more than +3) in size. It is recommended that an examiner use one technique and one system of documentation to maintain consistency across examinations.

The yield of the DRE is variable depending upon the indication for examination and the experience of the examiner. Although its importance as a screening tool for the diagnosis of prostate and colorectal cancer has been questioned [12–14], it is very useful in evaluating a man who presents with complaints related to urogenital tract. Although both left lateral and knee-elbow positions as described above have been reported to be comparable in patient discomfort, embarrassment, and completeness of examination [19], considerable inter-rater variability exists among examiners [20], as more experienced examiners are more likely to detect a significant abnormality [21].

Workup and Investigation

The extent of laboratory testing and radiographic imaging depends upon the data from the history and physical examination as described above. The AUA recommends routine baseline and follow-up evaluations of the PSA and urinalysis in patients with symptoms consistent with BPH and/or LUTS. It is reasonable to obtain baseline and follow-up serum blood urea nitrogen (BUN) and creatinine levels if symptoms have been insidious with gradual worsening or in cases of hematuria or urinary retention.

The urinalysis can provide a broad range of information to aid in confirming or ruling out a urinary tract infection (UTI); defining the presence of blood, protein, or glucose; or raising the possibility of other closely related urogenital conditions via the presence of crystals, casts, sediment, or leukocytes. Table 11.5 describes macroscopic features of the urinalysis and commonly associated conditions with these symptoms.

When present, a UTI should be appropriately treated before initiating chronic medical therapy for LUTS. Determination of a UTI can be straightforward in the presence of new onset dysuria, fever, and suprapubic tenderness; however, in many cases this may be complex and challenging to differentiate when caring for men with a history of chronic LUTS. In such cases, multiple findings on urinalysis can help to make diagnosis of UTI. Table 11.6 summarizes the validity and reliability of urinalysis parameters for the diagnosis of UTI [22].

The urine culture should be used to aid the determination of a proven UTI and to guide antibiotic therapy in men or nonpregnant patients (Fig. 11.3). A positive urine culture should always be treated in the presence of fever, fatigue, suprapubic pain, and/or flank tenderness [15]. In the absence of these classic features, it is recommended that positive urine culture be treated at least at the onset of medical therapy for LUTS or during a sudden worsening of symptoms.

Table 11.5 Macroscopic features and commonly associated conditions [15, 22]

Odor	• Ammonia-like	(Urea-splitting bacteria)
	• Foul, offensive	Old specimen, pus, or inflammation
	• Sweet	Glucose
	• Fruity	Ketones
	• Maple syrup-like	Maple syrup urine disease
Color	• Colorless	Diluted urine
	• Deep yellow	Concentrated urine, riboflavin
	• Yellow green	Bilirubin/biliverdin
	• Red	Blood/hemoglobin
	• Brownish red	Acidified blood (acute GN)
	• Brownish black	Homogentisic acid (melanin)
Turbidity	• Typically cells or crystals	
	• Cellular elements and bacteria will clear by centrifugation	
	• Crystals dissolved by a variety of methods (acid or base)	
	• Microscopic examination will determine which is present	

Table 11.6 Summary of the validity and reliability urinalysis parameters for diagnosis of UTI [15, 22]

Results	Sensitivity	Specificity	PPV	NPV
Positive leukocyte esterase	72–97	41–86	43–56	82–91
Presence of nitrites	19–48	92–100	50–83	70–88
Positive leukocyte esterase or presence of nitrites	46–100	42–98	52–68	78–98
≥3+ protein	63–83	50–53	53	82
≥1+ blood	68–92	42–46	51	88
Any of the above abnormalities	94–100	14–26	44	100
> 5 WBCs per HPF	90–96	47–50	56–59	83–95
> 5 RBCs per HPF	18–44	88–89	27	82
Bacteria (any amount)	46–58	89–94	54–88	77–86

All numerical values are expressed in percentage
UTI urinary tract infection, *PPV* positive predictive value, *NPV* negative predictive value, *WBC* white blood cells, *RBC* red blood cells

Fig. 11.3 Schematic flow diagram of positive urine culture based upon Infectious Disease Society of America (IDSA) guidelines [15]. *LUTS* lower urinary tract symptoms, *UA* urinalysis, *CFU* colony forming units, *HPF* high-powered field

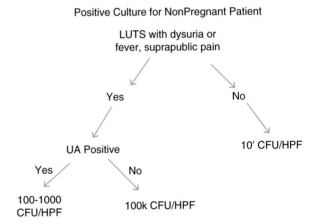

Serum prostate-specific antigen (PSA) levels are helpful in the initial workup and is routinely recommended by the AUA in all cases of LUTS and suspected BPH. Elevated levels (however, arbitrarily defined) still should raise suspicion for prostate cancer; however, these values should be interpreted with caution as elevated PSA levels may simply be the results of an increase in the volume of the prostate. Some studies have suggested a log-linear relationship between serum PSA levels and prostate volume [23, 24]. PSA density, which accounts for PSA ng/ml per gram of prostate volume, can be useful when determining appropriate or inappropriate elevations of PSA. Free PSA levels have been shown to have a better correlation with prostate volume than with predicting cancer risk [25]. In such cases, it is suggested that primary care clinicians consult a urologist to seek expert opinion on further workup and evaluation. Please see Chap. 14 for a further detailed discussion on abnormal PSA levels and prostate cancer risk.

Evaluation of Extent of Bladder Outlet Obstruction

Chronic bladder outlet obstruction may be suggested in men by obstructive LUTS and storage symptoms due to BPH, yet such symptoms do not quantify the extent of BOO. The AUA symptom score or the IPSS, both highlighted above, may provide further insight and help guide the goals of therapy [17]. The initial evaluation of the man with BPH and/or LUTS should assess the extent of BOO, which can be determined via post-void residual (PVR) volume, noninvasive uroflowmetry (UFM), or full urodynamic studies (UDS) for cystometrography (CMG).

Post-Void Residual

It is recommended by the European Association of Urology (EAU) for routine initial evaluation and monitoring of success of therapy [26]. It is a simple measure that can be obtained in the office setting via post-void urinary catheterization or ultrasonography. Post-void urinary catheterization is simple and cost-effective yet carries a risk of patient discomfort, embarrassment, and infection. Ultrasonography is also a very facile method to relatively assess post-void residual volume. While conventional ultrasonography requires radiologic training and expertise, bladder scanners are small handheld devices that require minimal training and expertise and can be easily performed in the office setting. Normal men without significant BOO usually have a PVR less than 12 ml of urine [16]. A significant controversy exists on the benefit of using PVR as a sole parameter to select surgical candidates [27]; hence, a full clinical picture, response to therapy, availability of procedural skills, and patient preference should all play a role when selecting patients for surgical therapy.

Noninvasive Uroflowmetry for Maximal Flow Cystometrography

CMG with real-time urodynamic pressure flow studies is considered to be the gold standard for examining voiding function [28]. This study can assess the static component of BOO as well as real-time bladder decompensation. This method, however, is invasive and involves a urinary catheter, rectal catheter, and infusion of fluid into the bladder. While cumbersome, this study is usually performed by urologists once a patient is refractory to treatment or has indications of bladder decompensation. Noninvasive UFM for maximal urine flow is, on the other hand, a relatively simple and harmless.

Since McConell's advocacy for the development of noninvasive parameters for above said purpose in 1994 [29], multiple studies [30, 31] have shown data in favor of using these measures. This leads to EAU recommendation for routine use of uroflowmetry in the management of LUTS, BPH, and BOO among men. Specifically for uroflowmetry to be useful, EAU standards require a pre-void volume of 250 ml with voided volume of at least 150 ml to make it to adequate uroflow study [26]. A maximal urinary flow rate of greater than 15 ml/s for a minimum voided volume of 150 ml has high negative predictive value for ruling clinically significant BOO [32]. A maximal urinary flow rate of less than 10 ml/s predicts better surgical outcome in BPH [31].

Treatment

Treatment for BPH causing significant LUTS is directed toward treating bothersome urinary symptoms to improve quality of life and preventing complications by early detection, behavioral modification, medical therapy, or surgical intervention. In the absence of significant BOO or any complication, initiation of medical therapy should be a shared decision between the patient and the physician to balance the quality of life and potential adverse effects from medications. The symptom severity of LUTS can easily be tracked semiquantitatively with an added quality of life question by using AUA symptoms index described above in the evaluation section [33].

Behavioral Modification

Behavioral modification should be considered when surgical intervention is not indicated and medical therapy is thought to be inappropriate either because of mild symptoms or side effects of the medications. Behavioral modification has been shown to be better than watchful waiting in mild (IPSS score less than 8) [34]. Examples include limiting caffeinated drinks, limiting fluid intake later in the day prior to bedtime, and performing timed voids to maximize bladder emptying.

Medical Therapy

Medical therapy is the mainstay of treatment in the absence of severe symptoms that indicate emergent evaluation, bladder outlet obstruction, and bladder decompensation. Medical therapy with a single agent should be the initial approach, yet some men may require combination therapy to adequate control LUTS and improve quality of life.

Alpha-1 blockers are the cornerstone of medical monotherapy for LUTS due to BPH. One large meta-analysis that combined RCTs and some comparative studies with over 7000 patients found a 30–40 % reduction of IPSS scores as compared to placebo [35]. The same study estimated a 16–25 % increase in maximal urinary flow rates as well. There are very few head-to-head trials [36, 37] to compare the efficacy of one alpha-1 blockers over another, as they are assumed to have similar efficacy yet may differ slightly in their adverse effect profile. Newer agents includ-

Table 11.7 Summary of routine dosing for alpha-1 blockers [38]

Terazosin	Dosage range is 1–10 mg PO QHS, starting with 1 mg, is titrated gradually to desired response over 7–8-week period for immediate release formulation while around 4-week period for longer acting formulation
Doxazosin	Dosage range is 1–8 mg PO QHS, starting with 1 mg, is titrated gradually to desired response over 7–8-week period for immediate release formulation while around 4-week period for longer acting formulation
Alfuzosin	Dose at 10 mg PO QHS initial and maintenance, no titration needed
Tamsulosin	Dose at 0.4 mg PO QHS initial and maintenance, may increase to 0.8 mg PO QHS if desired response not achieved in 2 weeks
Silodosin	Dose at 8 mg PO QHS initial and maintenance, no titration needed

Table 11.8 Common adverse reaction profile of alpha-blockers [39–42]

	Terazosin	Doxazosin	Alfuzosin	Tamsulosin	Silodosin
Hypotension	+++	+++	++	+	+
Ejaculatory dysfunction	+	+	−	+++	++
Headache, dizziness, syncope	++	++	++	+	+
Others	Other adverse reactions like floppy iris syndrome during cataract, etc. are equally distributed among these medications. Prazosin, not mentioned above, has cardiac adverse events and generally not used for BPH/LUTS				

The number of + signs indicates the commonality of occurrence of adverse events

ing alfuzosin and silodosin may have a slight advantage in efficacy yet also may be cost-prohibitive with certain healthcare plans. Standard dosing of alpha-1 blockers is summarized in Table 11.7, while Table 11.8 compares the side effect profile.

Five-alpha (5-α)-reductase inhibitors reduce prostate size slowly over months when taken regularly and in most cases reduce serum PSA values [43]. Although not considered to be as effective as alpha-1 blockers, they can be considered as initial monotherapy in cases where alpha-1 blockers are not well tolerated or contraindicated (e.g., those patients who will undergo ophthalmologic surgery due to risk of intraoperative floppy iris syndrome). Finasteride is dosed at 5 mg once daily, while dutasteride is ten times more potent and dosed at only 0.5 mg once daily. Since there is no risk of orthostatic hypotension with this class of medication, no titration is needed. Both finasteride and dutasteride are comparable in their efficacy and side effect profile and are FDA approved for treatment of BPH [43]. By convention, after a patient has been taking a 5-alpha-reductase inhibitor for 6 months, their PSA value should be doubled when followed.

There is some evidence that finasteride may be helpful in minimizing microscopic hematuria associated with BPH; however, this advantage is less clear with dutasteride [44, 45]. As mentioned in evaluation section, other causes of microscopic and gross hematuria should be excluded including bladder cancer with cystoscopy prior to commencement with 5-alpha-reductase therapy for the treatment of hematuria in BPH. In 2011, the US Food and Drug Administration (FDA) recommended

Table 11.9 Common adverse reactions of 5-alpha-reductase inhibitors

Sexual dysfunction	5-alpha reductase essential in testosterone metabolism, prostate growth and development, and adult prostate mass [47]. Its inhibition invariably causes some decreased libido, erectile dysfunction, and or ejaculatory dysfunction [47–49]
PSA levels and prostate cancer	With shrinkage of the prostate gland, PSA levels invariably decline with 5-alpha-reductase inhibitor treatment. Although the use of 5-alpha reductase decreases the incidence of prostate cancer, the declining levels of PSA may lead to detection of high-grade lesions in late stage in undiagnosed cases of prostate Ca. This leads FDA to issue a warning in 2011 [46]
Osteoporosis	Initial concern of osteoporosis and bone loss with 5-alpha-reductase inhibitors has been shown to be spurious. This is likely because estradiol has more effect on bone mass than testosterone itself [50]
Others	Nausea, headache, and other nonspecific adverse events have been described before; however, clinically these may not be that significant

evaluation for prostate cancer with DRE and PSA prior to initiating 5-alpha-reductase therapy, as this class has been shown to potentially decrease overall risk of prostate cancer yet has also been implicated in an increase in high-grade prostate cancer [46]. Four common significant adverse reactions of 5-alpha-reductase inhibitors are summarized in Table 11.9.

Phosphodiesterase type 5 inhibitors have inconsistent evidence showing beneficial effect on LUTS with BPH [51, 52]. This class of medication could be used as initial monotherapy in mild to moderate cases of men with severe symptoms or in combination with an alpha-blocker in men with erectile dysfunction. Caution and close monitoring for adverse effects are recommended initially because combination therapy may potentiate symptomatic orthostasis [53].

Anticholinergics can also be used as initial monotherapy for mild to moderate irritative LUTS along with symptoms commensurate with BOO. However, there should be no history of elevated PVRs (e.g., >150 ml) or frank urinary retention [54]. Table 11.10 summarizes the prescribing information and adverse effect profile of FDA-approved medications for treatment of overactive bladder. Significant caution should occur when using this class of medication in the geriatric population because anticholinergics can cause profound adverse effects on the central nervous, gastrointestinal, and musculoskeletal systems. Most of these effects are categorized as potentially inappropriate on The American Geriatric Society's Beers criteria list for use in older adults [33].

Combination Therapy

The MTOPS [55] and CombAT [56] trials have demonstrated safety and efficacy of the combination of alpha-blockers and 5-alpha-reductase inhibitors in the treatment of LUTS due to BPH. A combination of alpha-blockers and 5-alpha-reductase inhibitors should be considered later in treatment paradigms when treatment of LUTS causes moderate to severe functional disability (AUA score greater than 19

Table 11.10 FDA-approved anticholinergics for treatment of overactive bladder (OAB) which are on the Beers criteria list [33]

	Availability	Common significant adverse effects
Tolterodine	Oral immediate or extended release	Dizziness, drowsiness, nervousness, confusion, hypotension, edema, xeroderma, xerostomia, constipation, frequent UTIs, weakness, arthralgia
Oxybutynin	Oral immediate or extended release, transdermal	Xeroderma, xerostomia, dizziness, drowsiness, nervousness, confusion, hypotension, edema, arthralgias
Darifenacin	Oral immediate and extended release	Xerostomia, constipation, headache, dizziness, drowsiness, flu-like symptoms, weakness, arthralgias
Solifenacin	Oral and transdermal	Xerostomia, constipation, headache, dizziness, drowsiness, flu-like symptoms, weakness, arthralgias
Fesoterodine	Oral immediate and extended release	Xerostomia, constipation, headache, dizziness, drowsiness, weakness, myalgias
Trospium	Oral immediate and extended release	Xerostomia, constipation, headache, dizziness, drowsiness, weakness, myalgias

or IPSS score greater than 20). Some patients develop irritative voiding symptoms from detrusor irritability and continue to have high IPSS/AUA scores for LUTS despite adequate treatment with alpha-blocker monotherapy or alpha-blocker and 5-alpha-reductase inhibitor combination therapy. Addition of anticholinergic therapy should be considered in such cases. The NEPTUNE study group has shown long-term efficacy and safety of this combination in a single pill [57, 58].

Complementary and Alternative Treatments

A host herbal of products and agents from integrative medicine/complementary and alternative medicine have been presented as potential treatment for LUTS from BPH. Both the American Urological Association (AUA) [33] and National Institute for Healthcare and Clinical Excellence (NICE) [5, 59] do not recommend any dietary supplements, combination phytotherapy, homeopathic products, or any non-conventional therapies. Some of the common treatments are reviewed in Table 11.11. Multiple other unconventional therapies including acupuncture [70] and Chinese herbal saxifrage tablets [71] that have been presented by are ineffective or lack evidence in support of favorable outcome.

Monitoring Treatment and Evaluation for Complication

LUTS due to BPH are an ongoing, commonly progressive, phenomenon that requires continuous periodic monitoring once medical treatment is initiated. This is best conducted through routine follow-up evaluations with primary care clinicians that should focus on improving the lifestyle and minimizing risk of complications.

Table 11.11 Common herbal products used to treat LUTS

Product	Product info, active components	Mechanism of action	Safety and efficacy
Saw palmetto	*Serenoa repens, Sabal serrulata, Sabalis serrulatae*, sago palm	Unknown, may be alpha-adrenergic blockade [60, 61]	Inconsistent evidence in support of relief from LUTS [62], may have multiple interactions with routine meds [60, 61, 63]
Beta-sitosterol	One of the phytosterols found in Pygeum	Unclear	May be effective for mild to moderate LUTS [64, 65]
Pygeum africanum	African plum	Unknown	Poor quality evidence that it may or may not be safe and effective in mild to moderate LUTS [66, 67]
Pumpkin seed	Prosta fink forte	Unknown	Weak evidence from case series to improve LUTS, safety unclear [68]
Stinging nettle root	*Urtica dioica*	Unknown	May not be effective [67], may have multiple interactions
Rye products	Grass extract (*Secale cereale*), Cernilton		Weak evidence indicative that it may be effective in mild but no comparison [69]

This should be achieved with using the AUA-SI [17] or IPSS [18] longitudinally at each visit to look for objective improvement in symptom scores. Post-void residual (PVR) volume is also a valuable tool which should be used routinely and longitudinally to monitor the progress of treatment if the initial PVR is significant. The following conditions include common complications of LUTS/BPH and the suggested workup for each.

Urinary tract infection is common because of the change in dynamics of voiding and urostasis in the urinary bladder. This should be evaluated at the initial and subsequent visits via urinalysis and urine culture whenever dysuria or irritative LUTS are present or there is decline on the standardized symptoms scores.

Acute urinary retention refers to painful collection of residual urine in the bladder due to inability to voluntarily bladder. This is sometimes called ischuria or acute voiding dysfunction. Acute retention usually leads to up to 800 ml of residual urine. This may be superimposed to chronic retention described below which is an indication of acute-on-chronic bladder decompensation. Acute retention may be precipitated by variety of insults including as mild a thing as trying to hold urine voluntarily for a while if patients have underlying significant BPH [72]. Table 11.12 summarizes common precipitants of acute urine retention and further evaluation. All patients with suspected acute urine retention should be treated with urinary catheterization to relieve the obstruction. This is most commonly achieved by placing a Foley's catheter through urethra. Urinary catheterization can be significantly

Table 11.12 Common precipitants of urinary retention

Precipitant	Evaluation and treatment
UTI	Request urine culture, treat with antibiotics
Medications	Anticholinergics, TCAs, certain antiarrhythmics, antihistamines, dihydropyridine calcium channel blockers, hydralazine, antiparkinsonian, antipsychotics, benzodiazepines, sympathomimetics, muscle relaxants. Discontinue insulting med if possible [73]
Severe pain	Severe pain anywhere but more specifically pelvis, treat with pain killers
Large fluid challenge	May lead to acute bladder decompensation in BPH, treat with bladder drainage
General anesthesia	May lead to overdistension of the bladder and acute decompensation, treat with temporary catheterization

challenging in cases where prostate is very large volume. Expert (urologist) consultation with or without suprapubic catheterization is an alternative. Retention can lead to post-renal acute kidney injury and should be relieved promptly [74].

Chronic urinary retention usually refers to progressively increasing PVRs ultimately resulting in the inability to void or completely empty the bladder with voluntary effort. This condition may be preceded or accompanied by involuntary urine leakage, termed overflow incontinence. Chronic urinary retention is invariably associated with a large capacity bladder and commonly has a post-void residual of more than 500 ml of urine. Chronic urinary retention is usually painless [72], however, may be painful in cases with acute-on-chronic retention due to rapid distention, which may indicate bladder decompensation [73]. Urinary retention, if not relieved, may promptly lead additional complications including hydroureter and hydronephrosis [72, 74], venous congestion from bladder pushing on the vasculature [75], or rarely bladder rupture [76]. Chronic urinary retention is commonly associated with renal failure which should be quickly recognized, while other causes of chronic kidney disease should be excluded.

Urolithiasis in cases of chronic LUTS due to BPH causing BOO can lead to struvite stones due to urostasis. The most common site for stone formation is within bladder, yet this may occur at any location within the urinary tract. This may further aggravate LUTS because of decreasing bladder capacity and increasing irritative LUTS associated with the presence of a stone. A renal and bladder ultrasound can often diagnose stones, but if missed on this imaging modality and still highly suspected, a CT urogram should be obtained. Once detected, urologic consultation should be facilitated for possible extracorporeal shock wave lithotripsy (ESWL) or endoscopic cystolitholapaxy.

Neurogenic bladder may ultimately develop on account of bladder decompensation over time. This condition also manifests as an aggravation of LUTS and storage symptoms. The diagnosis should be made with urodynamic studies when suspected and if surgery is being considered. All efforts should be directed toward preventing this condition.

Referral to Urology for Evaluation for Surgery

Expert consultation with a urologist should be considered after any of the above complications are diagnosed. However, a single incidence of acute urinary retention can often be managed with catheterization followed by a combination of medical therapy and a trial of voiding without a catheter. This is especially true when a specific precipitant is identified and the offending agent is stopped. Other indications include (1) persistent progression to moderate to severe symptoms despite adequate treatment, (2) urinary retention refractory to conservative therapy (e.g., failure of trial of voiding without catheter), (3) multiple UTIs with retention events, (4) renal insufficiency attributable to BPH, and (5) the presence of an enlarged median lobe of the prostate that usually does not respond to medical therapy at all and requires surgery.

The enlargement of the median lobe refers to a configuration of prostate where a part of hyperplastic prostate tissue protrudes significantly into the lumen of the bladder near the bladder neck leading to mechanical obstruction of urinary outflow. This component of prostate tissue acts like a ball valve preventing outflow during normal voiding. In such cases, alpha-blockers, 5-alpha-reductase inhibitors, and phosphodiesterase type 5 inhibitors are ineffective because of the largely mechanical nature of the problem. Transurethral resection of the median lobe of the prostate should be strongly considered in these cases to prevent further obstructive complications.

Surgery remains the definitive treatment for BPH that has not responded to conservative and medical therapies, although LUTS may persist even after surgical treatment in many patients [6]. This result is largely due to the complex pathophysiology of LUTS, which commonly involves more than just pure mechanical obstruction from BPH [4–6]. LUTS related to BPH have a static component related to sheer volume and mechanical narrowing of the bladder neck as well as a dynamic component related to increased alpha-adrenergic muscle tone at the bladder neck. Moreover, these storage and irritative voiding symptoms are also complicated by some degree of detrusor dysfunction [4, 5]. Although all men who continue to have bothersome LUTS should be considered for surgical treatment, the decision for surgical treatment should be individualized based upon medical comorbidities, adequacy of medical therapy, the presence of a prominent and obstructive median lobe, bladder condition (e.g., decompensation), risk of development of postoperative complications, and patient preference for long-term undertaking of continuous daily medications. Clinical outcomes in terms of reduction in LUTS and improvement of lifestyle may not differ substantially between medical therapy and surgical treatments [5, 33, 59].

There are many current surgical options available for the treatment of BPH. Almost all of these methods are within most standards of care and involve transurethral procedures. These include (1) transurethral resection of prostate (TURP) with conventional electrical loop cautery, (2) TURP using bipolar cautery, (3) transurethral vaporization of prostate (TUVP), (4) transurethral HoLEP and ThuLEP procedures (which utilize various lasers), and (5) transurethral photoselective vaporization of prostate (TU-PVP). Urethral stenting and prostatic urethral lift are additional procedures that can be offered to patients who cannot have the defini-tive transurethral procedures due to medical comorbidities but are refractory to medical therapy. Not all of these procedures may be available at every community- or university-based hospital, and outcomes may be linked to experience of the urol-ogist relative to each surgical technique.

Painful Noncancerous Disorders of Prostate

Lower urinary tract symptoms (LUTS) in men can sometimes be associated with acute or chronic pain in the pelvis and perineum, which are usually a manifestation of benign disorders of prostate other than BPH. Most of these conditions are inflam-matory disorders; however, some patients with chronic symptoms may not show evidence of an inflammatory disorder. Pain and discomfort involving pelvic and perineum are the defining features of these disorders. Many different distinct clini-cal entities have been described including (1) acute bacterial prostatitis, (2) chronic bacterial prostatitis, and (3) chronic pelvic pain syndrome which could be either chronic inflammatory prostatitis or chronic noninflammatory prostatitis. The National Institute of Health (NIH) consensus guidelines describes another clinical entity "asymptomatic inflammatory prostatitis" as another distinct condition [77].

Acute Bacterial Prostatitis

Acute bacterial prostatitis refers to acute inflammation of the prostate due to bacte-rial infection manifesting as pain and significant LUTS. LUTS in such cases are commonly associated with systemic and constitutional symptoms including fever, chills, and malaise. Patients usually present as acutely ill with spiking fevers, rigors, dysuria, flank pain, myalgias, worsening LUTS which can lead to obstructive symp-toms, pain in the perineum or pelvis, and pyuria. The DRE usually reveals a firm, warm, edematous, and very tender prostate which is commonly described as a "painful and boggy prostate." Laboratory testing can reveal leukocytosis with a left shift, pyuria, bacteriuria, and sometimes positive blood cultures. Inflammatory markers including erythrocyte sedimentation rate (ESR) and C-reactive protein (CRP), although not routinely required for diagnosis, are also commonly moder-ately elevated. Rarely, acute bacterial prostatitis can present as sepsis with shock [78]. The PSA is commonly elevated and, if assayed, should be repeated 4–6 weeks after treatment and symptom resolution to document a return to baseline levels.

Acute bacterial prostatitis usually occurs when bacteria enter into the prostate from the urethra via the prostatic duct. The most common organisms are the same as other UTIs including urethritis, cystitis, or pyelonephritis. The most common organisms implicated in acute bacterial prostatitis include gram-negative organisms including *E. coli*, *Proteus mirabilis*, *Enterobacteriaceae* (including *Klebsiella*,

Enterobacter, and *Serratia* species), and *Pseudomonas aeruginosa* [79]. Rarely, in especially fulminant cases, gram-positive organisms including *Staphylococcus aureus* and *Streptococcus* or other *Staphylococcus* species have also been found. Due attention should be paid toward sexually transmitted infections (STIs) including chlamydia and gonorrhea in young sexually active patients who have risk factors, prior history of STIs, or any evidence to suggest epididymitis or orchitis [80].

Management of acute bacterial prostatitis includes prompt delivery of antibiotics and evaluation and treatment of any complications. Patients who have multiple comorbidities and have vital sign abnormalities or sepsis criteria should be admitted to the hospital for intravenous antibiotics and treatment monitoring. Hospitalized patients should be treated empirically to cover both gram-positive and gram-negative organisms, and antibiotic treatment should be narrowed after 48 h based upon culture results. Antibiotics with adequate penetration through the blood-prostate barrier should be used, including trimethoprim-sulfamethoxazole or fluoroquinolones like ciprofloxacin or levofloxacin. Acutely hospitalized patients should receive aminoglycosides in addition to fluoroquinolones. Gram-positive infections should be treated with cephalosporins or penicillinase-resistant penicillins including amoxicillin-clavulanic acid or dicloxacillin [80]. Methicillin-resistant *Staphylococcus aureus* (MRSA) should be treated with intravenous vancomycin or clindamycin [81]. A longer duration of treatment with antibiotics has been well supported. It is recommended that all cases of firmly diagnosed acute bacterial prostatitis should be treated with appropriate antibiotics for 6 weeks [81].

Complications, when suspected, should be promptly evaluated and expert opinion sought right away. Common complications include (1) *abscess* formation in the gland, (2) sepsis, (3) infective endocarditis, and (4) acute urinary retention.

Sepsis requires prompt hospitalization with an IV antibiotic treatment and aggressive fluid resuscitation. A *prostatic abscess* should be suspected if an adequate clinical response to antibiotic therapy is not achieved within 24–48 h. Usually a transrectal ultrasonogram or a CT scan of the pelvis is the choice for investigation and can reliably diagnose an abscess. Ultrasound, although relatively cheaper and radiation-free, may lead to further bacteremia from the prostatic message that happens with the ultrasound probe. A CT scan should be considered for patients who continue to spike fever or are unstable [82]. Abscess requires surgical drainage and expert consultation. It is more common among patients who are immunocompromised like HIV-AIDS, poorly controlled diabetes mellitus or using immunosuppressant medications [83, 84]. Prostatic abscess might need surgical drainage.

If a gram-positive organism like *Streptococcus* or *Staphylococcus aureus* is identified on blood cultures, then appropriate measures should be taken to evaluate for infective endocarditis, including a transesophageal echocardiogram.

Acute urinary retention secondary to acute bacterial prostatitis should be relieved promptly to avoid acute kidney injury from sepsis related to the acute infection and bacteremia. Commonly, it is more convenient to place a suprapubic catheter than to perform routine urinary catheterization. Suprapubic catheter not only promptly relieves the retention and acute blockage, but it also bypasses the possibility of prostatic message and increased bacteremia from the gland.

Chronic Bacterial Prostatitis

Chronic bacterial prostatitis should be suspected when a patient presents with chronic LUTS of more than 6–12 weeks duration with some component of pelvic or perennial pain. Such patients have normal-sized prostate glands which are as tender or "boggy" as found in acute bacterial prostatitis. These patients invariably have higher levels of bacteriuria and higher number of bacterial counts in prostatic fluid. Expression of prostatic fluid secretions for culture is the gold standard in diagnosis; however, it is very cumbersome and may be embarrassing for the patient to collect a specimen in routine clinical settings. Clinical data, especially (1) prolonged LUTS without significantly elevated PVRs, (2) prostate usually normal size rather than enlarged, (3) the presence of localized and pelvic pain, (4) positive urine cultures, and (5) recurrent treatments for UTIs and/or acute bacterial prostatitis, can be useful in making an accurate diagnosis of chronic bacterial prostatitis. Prolonged treatment with 6 weeks of appropriate antibiotics, as described above, in addition to nonsteroidal anti-inflammatory drugs (NSAIDs), is recommended.

Chronic Prostatitis-Chronic Pelvic Pain Syndrome

This syndrome refers to chronic symptoms of the urogenital tract without evidence of bacterial infection, BPH, or significant BOO. It can either be inflammatory or noninflammatory in etiology. In this sense, the term "prostatitis" may be a misnomer due to the extent and disability of the chronic pain [85].

Chronic prostatitis-chronic pelvic pain syndrome (CP-CPPS) is usually a diagnosis of exclusion. Patients often give a history of LUTS and should be asked about quality and duration of pain, any other related urinary complaints, sexual dysfunction, depressive symptoms or other mood disorders, and quality of life. Similar to the AUA-SI and IPSS for BPH, the NIH-based chronic prostatitis symptom index (NIH-CPSI) should be used to quantify symptoms and monitor treatment progress [86]. NIH-CPSI is shown in Fig. 11.4.

A firm diagnosis requires the exclusion of common causes of LUTS including BPH, prostate cancer, overactive bladder, detrusor-sphincter dyssynergia, bacterial prostatitis, recurrent UTIs, STIs, and bladder cancer. This requires a thorough history and physical examination including a DRE. Laboratory evaluation including urinalysis, urine culture, PVRs, uroflowmetry, and/or bladder ultrasound is recommended. However, tests of choice should be carefully selected based upon risk factors and history and physical examination. Routine PSA is not necessary; however, most clinicians will likely obtain this test to assess likelihood of concomitant prostate cancer.

Adequate treatment of CP-CPPS can be very challenging. Usual therapy includes an empiric trial of 6 weeks of antibiotic therapy, similar to that for acute or chronic bacterial prostatitis. This treatment should be followed by a trial of an alpha-blocker, a 5-alpha-reductase inhibitor, NSAIDs, or COX-2 inhibitors [87]. Phytotherapy

NIH-Chronic Prostatitis Symptom Index (NIH-CPSI)

Pain or Discomfort

1. In the last week, have you experienced any pain or discomfort in the following areas?

		Yes	No
a.	Area between rectum and testicles (perineum)	$\square_1$	$\square_0$
b.	Testicles	$\square_1$	$\square_0$
c.	Tip of the penis (not related to urination)	$\square_1$	$\square_0$
d.	Below your waist, in your pubic or bladder area	$\square_1$	$\square_0$

2. In the last week, have you experienced:

		Yes	No
a.	Pain or burning during urination?	$\square_1$	$\square_0$
b.	Pain or discomfort during or after sexual climax (ejaculation)?	$\square_1$	$\square_0$

3. How often have you had pain or discomfort in any of these areas over the last week?

   $\square_0$ Never
   $\square_1$ Rarely
   $\square_2$ Sometimes
   $\square_3$ Often
   $\square_4$ Usually
   $\square_5$ Always

4. Which number best describes your AVERAGE pain or discomfort on the days that you had it, over the last week?

   $\square$ $\square$ $\square$ $\square$ $\square$ $\square$ $\square$ $\square$ $\square$ $\square$ $\square$
   0   1   2   3   4   5   6   7   8   9   10
   NO   PAIN AS
   PAIN   BAD AS
                                              YOU CAN
                                              IMAGINE

Urination

5. How often have you had a sensation of not emptying your bladder completely after you finished urinating, over the last week?

   $\square_0$ Not at all
   $\square_1$ Less than 1 time in 5
   $\square_2$ Less than half the time
   $\square_3$ About half the time
   $\square_4$ More than half the time
   $\square_5$ Almost always

6. How often have you had to urinate again less than two hours after you finished urinating, over the last week?

   $\square_0$ Not at all
   $\square_1$ Less than 1 time in 5
   $\square_2$ Less than half the time
   $\square_3$ About half the time
   $\square_4$ More than half the time
   $\square_5$ Almost always

Impact of Symptoms

7. How much have your symptoms kept you from doing the kinds of things you would usually do, over the last week?

   $\square_0$ None
   $\square_1$ Only a little
   $\square_2$ Some
   $\square_3$ A lot

8. How much did you think about your symptoms, over the last week?

   $\square_0$ None
   $\square_1$ Only a little
   $\square_2$ Some
   $\square_3$ A lot

Quality of Life

9. If you were to spend the rest of your life with your symptoms just the way they have been during the last week, how would you feel about that?

   $\square_0$ Delighted
   $\square_1$ Pleased
   $\square_2$ Mostly satisfied
   $\square_3$ Mixed (about equally satisfied and dissatisfied)
   $\square_4$ Mostly dissatisfied
   $\square_5$ Unhappy
   $\square_6$ Terrible

Scoring the NIH-Chronic Prostatitis Symptom Index Domains

Pain: Total of items 1a, 1b, 1c,1d, 2a, 2b, 3, and 4   = _____

Urinary Symptoms: Total of items 5 and 6   = _____

Quality of Life Impact: Total of items 7, 8, and 9   = _____

Fig. 11.4 National Institute of Health Chronic Prostatitis Symptom Index (NIH-CPSI) [86]

with pollen extract like Cernilton [88] and bioflavonoids like quercetin [89] also has some evidence of success in reducing symptom index. Referral for expert consultation should be sought if there is inadequate initial response to treatment as outlined above.

Conclusion

Men commonly experience various lower urinary tract symptoms due to benign prostatic enlargement with or without some degree of obstruction. Standard medical therapy helps most men to achieve improvement in quality of life and urinary function. More severe cases require intraurethral resection procedures. Utilization of various symptomatic assessment scores can help to track severity and improvement of symptoms over time. Referral to a urologist for consultation should occur when medical therapies fail and when evidence of severe bladder outlet obstruction is imminent.

References

1. Abrams P. New words for old: lower urinary tract symptoms for "prostatism". Br Med J. 1994;69:929–30.
2. Abrams P. LUTS, BPH, BPE, BPO; A plea for the logical use of correct terms. Rev Urol. 1999;1(2):65.
3. Abrams P, Cardozo L, Fall M, et al. The standardization of terminology of lower urinary tract function: report from the Standardization Sub-committee of the International Continence Society. Neurourol Urodyn. 2002;21:167–78.
4. Warren K, Burden H, Abrams P. Lower urinary tract symptoms: still too much focus on prostate. Curr Opin Urol. 2014;24:3–9.
5. Jones C, Hill J, Chapple C, Guideline Development Group. Management of lower urinary tract symptoms in men: summary of NICE guidance. BMJ. 2010;340:c2354.
6. Taylor BC, Wilt TJ, Lambert LC, et al. Prevalence, severity, and health correlates of lower urinary tract symptoms among older men: the MrOS study. Urology. 2006;68:804–9.
7. Parsons JK, Bergstrom J, Silberstein J, et al. Prevalence and characteristics of lower urinary tract symptoms in men aged > or = 80 years. Urology. 2008;72(2):318–21.
8. Leissner KH, Tisell LE. The weight of the human prostate. Scan J Urol Nephrol. 1979; 13(2):137–42.
9. Berry SJ, Coffey DS, Walsh PC, et al. The development of human benign prostatic hyperplasia with age. J Urol. 1984;132(3):474.
10. Chute CG, Panser LA, Girman CJ, et al. The prevalence of prostatism: a population based survey of urinary symptoms. J Urol. 1993;150(1):85.
11. Bosch JL, Hop WC, Kirkels WJ, et al. Natural History of benign prostatic hyperplasia: appropriate case definition and estimation of its prevalence in the community. Urology. 1995;46(Suppl 3A):34.
12. Epstein JI. Pathology of prostate neoplasia. In: Walsh PC, editor. Campbell's urology. 8th ed. Philadelphia: Saunders; 2002.
13. Chodak GW, Keller P, Schoenberg HW. Assessment of screening for prostate cancer using the digital rectal examination. J Urol. 1989;141(5):1136.
14. Krahn MD, Mahoney JE, Eckman MH, et al. Screening for prostate cancer. A decision analytic view. JAMA. 1994;272(10):773.
15. Rubin RH, Shapiro ED, Andriole VT, et al. Evaluation of new anti-infective drugs for the treatment of urinary tract infection (IDSA guidelines). Clin Infec Dis. 1992;15 Suppl 1:S216–27.
16. Dimare JR, Fish SR, Harper JM, et al. Residual urine in normal male subjects. J Urol. 1963;96:180.

17. Barry MJ, Fowler Jr FJ, O'Leary MP, et al. The American Urologic Association Symptom Index for benign prostatic hyperplasia. The measurement committee of the American Urologic Association. J Urol. 1992;148(5):1549–57.
18. Wadie BS, Ibrahim EH, de la Rosette JJ, et al. The relationship of the international prostate symptoms score and objective parameters for diagnosing bladder outlet obstruction. Part-1: when statistics fail. J Urol. 2001;65(1):32.
19. Frank J, Thomas K, Oliver S, et al. Couch or crouch? Examining the prostate: a randomized study comparing the knee elbow and left lateral position. BJU Int. 2001;87:331–4.
20. Smith DS, Catalona WJ. Inter-examiner variability of digital rectal examination in detecting prostate cancer. Urology. 1995;45(1):70.
21. Balkissoon R, Blossfield K, Salud L, et al. Lost in translation: unfolding medical students' misconceptions of how to perform a clinical digital rectal examination. Am J Surg. 2009;197(4):525–32.
22. Simerville JA, Maxted WC, Pahira JC. Urinalysis: a comprehensive review. Am Fam Physician. 2005;71(6):1153–62.
23. Roehrborn CG, Boyle P, Gould AL, et al. Serum prostate specific antigen as a predictor of prostate volume in men with benign prostatic hyperplasia. Urology. 1999;53(3):581.
24. Hochberg DA, Armenakas NA, Fracchia JA. Relationship of prostate specific antigen and prostate volume in patients with biopsy proven benign prostatic hyperplasia. Prostate. 2000;45(4):315.
25. Mao Q, Zheng X, Jia X, et al. Relationship between total/free prostate specific antigen and prostate volume in Chinese men with biopsy-proven benign prostatic hyperplasia. Int Urol Nephrol. 2009;41(4):761.
26. Madersbacher S, Alivizatos G, Nordling J, et al. EAU 2004 guidelines on assessment, therapy and follow-up of men with lower urinary tract symptoms suggestive of benign prostatic obstruction (BPH guidelines). Eur Urol. 2004;46(5):547.
27. Wasson JH, Dj R, Bruskewtiz RC, et al. A comparison of transurethral surgery with watchful waiting for moderate symptoms of benign prostatic hyperplasia. The Veterans Affairs Cooperative Study Group on Transurethral Resection of the Prostate. N Engl J Med. 1995;322(2):75.
28. Nitti VW. Pressure flow urodynamic studies: the Gold Standard for Diagnosing Bladder Outlet Obstruction. Rev Urol. 2005;7 Suppl 6:14–21.
29. McConnell JD. Why pressure flow studies should be optional and not mandatory for evaluating men with Benign Prostatic Hyperplasia. Urology. 1994;44:156–8.
30. Kang MY, Ku JH, Oh SJ. Non-invasive parameters predicting bladder outlet obstruction in Korean men with lower urinary tract symptoms. J Korean Med Sci. 2010;25:272–5.
31. Porru D, Jallous H, Cavalli V, et al. Prognostic value of a combination of IPSS, flow rate and residual urine volume compared to pressure-flow studies in the preoperative evaluation of symptomatic BPH. Eur Urol. 2002;41(3):246.
32. Dicuio M, Vesely S, Knutson T, et al. Is it possible to predict post-residual voided urine by bladder scan before uroflowmetry — a useful and timesaving test to reduce the number of non-evaluable uroflow measurements? Arch Ital Urol Androl. 2010;82(2):100.
33. McVary KT, Roehrborn CG, Avins AL, et al. Update on AUA guideline on the management of benign prostatic hyperplasia. J Urol. 2011;185(5):1793.
34. Brown CT, Yap T, Cromwell DA, et al. Self-management for men with lower urinary tract symptoms: randomised controlled trial. BMJ. 2007;334(7583):25.
35. Djavan B, Marberger M. A meta-analysis on the efficacy and tolerability of alpha1-adrenoceptor antagonists in patients with lower urinary tract symptoms suggestive of benign prostatic obstruction. Eur Urol. 1999;36(1):1.
36. MacDonald R, Wilt TJ, Howe RW. Doxazosin for treating lower urinary tract symptoms compatible with benign prostatic obstruction: a systematic review of efficacy and adverse effects. BJU Int. 2004;94(9):1263.
37. MacDonald R, Wilt TJ. Alfuzosin for treatment of lower urinary tract symptoms compatible with benign prostatic hyperplasia: a systematic review of efficacy and adverse effects. Urology. 2004;66(4):780.

38. Rees J, Bultitude M, Challacombe B. The management of lower urinary tract symptoms in men. BMJ. 2014;348:g3861.
39. Lee M. Tamsulosin for the treatment of benign prostatic hyperplasia. Ann Pharmacother. 2000;43(2):188.
40. Roehrborn CG, Van Kerrebroeck P, Nording J. Safety and efficacy of alfuzosin 10 mg once-daily in the treatment of lower urinary tract symptoms and clinical benign prostatic hyperplasia: a pooled study of double-blinded randomized controlled trials. BJU Int. 2003;92(3):257.
41. Marks LS, Gittelman MC, Hill LA, et al. Rapid efficacy of the highly selective alpha1A-adrenoceptor antagonist silodosin in men with signs and symptoms of benign prostatic hyperplasia: pooled results of 2 phase-3 studies. J Urol. 2009;181(6):2634.
42. Wilt TJ, Macdonald R, Rutks I. WITHDRAWN: Tamsulosin for benign prostatic hyperplasia. Cochrane Database Syst Rev. 2011;9, CD002081.
43. Nickle JC, Gilling P, Tammela TL, et al. Comparison of dutasteride and finasteride for treating benign prostatic hyperplasia: the Enlarged Prostate International Comparator Study (EPICS). BJU Int. 2011;108(3):388–94.
44. Foley SJ, Soloman LZ, Wedderburn AW, et al. A prospective study of the natural history of hematuria associated with benign prostatic hyperplasia and effect of finasteride. J Urol. 2000;163(2):496.
45. Miller MI, Punchner PJ. Effects of finasteride on hematuria associated with benign prostatic hyperplasia: long term follow up. Urology. 1998;51(2):237.
46. http://www.fda.gov/Safety/MedWatch/SafetyInformation/SafetyAlertsforHumanMedicalProducts/ucm258529.htm.
47. Randall VA. Role of 5-alpha reductase inhibitor in health and disease. Ballieres Clin Endocrinol Metab. 1994;8(2):405–31.
48. Gacci M, Ficarra V, Sebastianelli A, et al. Impact of medical treatments for male lower urinary tract symptoms due to benign prostatic hyperplasia on ejaculatory function: a systematic review and meta-analysis. J Sex Med. 2014;11(6):1554–66.
49. Wessells H, Roy J, Bannow J, Grayhack J, et al. Incidence and severity of sexual adverse experiences in finasteride and placebo-treated men with benign prostatic hyperplasia. Urology. 2003;61(3):579.
50. Jacobsen SJ, Cheetham TC, Haque R, et al. Association between 5-alpha reductase inhibition and risk of hip fracture. JAMA. 2008;300(14):1660.
51. Liu L, Zheng S, Han P, et al. Phosphodiesterase-5 inhibitors for lower urinary tract symptoms secondary to benign prostatic hyperplasia: a systematic review and meta-analysis. Urology. 2011;77(1):123–9.
52. Laydner HK, Oliveira P, Oliveira CR, et al. Phosphodiesterase 5 inhibitors for lower urinary tract symptoms secondary to benign prostatic hyperplasia: a systematic review. BJU Int. 2011;107(7):1104–9.
53. Schwartz BG, Kloner RA. Drug interactions with phosphodiesterase-5 inhibitors used for the treatment of erectile dysfunction or pulmonary hypertension. Circulation. 2010;122(1):88–95.
54. http://www.americangeriatrics.org/health_care_professionals/clinical_practice/clinical_guidelines_recommendations/.
55. McConnell JD, Roehrborn CG, Bautista OM, et al. The long-term effect of doxazosin, finasteride, and combination therapy on the clinical progression of benign prostatic hyperplasia. N Engl J Med. 2003;349(25):2387.
56. Roehrborn CG, Siami P, Barkin J, et al. The effects of combination therapy with dutasteride and tamsulosin on clinical outcomes in men with symptomatic benign prostatic hyperplasia: 4-year results from the CombAT study. Eur Urol. 2010;57(1):123–31.
57. Kerrebroeck VP, Chapple C, Drogendijk T, et al. Combination therapy with solifenacin and tamsulosin oral controlled absorption system in a single tablet for lower urinary tract symptoms in men: efficacy and safety results from the randomised controlled NEPTUNE trial. Eru Urol. 2013;64(6):1003–12.
58. Drake MJ, Chapple C, Sokol R, et al. Long-term safety and efficacy of single-tablet combinations of solifenacin and tamsulosin oral controlled absorption system in men with storage and

voiding lower urinary tract symptoms: results from the NEPTUNE Study and NEPTUNE II open-label extension. Eur Urol. 2015;67(2):262–70.

59. http://www.nice.org.uk/guidance/CG97.

60. Barrette EP. Use of saw palmetto extract for benign prostatic hyperplasia. Altern Med Alert. 1998;1:1–4.

61. ACP Journal Club. Review: β-sitosterols improve urinary symptoms in the short term in men with benign prostatic hyperplasia. ACP J Club. 2000;132(3):94.

62. Tacklind J, MacDonald R, Rutks I, et al. Serenoa repens for benign prostatic hyperplasia. Cochrane Database Syst Rev. 2012;12, CD001423.

63. Feifer AH, Fleshner NE, Klotz L. Analytical accuracy and reliability of commonly used nutritional supplements in prostate disease. J Urol. 2002;168(1):150–4.

64. Wilt T, Ishani A, MacDonald R, et al. Beta-sitosterol for benign prostatic hyperplasia. Cochrane Database Syst Rev. 2000;2, CD001043.

65. Berges RR, Kassen A, Senge T. Treatment of symptomatic benign prostatic hyperplasia with beta-sitosterol: an 18-month follow up. BJU Int. 2000;85(7):842.

66. Wilt T, Ishani A, MacDonald R, et al. Pygeum africanum for benign prostatic hyperplasia. Cochrane Database Syst Rev. 2002;1, CD001044.

67. Melo EA, Bertero EB, Rios LA, et al. Evaluating the efficiency of a combination of Pygeum africanum and stinging nettle roots (Urtica Dioica) extracts in treating benign prostatic hyperplasia (BPH): double-blinded, randomized controlled trial. Int Braz J Urol. 2002;28(5):418–25.

68. Friederich M, Theurer C, Schiebel-Schlossor G. Prosta Prink Forte capsules in the treatment of benign prostatic hyperplasia: multicentric surveillance study in 2245 patients. Forsch Komplementamed Naturheilkd. 2000;7(4):200–4.

69. Wilt T, Ishani A, MacDonald R, et al. WITHDRAWN: Cernilton for benign prostatic hyperplasia. Cochrane Database Syst Rev. 2011;5, CD001042.

70. Johnstone PA, Bloom TL, Niemtzow RC, et al. A prospective, randomized pilot trial of acupuncture of the kidney-bladder distinct meridian for LUTS. J Urol. 2003;169(3):1037–9.

71. Li S, Lu A, Wang Y. Symptomatic comparison in efficacy on patients with benign prostatic hyperplasia treated with no therapeutic approaches. Complement Ther Med. 2010;18(1):21–7.

72. Selius BA, Subedi R. Urinary retention in adults: diagnosis and initial management. Am Fam Physician. 2008;77(5):643–50.

73. Reynard JM, Shearer RJ. Failure to void after transurethral resection of prostate and mode of presentation. Urology. 1999;53(2):336–9.

74. Roehrborn CG. Acute urinary retention: risks and management. Rev Urol. 2005;7 Suppl 4:S31–41.

75. Evans JM, Owens Jr TP, Zerbe DM, et al. Venous obstruction due to distended urinary bladder. Mayo Clin Proc. 1995;70(11):1077–9.

76. Duenas-Garcia OF, Rico H, Gorbea-Sanchez V, et al. Bladder rupture caused by post partum urinary retention. Obstet Gynecol. 2008;112(2 Pt 2):481–2.

77. Kreiger JN, Nyberg Jr L, Nickel JC. NIH consensus definition and classification of prostatitis. JAMA. 1999;282(3):236.

78. Etienne M, Pestel-Caron M, Chapuzet C, et al. Should blood cultures be performed for patients with acute prostatitis? J Clin Microbiol. 2010;48(5):1935–8.

79. Cornia PB, Takahashi TA, Lipsky BA. The microbiology of bacteriuria in men: a 5-year study at a Veterans' Affairs hospital. Diagn Microbiol Infect Dis. 2006;56(1):25.

80. Etienne M, Chavanet P, Sibert L, Michel F, et al. Acute bacterial prostatitis: heterogeneity in diagnostic criteria and management. Retrospective multicentric analysis of 371 patients diagnosed with acute prostatitis. BMC Infect Dis. 2008;8:12.

81. Wagenlehner FM, Weidner W, Naber KG. Therapy for prostatitis with emphasis on bacterial prostatitis. Expert Opin Pharmacother. 2007;8(11):1667.

82. Chia JK, Longfield RN, Cook DH, et al. Computed axial tomography in the early diagnosis of prostatic abscess. Am J Med. 1986;81(5):942.

83. Ludwig M, Schroeder-Printzen I, Schiefer HG, et al. Diagnosis and therapeutic management of 18 patients with prostatic abscess. Urology. 1999;53(2):340–5.
84. Trauzzi SJ, Kay CJ, Kaufman DG, et al. Management of prostatic abscess in patients with human immunodeficiency syndrome. Urology. 1994;43(5):729.
85. Potts JM. Chronic pelvic pain syndrome: a non-prostatocentric perspective. World J Urol. 2003;21(2):54.
86. Turner JA, Ciol MA, Von Korff M, et al. Validity and responsiveness of the national institutes of health chronic prostatitis symptom index. J Urol. 2003;169(2):580.
87. Anothaisintawee T, Attia J, Nickel JC, et al. Management of chronic prostatitis/chronic pelvic pain syndrome: a systematic review and network meta-analysis. JAMA. 2011;305(1):78.
88. Wagenlehner FM, Schneider H, Ludwig M, et al. A pollen extract (Cernilton) in patients with inflammatory chronic prostatitis-chronic pelvic pain syndrome: a multicentre, randomised, prospective, double-blind, placebo-controlled phase 3 study. Eur Urol. 2009;56(3):544.
89. Shoskes DA, Zeitlin SI, Shahed A, et al. Quercetin in men with category III chronic prostatitis: a preliminary prospective, double-blind, placebo-controlled trial. Urology. 1999;54(6):960.

Chapter 12
Testicular, Scrotal, and Penile Disorders

Michael A. Malone and Ahad Shiraz

Conditions Presenting with Acute Scrotal Pain

The most common causes of acute scrotal pain in adults are testicular torsion and epididymitis. Other conditions that should be considered in patients presenting with acute scrotal pain include Fournier's gangrene, torsion of the appendix testis, trauma, testicular cancer, inguinal hernia, vasculitis, mumps, and referred pain from the lower abdomen or groin. The evaluation of acute scrotal pain can be challenging, because laboratory and physical examination in conditions causing acute scrotal pain may be limited by patient guarding, and physical findings can overlap with other condition. If the history, examination, and imaging do not supply a clear diagnosis, then surgical exploration is mandatory [1].

Torsion of the Appendix Testis

Torsion of the appendix testis is the leading cause of acute scrotal pathology in childhood and most cases occur between the ages of 7 and 14 years [2, 3]. Torsion of the appendix testis rarely occurs in adults [4]. The onset of testicular pain from torsion of the appendix testis ranges from mild to severe and generally has a more gradual onset than testicular torsion.

M.A. Malone, MD (✉) • A. Shiraz, MD
Department of Family and Community Medicine, Penn State College of Medicine,
Hershey, PA, USA
e-mail: mmalone@hmc.psu.edu; ashiraz@hmc.psu.edu

© Springer International Publishing Switzerland 2016
J.J. Heidelbaugh (ed.), *Men's Health in Primary Care*, Current Clinical Practice,
DOI 10.1007/978-3-319-26091-4_12

225

On physical examination, a reactive hydrocele is commonly present that may transilluminate, and tenderness can often be localized to the appendix testis on the anterosuperior testis. Careful inspection of the scrotal wall at this location may detect the classic "blue dot" sign, caused by infarction and necrosis of the appendix testis [5]. If the diagnosis is unclear after the exam, then a testicular ultrasound can be performed that will show the torsed appendage as a lesion of low echogenicity and normal blood flow to the testis.

Management of acute torsion of the appendix testis usually includes conservative treatment, which includes rest, ice, and nonsteroidal anti-inflammatory drugs (NSAIDs) [6]. Recovery is generally slow with this approach, and pain may last for several weeks to months. Surgical excision of the appendix testis is reserved for patients who have persistent pain.

Fournier's Gangrene (Necrotizing Fasciitis of the Perineum)

Fournier's gangrene is a necrotizing fasciitis of the perineum caused by a mixed aerobic and anaerobic bacterial infection [7]. The overall incidence is about 1.6/100,000 males, and it typically presents with severe pain that starts on the anterior abdominal wall that migrates into the gluteal muscles and onto the scrotum and penis. Pain is accompanied by edema, blisters, bullae, fever, tachycardia, and hypotension. Computerized tomography (CT) and magnetic resonance imaging (MRI) may be helpful in showing air along the fascial planes or deeper tissue involvement [8] (see Fig. 12.1). Treatment of necrotizing fasciitis consists of early and aggressive surgical debridement, antibiotic therapy, and hemodynamic support as needed [7].

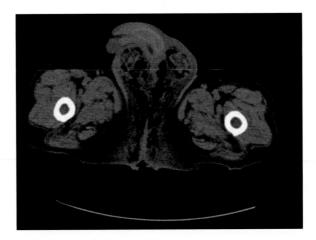

Fig. 12.1 CT scan of a patient with Fournier's gangrene showing emphysematous gangrene of perineum and scrotum. http://openi.nlm.nih.gov/detailedresult.php?img=3867231_mjhid-5-1-e2013067f1&query=fournier%27s%20gangrene&it=xg&req=4&npos=80

Treatment of Fournier gangrene includes broad spectrum antibiotics to cover gram positives, gram negatives, and anaerobes. A quinolone and clindamycin or an extended spectrum IV penicillin in combination with clindamycin or metronidazole can be used empirically.

Orchitis

Orchitis is an acute inflammatory reaction of one or both testicles. It is usually caused by a coliform bacterial infection or by the mumps virus. Bacterial orchitis can also be caused by sexually transmitted infections (STIs), particularly gonorrhea or chlamydia [9]. With the exception of mumps orchitis, isolated orchitis without epididymitis is uncommon, particularly in adults. Orchitis is a common complication of mumps infection with fever and parotitis preceding the onset of orchitis [10]. Patients often report severe unilateral or bilateral testicular pain, as well as scrotal swelling and erythema. Patients with orchitis are treated symptomatically with ice packs, scrotal elevation, and NSAIDs [10].

For suspected bacterial orchitis, pathogens are similar to those in epididymitis, and a single 250 mg IM dose of ceftriaxone and 100 mg of doxycycline twice daily for 10 days would be recommended. If epididymitis is thought to be caused by coliform bacteria, treatment should include ofloxacin 300 mg twice daily for 10 days or levofloxacin 500 mg daily for 10 days [9].

Epididymitis

Introduction Epididymitis is one of the most common causes of scrotal pain in the outpatient setting, and there are approximately 600,000 cases per year diagnosed in the USA [9]. In a study with 121 patients diagnosed in the outpatient setting with acute epididymitis, a bimodal distribution was seen with peak incidence occurring in men 16–30 years old and then between the ages of 51 and 70 years [11]. In younger men, epididymitis is typically caused by sexually transmitted infections (STIs) such as *Neisseria gonorrhoeae* or *Chlamydia trachomatis*. In patients younger than 14 years or greater than 35 years, the usual pathogen involved is *E. coli*.

Clinical Presentation The common presenting history provided by the patient will describe a steady and gradual increase in testicular pain that may radiate to the lower abdomen. Symptoms typical of urinary tract infection (UTI) such as fever, increased frequency, dysuria, and hematuria may also be present [9].

Physical Exam It is important to examine the patient while he is in a standing position. Key findings on exam include tenderness to palpation of the affected testicle, epididymis, or the spermatic cord [12]. There may also be swelling and induration of the testicle at the epididymis [9]. Pain relief with testicular elevation (Prehn's sign) and a normal cremasteric reflex are important physical exam findings which aid in differentiating from testicular torsion.

Evaluation A proper evaluation should include a urinalysis and urine culture, in addition to nucleic acid amplification testing (NAAT), and a gram stain and culture of the urethral discharge [9, 12].

Treatment A combination of antibiotics (if the cause is determined to be infectious), NSAIDs, and scrotal elevation is the standard treatment [13]. Empiric treatment should not be delayed yet should be initiated based on the most likely pathogen(s). For patients younger than 35 years of age, gonococcal or chlamydial infections are the usual pathogens and should be treated with 250 mg of ceftriaxone IM and a single dose of 1 g azithromycin or alternatively doxycycline 100 mg daily for 10 days [9]. If enteric organisms are suspected or if the patient is either greater than 35 years of age, younger than 14 years of age, or a male who practices insertive anal intercourse, then fluoroquinolones such as ofloxacin 300 mg twice daily for 10 days or levofloxacin 500 mg daily for 10 days, along with ceftriaxone IM, should be prescribed [2, 3].

Testicular Torsion

Testicular torsion generally presents with the abrupt onset of severe testicular pain and should be considered in all patients presenting with acute scrotal pain. Testicular torsion results from inadequate fixation of the testis to the tunica vaginalis causing the testis to twist on the spermatic cord. Testicular torsion often occurs within a few hours after an inciting traumatic event or can occur spontaneously. There may be associated nausea and vomiting. Another typical presentation, particularly in children, is awakening with scrotal pain in the middle of the night or in the morning, likely related to cremasteric contraction with nocturnal sexual stimulation during the rapid eye movement (REM) sleep cycle.

Epidemiology Testicular torsion is a urologic emergency that is more common in neonates and postpubertal young men but can occur at any age [14]. In one retrospective review, approximately 40 % of the cases of testicular torsion occurred in men aged 21 years and older [15]. The prevalence of testicular torsion in adult patients hospitalized with acute scrotal pain is approximately 25–50 % [14, 16].

Exam A physical exam is useful in the evaluation of testicular torsion but is not always definitive. Profound testicular swelling occurs early in the course of torsion, while a reactive hydrocele and overlying erythema of the scrotal wall are typically later findings (>12 h). On exam, the testis is typically tender and retracted (see Fig. 12.2a). The cremasteric reflex is almost always absent, which helps to distinguish testicular torsion from epididymitis which typically has an intact cremasteric reflex. The cremasteric reflex should be assessed by stroking or gently pinching the skin of the upper thigh while observing the ipsilateral testis. A normal response is cremasteric contraction with elevation of the ipsilateral testis, while the examiner strokes or gently pinches the skin of the upper thigh. The classic finding on physical examination is an asymmetrically high-riding testis on the affected side with the long axis of the testis oriented transversely instead of longitudinally secondary to shortening of the spermatic cord from the torsion, also called the "bell clapper deformity." [17] While an abnormal testicular lie is helpful when present, it occurs in fewer than 50 % of cases [17].

It may be possible to detorse a testis during examination by gentle rotation. The classic teaching is that the testis usually rotates medially during torsion and can be detorsed by rotating it outward toward the thigh. However, lateral rotation can occur in up to one-third of cases. The degree of twisting of the testis may range from 180° to 720°, requiring multiple rounds of detorsion [18]. Successful detorsion is suggested by relief of pain, resolution of the transverse lie of the testis to a longitudinal orientation, lowering the position of the testis in the scrotum, and the return of normal blood flow detected with a color Doppler study [19]. However, almost all patients will re-torse after manual detorsion, so this maneuver is only useful to allow for an urgent rather than emergent definitive surgical fixation.

Diagnosis The diagnosis of testicular torsion is usually determined by acute onset of severe testicular pain, abnormal testicular lie, and an absent cremasteric reflex. An ultrasound evaluation is necessary in equivocal cases.

Imaging/Evaluation If the etiology of an acute scrotal process is equivocal after history and physical examination, then color Doppler ultrasonography is the diagnostic test of choice to differentiate testicular torsion from other causes, including epididymitis [1]. Doppler ultrasonography has a sensitivity and specificity of 82 and 100 %, respectively, for the diagnosis of testicular torsion [20]. Subsequent studies have confirmed the high sensitivity and specificity of ultrasound in the diagnosis of

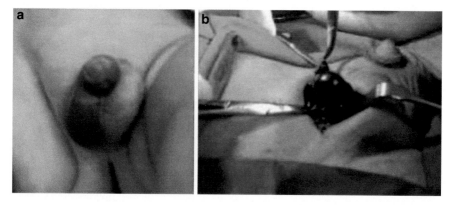

Fig. 12.2 Testicular torsion. (**a**) Erythema of the scrotum over torted testis. (**b**) Intraoperative photo showing torted gangrenous testis. http://openi.nlm.nih.gov/detailedresult.php?img=3564080_IJPD-22-281-g004&query=testicular%20torsion&it=xg&req=4&npos=3

testicular torsion, yet results may depend on the individual ultrasound technique [21]. If there is no immediate access to ultrasound or if ultrasound does not exclude testicular torsion, then prompt surgical exploration is required [1].

Treatment Patients suspected of having testicular torsion should be sent immediately to an emergency room for urological surgical evaluation. Treatment for suspected testicular torsion is immediate surgical exploration with intraoperative detorsion and fixation of the testes. Detorsion and fixation of both the involved testis and the contralateral uninvolved testis should be performed since inadequate gubernacular fixation is usually a bilateral defect [18]. Delay in detorsion of a few hours may lead to progressively higher rates of non-viability of the testis. If surgical treatment is not immediately available, then manual detorsion should be performed. Surgical exploration is necessary even after clinically successful manual detorsion to prevent recurrence, and residual torsion may be present that can be further relieved [22]. The testicular salvage rate for surgery appears to be better in children than in adults, although part of this may be related to more extensive twisting in adults with torsion [15].

Complications Potential complications of testicular torsion include ischemia from reduced arterial inflow and venous outflow obstruction (see Fig. 12.2b). It is generally felt that the testis suffers irreversible damage after 12 h of ischemia due to testicular torsion [23]. Infertility may result, even with a normal contralateral testis, because the exposure of sperm to the bloodstream can lead to the development of antisperm antibodies [24].

Painless Scrotal Mass/Swelling

Varicocele

Introduction A varicocele is an external manifestation of a collection of dilated and tortuous spermatic veins (see Figs. 12.3 and 12.4). It is thought that this is a result of increased hydrostatic pressure of incompetent valves in the testicular venous system resulting in reflux [25]. Most varicoceles are left sided, due to right angle insertion of the left testicular vein into the left renal vein [26]. The overall incidence of varicocele in the healthy male population is between 10 and 15 % and typically appears soon after puberty [27]. The clinical importance of a varicocele is its association with infertility, but the impact of varicocele on fertility and the benefits of treatment remain controversial [26].

Clinical Presentation Males with varicocele are often asymptomatic and it is recognized on routine physical examination [27].

Physical Exam The patient should first be examined in the standing position so that the examiner can inspect the scrotum [27]. On palpation a varicocele has been

Fig. 12.3 Varicocele: photograph of a large left grade III varicocele that can be seen through the scrotal skin. http://openi.nlm.nih.gov/detailedresult.php?img=3093801_cln-66-04-691-g002&query=varicocele&it=xg&req=4&npos=17

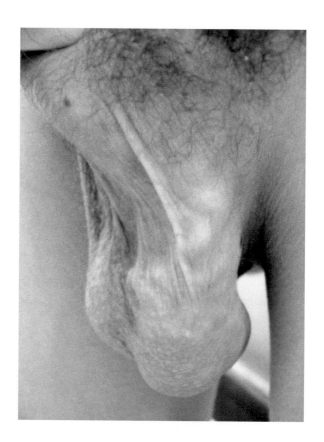

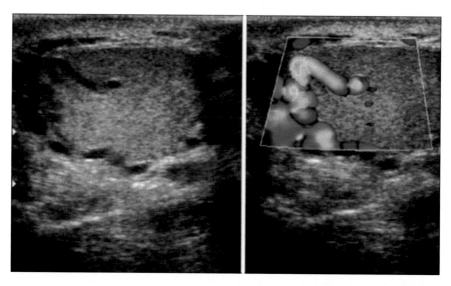

Fig. 12.4 Ultrasonography (*left*) and color Doppler study (*right*) show subcapsular and mediastinal location of intratesticular varicocele. https://openi.nlm.nih.gov/detailedresult.php?img=3761996_NJS-18-92-g003&query=varicocele&it=xg&req=4&npos=2

classically described as a "bag of worms" but may also feel like a thickened, asymmetric cord if it is subtle [27]. There are various grades of varicocele that can be distinguished:

Grade 1: palpable with Valsalva maneuver only
Grade 2: palpable at rest but not visible
Grade 3: palpable and visible at rest [26]

Idiopathic varicocele is more apparent in the upright position and disappears when the patient is supine [27]. The examiner may also not be able to note any abnormality at rest or with Valsalva; however, an ultrasound may discover a subclinical varicocele as well [26].

Evaluation An ultrasound of the scrotum is a widely used test to assess for a varicocele [25]. In men with varicoceles and an abnormal semen analysis, it is recommended that an endocrine work-up be performed with serum testosterone and follicle-stimulating hormone (FSH) levels [26]. Furthermore, a referral should be made to a urologist and/or reproductive endocrine and infertility specialist.

Treatment There are many available treatment modalities for varicoceles, and they depend on the severity of the varicocele. There are a variety of operative and nonoperative techniques such as percutaneous radiological, open surgical, laparoscopic, and microsurgical techniques. The goal of the surgery is to ligate the veins contributing to the varicocele formation while at the same time leaving some veins patent to drain [25]. Interestingly, a 2001 Cochrane review of the effect of varicocelectomy or embolization on fertility was inconclusive [26].

   Current literature suggests surgical treatment to be offered to adolescents that meet the following criteria [25]:

1. Testicular growth arrest, defined as 2 SD from normal testicular growth curves, more than 2 mL difference between left and right testicles
2. Those with abnormal semen analysis with high-grade varicocele
3. Those with symptoms such as pain, heaviness, and swelling
4. Bilateral varicoceles

Epididymal Cysts and Spermatoceles

Spermatoceles and epididymal cysts are typically painless, fluid-filled cysts of the head of the epididymis. Epididymal cysts are often grouped with spermatoceles and the two may be impossible to differentiate based on gross anatomy [28]. A distinction between spermatoceles and epididymal cysts is that spermatocele fluid typically contains sperm. Spermatoceles are also typically larger than epididymal cysts [28]. Spermatoceles and epididymal cysts rarely cause symptoms such as pain and are often discovered incidently by the examiner or patient. Although the cause of a spermatocele is often unknown, it may be caused by obstruction of the epididymal ducts. There is an increased risk of epididymal cysts and spermatoceles in those with DES exposure in utero and with Von Hippel-Lindau disease [29]. Differential diagnoses include hydrocele, varicocele, hernia, and neoplasm.

Exam On physical exam, spermatoceles and epididymal cysts usually feel smooth, soft, well-circumscribed, and transilluminate (see Fig. 12.5). Failure to transilluminate suggests a solid lesion, which warrants further evaluation, including scrotal ultrasonography and possible inguinal exploration [30]. Spermatoceles and epididymal cysts are palpated as distinct from the testis, which differentiates them from hydroceles and testicular cancer.

Evaluation Spermatoceles and epididymal cysts are often easily differentiated from other scrotal pathology based on history and exam. However, if there is uncertainty, they can be diagnosed by scrotal ultrasonography [30].

Treatment Treatment of spermatoceles and epididymal cysts is typically reassurance and surveillance. Occasionally, patients require surgical excision for chronic pain related to a spermatocele.

Fig. 12.5 (**a**) Ultrasonic and (**b**) intraoperative images: the paratesticular mass, found to be an epididymal cyst was excised. Ref: http://openi. nlm.nih.gov/legacy/ detailedresult. php?img=3135104_ CRIM2011- 389857.002&query=epidid ymalcyst&req=4&npos=2 &prt

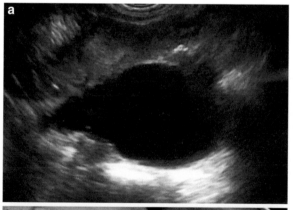

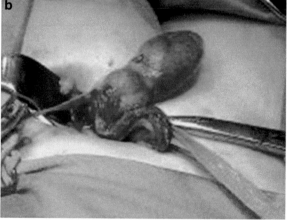

Hydrocele

A hydrocele is a collection of peritoneal fluid in the scrotum between the parietal and visceral layers of the tunica vaginalis [31]. Hydroceles are believed to arise from an imbalance of secretion and reabsorption of fluid from the tunica vaginalis [32]. Symptoms of pain and disability generally increase with size, and hydroceles can range from small collections of fluid to several liters. Hydroceles may be communicating or noncommunicating. Communicating hydroceles usually develop as a result of the failure of the processus vaginalis to close during development, while in noncommunicating hydroceles, the processus vaginalis is not patent. Noncommunicating hydroceles have no connection to the peritoneum; the fluid comes from the mesothelial lining of the tunica vaginalis [32]. Hydroceles are common in newborns, and whether communicating or noncommunicating, hydroceles usually resolve spontaneously by the first birthday, unless they are accompanied by an inguinal hernia [31, 32].

Causes Idiopathic hydroceles are the most common type of hydrocele and usually arise over a significant period of time. Idiopathic hydroceles are often asymptomatic, despite considerable scrotal enlargement. Other conditions such as inflammatory disorders of the scrotum (e.g., epididymitis, torsion, appendiceal torsion), trauma, and testicular cancer can produce an acute reactive hydrocele, which often resolves with treatment or resolution of the underlying condition [31]. Conditions resulting in generalized edema such as protein losing enteropathy, hepatic cirrhosis, and nephrotic syndrome can also cause a hydrocele.

Clinical Presentation Patients with hydroceles often present with a painless swelling or mass which may appear unilateral or bilateral in the scrotum. Patients may also report a sensation of heaviness in the scrotum. Significant discomfort should alert the clinician to consider a reactive hydrocele from another cause.

Exam Examination of patients with hydroceles should include palpation of the entire testicular surface for findings of epididymal tenderness, testicular torsion, trauma, or mass/tumor as the primary etiology [33]. Hydrocele fluid in the scrotal sac transilluminates well, which differentiates the process from hematocele, hernia, or solid mass (see Fig. 12.6). A hydrocele that communicates with the peritoneal cavity may increase in size with the Valsalva maneuver. Hydroceles discovered in infancy are usually communicating and usually disappear in the recumbent position, and an indirect hernia is often appreciated on exam. Communicating hydroceles are usually reducible, while noncommunicating hydroceles are not reducible.

Diagnosis The diagnosis of hydrocele can be made by physical examination and transillumination of the scrotum demonstrating a cystic fluid collection. A scrotal ultrasound should be performed if the diagnosis is in question since a reactive hydrocele can occur in the presence of a testicular neoplasm or with acute inflammatory scrotal conditions.

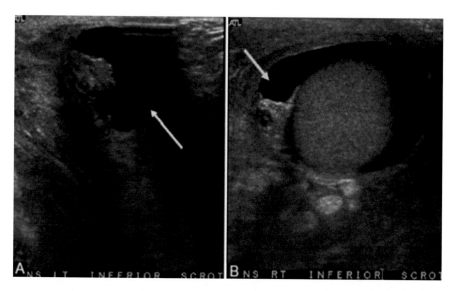

Fig. 12.6 *Left* (**a**) and *right* (**b**) transverse images demonstrate bilateral hydroceles (*arrows*) in a patient with blunt scrotal trauma. http://openi.nlm.nih.gov/detailedresult.php?img=3698892_IJRI-22-293-g004&query=hydrocele&it=xg&req=4&npos=26

Management/Treatment In adults, no therapy is needed unless the hydrocele causes discomfort and compromises scrotal skin integrity from chronic irritation or if there is an underlying cause that required treatment [31, 34]. The management of hydrocele in a neonate or child younger than 1 year of age usually is supportive [31]. In children, surgical repair is indicated for hydroceles in newborns that persist beyond 1 year of age, for communicating hydroceles, and for other symptomatic hydroceles that are enlarging [31]. Reactive hydroceles usually resolve with treatment of the underlying condition. If surgical repair is required, the most common treatment is surgical excision of the hydrocele sac. Simple aspiration of a hydrocele is generally unsuccessful due to rapid re-accumulation of fluid.

Complications Communicating hydroceles in older men rarely resolve and pose a risk for the development of an incarcerated inguinal hernia [31, 33, 34].

Testicular Cancer

Testicular cancer accounts for only 1 % of all cancers in men, but it is the most common solid malignancy affecting males between the ages of 18 and 40 years [35]. The age-adjusted incidence and death rates of testicular cancer were 5.5 cases and 0.2 deaths per 100,000 men per year. Worldwide, the incidence and death rates for testicular cancer were similar: 4.6 cases and 0.3 deaths per 100,000 men per year [36].

In the USA, more than 95 % of men diagnosed with testicular cancer were alive 5 years later [37]. Greater than 90 % of testicular cancers are *germ cell tumors*, and these are divided evenly between seminomas and non-seminomatous germ cell tumors [38, 39]. Many testicular cancers contain both seminoma and non-seminoma cells. There are two main subtypes of seminoma tumors: classical seminomas and spermatocytic seminomas. Non-seminomatous subtypes include embryonal carcinomas, teratomas, yolk sac tumors, and choriocarcinomas. Testicular germ cell tumors are one of the most curable solid neoplasms, with an overall cure rate greater than 90 % [40].

Risk Factors There are a number of known risk factors for testicular neoplasia, including cryptorchidism, a personal or family history of testicular cancer, infertility or subfertility, hypospadias, white males, family history, and HIV infection [41–45]. Studies investigating the contribution of prenatal and later environmental exposures, such as endocrine disruptors and estrogen/antiandrogen components, to testicular cancer risk have yielded inconsistent results [42, 46]. It has been suggested that vasectomy may increase the risk of testicular cancer, but data does not support this association [47]. Men who are at high risk for testicular cancer should consider regular testicular exams with a healthcare provider and self-examination. However, the US Preventive Services Task Force (USPSTF) recommends against testicular cancer screening in the general population [48]. This recommendation is based on inadequate evidence that screening asymptomatic patients by means of self-examination or clinician examination has greater yield or accuracy for detecting testicular cancer at more curable stages and potential harms of false-positive results, anxiety, and harms from diagnostic tests or procedures. The USPSTF notes, "Screening by self-examination or clinician examination is unlikely to offer meaningful health benefits, given the very low incidence and high cure rate of even advanced testicular cancer" [48].

Clinical Presentation Testicular cancer usually presents as a painless mass discovered by the patient or clinician on physical examination. However, in approximately 10 % of cases, rapidly growing germ cell tumors may cause acute scrotal pain secondary to hemorrhage and infarction. Other presenting symptoms include testicular firmness, swelling, an aching in the lower abdomen, and scrotal heaviness. In approximately 10 % of cases, the presenting manifestations of testicular cancer are attributable to metastatic disease including gynecomastia, gastrointestinal symptoms such as dull abdominal pain that can radiate to the groin area, or respiratory symptoms such as cough, chest pain, and shortness of breath [38, 49]. Rare presentations include those of Leydig cell tumors, which account for 2 % of testicular tumors and have a clinical presentation dominated by symptoms of excess estrogen and reduced testosterone such as gynecomastia, breast tenderness, fatigue, and decreased sexual drive. Sertoli cell tumors are even less common and also present with symptoms of excess estrogen [38].

Exam The initial evaluation of a man with a suspected testicular tumor should include a detailed and thorough physical examination of the scrotum. Small, benign calcifications on the surface of the testis are relatively commonly detected on

Fig. 12.7 An 8-year-old
black male with testicular
cancer. http://phil.cdc.gov/
phil/details.aspID#4411

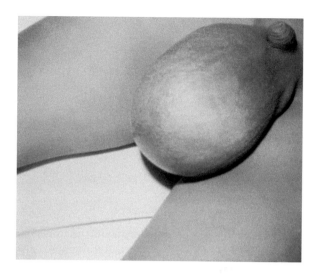

physical examination and are not cause for alarm but should be well documented and followed on repeat examinations to document stability. Intrascrotal malignancies are usually firm, non-tender, nonmobile masses that *do not transilluminate*, although a reactive hydrocele may be evident with transillumination (see Fig. 12.7). Some patients may have accompanying gynecomastia resulting from excess estrogen production with various tumors.

Diagnosis The diagnostic evaluation of men with suspected testicular cancer includes scrotal ultrasound, measurement of serum tumor markers including alpha fetoprotein and beta human chorionic gonadotropin, radical inguinal orchiectomy, and in some cases, retroperitoneal lymph node dissection. Scrotal ultrasound is the initial test of choice to diagnose testicular cancer [50]. Although pathology is the definitive diagnostic test, scrotal ultrasound may help to distinguish intrinsic from extrinsic testicular lesions. Several conditions may mimic neoplasia on ultrasound, including inflammation, hematoma, infarction, fibrosis, and tubular ectasia. In cases in which the ultrasound is inconclusive, MRI may help differentiate benign from malignant lesions [51].

Testicular biopsy is commonly not performed as part of the evaluation due to concern that it may result in tumor seeding into the scrotal sac or metastatic spread of tumor into the inguinal nodes. A high-resolution CT scan of the abdomen and pelvis and a chest radiograph should be performed to evaluate for possible metastatic disease. A chest CT is recommended if the chest radiograph is abnormal or if metastatic disease involving the thorax is strongly suspected [52]. CT or MRI of the brain is performed if brain metastases are suspected. Men suspected of having a testicular cancer should have serum levels of alpha fetoprotein (AFP) and the beta subunit of human chorionic gonadotropin (beta-hCG) measured, as above. Although serum tumor markers can be helpful at the time of initial diagnosis of a testicular cancer and for prognostication, their main utility is for subsequent follow-up of disease status after treatment.

Treatment Men diagnosed with testicular tumors should be referred to a urologist for appropriate treatment based on the type of tumor and disease stage. Treatment of testicular cancer involves radical orchiectomy to provide local tumor control but may also include radiation, chemotherapy, or retroperitoneal lymph node dissection. Prior to definitive treatment, the possible need for cryopreservation of sperm should also be considered.

Penile Disorders

Phimosis/Paraphimosis

Introduction Phimosis is defined as the inability to withdraw the penile foreskin or prepuce behind the glans. Approximately 96 % of males are noted at birth to have phimosis which is physiologic and considered to be normal at that time in life [53]. The foreskin gradually becomes more retractable over a period of time that ranges from birth to 18 years old aided by naturally occurring erections and keratinization of inner epithelium [53]. Paraphimosis is a urologic emergency that occurs when the foreskin is retracted, often forcibly, but cannot be reduced back due to venous and lymphatic congestion [54]. This is considered to be an emergency because it can cause a lack of blood flow to the glans penis and result in tissue necrosis and permanent damage. In the young infant or toddler, this condition is often caused by parents attempting to clean the infant's penis. In the adolescent or sexually active male, it may be caused by intercourse or improper manipulation such as catheter insertion. Patients with paraphimosis often present with marked penile pain and swelling, as well as significant concern over the condition.

Physical Exam With physiologic phimosis, the prepuce puckers on gentle traction and the overlying tissue appears pink and healthy. If there is a pathologic phimosis with inflammation or infection, there is usually a history of pain, skin irritation, local infection, bleeding, dysuria preputial pain, frequent UTIs, painful erections and intercourse, and weak urinary stream [53]. On exam, there is typically swelling and tenderness of the glans penis, as well as tenderness and swelling of the retracted foreskin. The shaft of the penis will be unaffected [55] (see Fig. 12.8).

Evaluation The diagnosis of phimosis is classically a clinical diagnosis that does not necessitate any specific laboratory or diagnostic imaging. However, if there are recurrent UTIs or local skin infections, then pertinent laboratory data should be collected including a complete blood count (CBC) [53]. Paraphimosis is a urological emergency that should necessitate an urgent urology consultation; however, the diagnosis is also clinical in nature as indicated by history and physical exam findings.

Fig. 12.8 Acquired
phimosis with tight scar.
Ref: http://openi.nlm.nih.
gov/legacy/detailedresult.
php?img=3954356_
rcse9406-e186-02&query=
phimoses&req=4&npos=2
&prt

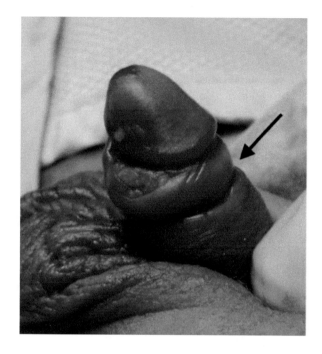

Treatment The management of physiologic phimosis is purely conservative. Along
with reassurance that it is normal for the child's age group, parents should be
instructed on how to properly clean the foreskin and glans. Over time, this practice
will aid in making the foreskin more retractile. Topical corticosteroids have been
utilized with efficacy reported between 65 and 95 % for pathological phimosis.
Another treatment modality is nonsurgical adhesiolysis in the outpatient setting
which is also quite effective in yielding resolution. There are multiple methods for
stretching, but one method is to grasp the foreskin opening and gently pull on each
side until it feels uncomfortably stretched but not actually painful. In this practice,
the foreskin is gently stretched and dilated over the course of numerous visits, and
finally circumcision for definitive therapy [53].

Treatment of paraphimosis revolves around swift recognition and reduction. It is
recommended to take the least invasive to most invasive approach in treatment.
Adequate analgesia is the first step via application of ice to the area if there are no
signs of penile ischemia, as this commonly aids in the reduction of swelling [56]. In
addition, compression wraps [57] and application of osmotic agents such as granulated sugar or 50 % dextrose-soaked gauze over the edematous skin region can be
applied [58, 59]. If these modalities are effective, then the clinician may proceed
with manual reduction of the edematous foreskin. If these conservative measures
fail, then an emergent urology consultation should be obtained.

Priapism

Introduction Priapism is generally defined as a painful erection persisting for four or more hours that is unrelated to sexual stimulation. There are two basic types of priapism that are discussed in the literature, namely, ischemic and nonischemic. Ischemic priapism has been described as a compartment syndrome of the penis that may lead to irreversible tissue damage and necrosis and erectile dysfunction [60]. It may occur because of either inability of blood to flow out of the penis through penile veins and/or the failure of the smooth muscle within the spongy erectile tissue to contract appropriately [60]. Mixed venous blood is unable to adequately flow out of the penis causing increased pressure and ischemia within the corporal bodies [61]. Nonischemic priapism, also known as "high-flow" priapism, is more uncommon and is usually a result of trauma. It occurs with unregulated arterial blood flow into the corpora cavernosa due to rupture of a branch of the cavernosal artery [60]. The incidence of priapism has been reported to be approximately 1.5 cases per 100,000 men and can occur at any age, from newborn to the elderly. There appears to be a bimodal distribution in incidence in children from ages 5 to 10 years and in adults ages 20 to 50 years [62].

Physical Exam On physical examination, the extent of penile tumescence and rigidity in addition to corporal body involvement and tenderness is essential to note and document [61]. In ischemic priapism, the corpora cavernosa are rigid and very tender to palpation [61]. Nonischemic priapism should be suspected when there is minimal to no pain upon history gathering, and on exam the penis is engorged or partially erect [60]. In cases of nonischemic priapism, there is often a clear history of trauma to the perineum or penis [60, 62].

Evaluation A thorough evaluation of the man with suspected priapism should include a complete blood count with differential (CBCPD). A hemoglobin electrophoresis should be considered in all men to assess for sickle cell disease, sickle cell trait, or any other hemoglobinopathies [63]. A urine toxicology screen may be useful if medications are suspected that can cause priapism, specifically trazodone [60, 63]. Phlebotomy directly from the corpus cavernosum of a patient with ischemic priapism for venous blood gas analysis will display dark and hypoxic blood with a low PO2 and elevated PCO2; the blood gas analysis will be normal in the patient with nonischemic priapism [60–63]. In addition, a color duplex Doppler ultrasound is useful in differentiating ischemic from nonischemic priapism. In cases of ischemic priapism, there is minimal or absent blood flow to the corpora cavernosa observed, whereas normal to high blood flow velocities are seen in nonischemic priapism [60–63].

Treatment First-line management of ischemic priapism includes aspiration of blood from one of the corpora cavernosa followed by irrigation with normal saline [60–63]. This first-line therapy is successful 24–36 % of cases according to one study [61]. If there is no relief of pressure and pain, then direct application of an alpha-1 adrenergic agonist such as phenylephrine is highly effective in achieving complete penile detumescence and can be applied every 5 min [60, 62, 63]. One study determined that there is approximately 100 % resolution of the acute event if treated in this manner within the first 12 h of onset of symptoms [60, 62].

First-line treatment of nonischemic priapism should be close clinical surveillance. In some cases rest (lying supine, avoidance of sexual activity), ice packs, and time have been shown to lead to spontaneous resolution in most cases [60]. Current evidence also shows that there is a lack of significant pathological damage and maintenance of good erectile function even with long-standing cases [62]. If, however, after discussing risks and benefits of intervention, the patient desires definitive resolution, then one option is super-selective embolization of the implicating vessel via interventional radiology [60–63].

Peyronie's Disease

Introduction Peyronie's disease is an acquired disorder of the penis in which there is penile tissue fibrosis of the tunica albuginea, a curved deformity with erections, pain, and an association with erectile dysfunction. The pathophysiology and causative factors of Peyronie's disease are not completely understood but are thought to be benign in nature and without systemic sequelae. The most plausible proposed etiology of this disorder stems from repeated minor trauma to the penis and aberrant wound healing [64–66]. Considering that this condition is in essence a disorder of fibrosis, collagen synthesis is abnormally increased in respect to collagen breakdown [65]. The condition predominantly affects men aged 40–60 years with an incidence of approximately 0.3–3 % over the man's life [67].

History/Physical Exam History questions oriented toward duration of illness, presence or absence or resolution of pain, an estimation of degree of penile deformity (some men may show the clinician pictures for documentation), and orientation of the bend [64]. Presenting symptoms may include penile curvature or shortening during erection, penile pain, and erectile and/or ejaculatory dysfunction [66]. On exam, there may be a palpable plaque or area of induration, commonly on the dorsal aspect and less common on the lateral or ventral aspects of the penis [66].

Evaluation Although diagnosis of priapism is usually based on clinical exam, an evaluation of the patient often includes ultrasonography to image and quantifies calcified and soft tissue. A duplex Doppler is also utilized for assessing vascular status if a reconstructive procedure is being considered [66]. MRI has recently been a new modality used to evaluate penile morphology in individuals with Peyronie's disease, which can provide insight into active or non-active status of the disease [67].

Treatment There are numerous medications and modalities that are used to treat Peyronie's disease. However, there are only a few prospective, blinded, randomized, placebo-controlled studies with standardized outcomes of sufficient power to evaluate any of the therapies [64]. It has been proposed that the antioxidant role of Vitamin

E could reverse or stabilize pathologic changes in the tunica albuginea [65]. Vitamin E was the first oral therapy for Peyronie's disease and is currently first-line therapy at a recommended dose of Vitamin E is 400 IU per day [66]. There are other oral medications that can be tried, without significant efficacy data. Colchicine is an oral anti-microtubule agent that inhibits collagen secretion and is administered at a dose of 0.6–1.2 mg that is titrated up to a dose of 2.4 mg/day divided in multiple doses for up to 3 months of therapy, but data for efficacy is lacking, and renal function needs to be closely monitored [64, 65].

Potassium para-aminobenzoate (Potaba) is an anti-fibrotic agent that is also used but is not considered to be first-line treatment as it is poorly tolerated and expensive, and data for reduction in curvature is lacking [64, 66]. Oral tamoxifen is also an option for treatment, but efficacy has not been demonstrated in controlled trials to date [66]. Intralesional therapies, such as verapamil, also exist for treatment of plaques [65, 66]. A recent prospective study with 156 participants demonstrated that intralesional verapamil led to 60 % of the participants having decreased penile curvature, 80 % had an increase in rigidity dorsal to the plaque, and 71 % had an increase in sexual function [64]. Other medications that are being used or studied in the clinical setting include oral carnitine and pentoxifylline [66]. Other modalities of therapy include iontophoresis and extracorporeal shockwave lithotripsy and radiation.

Penile Cancer

Cancers of the penis are rare in the USA and other industrialized countries but occur at a higher frequency in developing countries. The overall survival of men with penile cancer is high [68]. In the USA, penile carcinoma accounts for less than 1 % of cancers in men and less than 300 deaths annually [35]. In Africa, Asia, and South America, penile cancer is much more common accounting for about 10–20 % of all malignancies in men [69]. Penile cancer is typically a disease of older men, with the average age at diagnosis about 60 years old, but men of any age can be affected [68].

Squamous cell carcinoma (SCC) is the most common histology of penile cancer, accounting for 95 % of cases. Non-squamous cell cancers that may involve the penis include melanoma, basal cell carcinoma, lymphoma, and sarcoma [70]. Risk factors associated with an increased risk of penile cancer include previous penile tear or injury, urethral stricture, chronic penile rash, phimosis, human papillomavirus (HPV) infection, tobacco abuse, lack of circumcision, and HIV infection [71, 72]. In the USA, key risk factors for excessive incidence of penile cancer include Hispanic ethnicity, residence in the south, and low socioeconomic status [73]. Risks for excess mortality include these key factors in addition to black race [73].

Presentation In a series of 243 men with newly diagnosed penile cancer, the most common signs were a painless penile lump or ulcer [74]. Inguinal lymphadenopathy is present in up to 60 % of men at diagnosis, yet malignant infiltration of the

Fig. 12.9 Penile cancer.
http://phil.cdc.gov/Phil/
quicksearch.asp

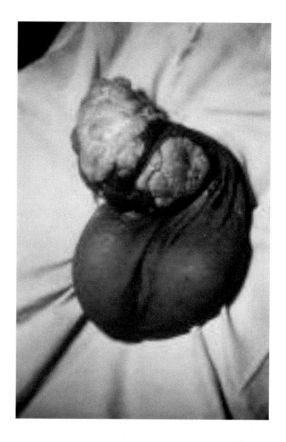

lymph nodes is demonstrated in only approximately one-half of these cases [75] (See Fig. 12.9).

Exam All men with penile cancer require a detailed examination of the penis for lesions and the inguinal region for the presence or absence of lymphadenopathy. The majority of cancers arise on the glans, in the coronal sulcus, or on the prepuce as either a mass or ulceration and may be associated with a secondary infection [74].

Evaluation Biopsy should be considered for all men presenting with a penile lesion and should be done immediately for a highly suspicious lesion or those with notable lymphadenopathy [76]. If a biopsy result is positive for malignancy, then inguinal ultrasound with fine needle aspiration of the involved lymph nodes is recommended [76].

Survival of penile cancer is related to stage, so early diagnosis is critical toward obtaining a favorable treatment outcome [70]. The presence of organomegaly, cachexia, or altered mental status may indicate the presence of metastatic disease and identify patients who require imaging and further laboratory evaluation in addition to biopsy. Imaging by ultrasound, CT, or MRI is suggested for patients presenting with clinical lymphadenopathy or those with an elevated body mass index (BMI) above 30.

Treatment If there is significant erythema, swelling, discharge, or other history and exam findings suggestive of infection and an otherwise low suspicion for penile cancer, then a 6-week course of antifungal or antibiotic medication such as a cephalosporin, Bactrim, or doxycycline may be reasonable. However, lesions that do not resolve after that time or progress rapidly should be biopsied [70].

Men with a positive penile biopsy result and/or lymphadenopathy should be promptly referred to urologic oncologist. For low-risk disease, surveillance, rather than nodal dissection, may be reasonable. The presence and extent of inguinal lymph node metastases is the strongest predictor of cancer-specific survival. There is a clear benefit for early lymphadenectomy in men with positive nodal disease, but identifying who will benefit from prophylactic lymphadenopathy remains a challenge [68]. In a study of penile cancer presenting with lymphadenopathy, 82 % of patients underwent unnecessary prophylactic lymphadenectomy [68]. Overall, the choice of further evaluation and treatment methods should be based on local expertise and consideration of patient preferences.

Conclusion

Multiple conditions can present with acute scrotal pain. Conditions that should be considered include epididymitis, orchitis, testicular torsion, torsion of the appendix testis, and Fournier's gangrene. Epididymitis is one of the most common causes of scrotal pain in the outpatient setting and a patient with a classical presentation will describe a steady and gradual increase in testicular pain that may radiate to the lower abdomen with or without symptoms typical of urinary tract infection (UTI) such as fever, increased frequency, dysuria, and hematuria. Epididymitis typically has tenderness to palpation of the affected testicle, epididymis, or the spermatic and pain relief with testicular elevation a normal cremasteric reflex. *Treatment* of epididymitis includes a combination of antibiotics, NSAIDs, and scrotal elevation.

Testicular torsion generally presents with the abrupt onset of severe testicular pain and should be considered in all patients presenting with acute scrotal pain. The diagnosis of testicular torsion is usually determined by acute onset of severe testicular pain, abnormal testicular lie, and an absent cremasteric reflex. An ultrasound evaluation is necessary in equivocal cases. Treatment of testicular torsion is surgical and all suspected cases should be sent immediately to an emergency room for urological surgical evaluation. If surgical treatment is not immediately available, manual detorsion should be performed until surgical treatment can be obtained.

Painless scrotal masses and swelling can occur from a variety of conditions including varicocele, hydrocele, epididymal cysts, spermatoceles, and testicular cancer. Testicular cancer usually presents as a painless mass, with associated symptoms such as testicular firmness and swelling, an aching in the lower abdomen, and scrotal heaviness. Some patients may have accompanying gynecomastia resulting from excess estrogen production with various tumors.

The diagnostic evaluation of men with suspected testicular cancer includes scrotal ultrasound, measurement of serum tumor markers including alpha fetoprotein and beta human chorionic gonadotropin, radical orchiectomy, and in some cases, retroperitoneal lymph node dissection.

Penile disorders include phimosis, paraphimosis, priapism, Peyronie's disease, and penile cancer. Priapism is divided into ischemic and nonischemic types. A color duplex Doppler ultrasound is useful in differentiating ischemic from nonischemic priapism. First-line management of ischemic priapism includes aspiration of blood from one of the corpora cavernosa followed by irrigation with normal saline. If there is no relief of pressure and pain, then direct application of an alpha-1 adrenergic agonist such as phenylephrine can be applied every 5 min. First-line treatment of nonischemic priapism should be close clinical surveillance. In some cases rest (lying supine, avoidance of sexual activity), ice packs, and time have been shown to lead to spontaneous resolution in most cases.

Penile cancer is rare in the USA but is much more common in developing countries.

The most common presentation is a painless penile lump or ulcer, and presenting patients often also have inguinal lymphadenopathy. Biopsy should be considered for all men presenting with a penile lesion and should be done immediately for a highly suspicious lesion or those with notable lymphadenopathy. If a biopsy result is positive for malignancy, then inguinal ultrasound with fine needle aspiration of the involved lymph nodes is recommended.

Survival of penile cancer is related to stage, so early diagnosis is critical toward obtaining a favorable treatment outcome. Men with a positive penile biopsy result and/or lymphadenopathy should be promptly referred to urologic oncologist. There is a clear benefit for early lymphadenectomy in men with positive nodal disease, but identifying who will benefit from prophylactic lymphadenopathy remains a challenge. Overall, the choice of further evaluation and treatment methods should be based on local expertise and consideration of patient preferences.

References

1. Liguori G, Bucci S, Zordani A, Benvenuto S, Ollandini G, Mazzon G, Bertolotto M, Cacciato F, Siracusano S, Trombetta C. Role of US in acute scrotal pain. World J Urol. 2011;29(5):639.
2. Workowski KA, Berman S, Centers for Disease Control and Prevention (CDC). Sexually transmitted diseases treatment guidelines, 2010. MMWR Recomm Rep. 2010;59:1.
3. Fisher R, Walker J. The acute paediatric scrotum. Br J Hosp Med. 1994;51(6):290.
4. Palestro CJ, Manor EP, Kim CK, Goldsmith SJ. Torsion of a testicular appendage in an adult male. Clin Nucl Med. 1990;15(7):51.
5. Teague RE. Testicular torsion. Am Fam Physician. 2006;74(10):1739.

6. Holland JM, Graham JB, Ignatoff JM. Conservative management of twisted testicular appendages. J Urol. 1981;125(2):213–4.
7. Benizri E, Fabiani P, Migliori G, et al. Gangrene of the perineum. Urology. 1996; 47(6):935–9.
8. Sherman J, Solliday M, Paraiso E, Becker J, Mydlo JH. Early CT findings of Fournier's gangrene in a healthy male. Clin Imaging. 1998;22(6):425–7.
9. Trojian TH, Lishnak TS, Heiman D. Epididymitis and orchitis: an overview. Am Fam Physician. 2009;79(7):583–7.
10. Lane TM, Hines J. The management of mumps orchitis. BJU Int. 2006;97(1):1–2.
11. Kaver I, Matzkin H, Braf ZF. Epididymo-orchitis: a retrospective study of121 patients. J Fam Pract. 1990;30(5):548–52.
12. Stewart A, Ubee SS, Davies H. 10-minute consultation epididymo-orchitis. BMJ. 2011;342:d1543.
13. Tracy CR, Steers WD, Costabile R. Diagnosis and management of epididymitis. Urol Clin N Am. 2008;35:101–8.
14. Molokwu CN, Somani BK, Goodman CM. Outcomes of scrotal exploration for acute scrotal pain suspicious of testicular torsion: a consecutive case series of 173 patients. BJU Int. 2011;107(6):990.
15. Cummings JM, Boullier JA, Sekhon D, Bose K. Adult testicular torsion. J Urol. 2002;167(5):2109.
16. Tajchner L, Larkin JO, Bourke MG, Waldron R, Barry K, Eustace PW. Management of the acute scrotum in a district general hospital: 10-year experience. ScientificWorldJournal. 2009;9:281.
17. Schmitz D, Safranek S. Clinical inquiries. How useful is a physical exam in diagnosing testicular torsion? J Fam Pract. 2009;58(8):433.
18. Sessions AE, Rabinowitz R, Hulbert WC, Goldstein MM, Mevorach RA. Testicular torsion: direction, degree, duration and disinformation. J Urol. 2003;169(2):663.
19. Perron CE. Pain–Scrotal. In: Fleisher GR, Ludwig S, editors. Textbook of pediatric emergency medicine. 4th ed. Philadelphia: Lippincott, Williams and Wilkins; 2000. p. 473.
20. Wilbert DM, Schaerfe CW, Stern WD, Strohmaier WL, Bichler KH. Evaluation of the acute scrotum by color-coded Doppler ultrasonography. J Urol. 1993;149(6):1475.
21. Kapasi Z, Halliday S. Best evidence topic report. Ultrasound in the diagnosis of testicular torsion. Emerg Med J. 2005;22(8):559.
22. Cornel EB, Karthaus HF. Manual derotation of the twisted spermatic cord. BJU Int. 1999;83(6):672.
23. Wampler SM, Llanes M. Common scrotal and testicular problems. Prim Care. 2010;37(3):613.
24. Jarow JP, Sanzone JJ. Risk factors for male partner antisperm antibodies. J Urol. 1992;148(6):1805.
25. Paduch DA, Skoog SJ. Current management of adolescent varicocele. Rev Urol. 2001;3(3):120–33.
26. Will MA, Swain J, Fode M, Sonksen J, Christman GM, Ohl D. The great debate: varicocele treatment and impact on fertility. Fertil Steril. 2011;95(3):841–52.
27. Woo SC, Soo WK. Current issues in varicocele management: a review. World J Men's Health. 2013;31(1):12–20.
28. Davis RS. Intratesticular spermatocele. Urology. 1998;51(5A Suppl):167–9.
29. Choyke PL, Glenn GM, Wagner JP, Lubensky IA, Thakore K, Zbar B, Linehan WM, Walther MM. Epididymal cystadenomas in von Hippel-Lindau disease. Urology. 1997;49(6):926.
30. Rubenstein RA, Dogra VS, Seftel AD, Resnick MI. Benign intrascrotal lesions. J Urol. 2004;171(5):1765–72.
31. Barthold JS, Kass EJ. Abnormalities of the penis and scrotum. In: Belman AB, King LR, Kramer SA, editors. Clinical pediatric urology. 4th ed. London: Martin Dunitz Ltd; 2002. p. 1093.
32. Baskin LS, Kogan AB. Hydrocele/Hernia. In: Gonzales ET, Bauer SB, editors. Pediatric urology practice. Philadelphia: Lippincott Williams and Wilkins; 1999. p. 649.

33. Rohn RD. Male genitalia: examination and findings. In: Friedman SB, Fisher M, Schonberg SK, et al., editors. Comprehensive adolescent health care. St. Louis: Mosby-Yearbook; 1998. p. 1078.

34. Anderson MM, Neinstein LS. Scrotal disorders. In: Neinstein LS, editor. Adolescent health care: a practical guide. Baltimore: Williams and Wilkins; 1996. p. 464.

35. Siegel RL, Miller KD, Jemal A. Cancer statistics, 2015. CA Cancer J Clin. 2015;65(1):5.

36. Jemal A, Bray F, Center MM, Ferlay J, Ward E, Forman D. Global cancer statistics. CA Cancer J Clin. 2011;61(2):69.

37. Howlader N, Noone AM, Krapcho M, et al. SEER cancer statistics review, 1975-2008. Bethesda, MD: National Cancer Institute; 2011. Available at http://seer.cancer.gov/statfacts/html/testis.html. Accessed 1 May 2015.

38. American Cancer Society. What is testicular cancer? Available at http://www.cancer.org/cancer/testicularcancer/detailedguide/testicular-cancer-what-is-testicular-cancer. Accessed 11 May 2015.

39. Walsh TJ, Grady RW, Porter MP, Lin DW, Weiss NS. Incidence of testicular germ cell cancers in U.S. children: SEER program experience 1973 to 2000. Urology. 2006;68(2):402.

40. van Dijk MR, Steyerberg EW, Habbema JD. Survival of non-seminomatous germ cell cancer patients according to the IGCC classification: an update based on meta-analysis. Eur J Cancer. 2006;42(7):820.

41. Dieckmann KP, Pichlmeier U. Clinical epidemiology of testicular germ cell tumors. World J Urol. 2004;22(1):2.

42. Walsh TJ, Croughan MS, Schembri M, Chan JM, Turek PJ. Increased risk of testicular germ cell cancer among infertile men. Arch Intern Med. 2009;169(4):351.

43. Eifler Jr JB, King P, Schlegel PN. Incidental testicular lesions found during infertility evaluation are usually benign and may be managed conservatively. J Urol. 2008;180(1):261.

44. Richiardi L, Akre O, Montgomery SM, Lambe M, Kvist U, Ekbom A. Fecundity and twinning rates as measures of fertility before diagnosis of germ-cell testicular cancer. J Natl Cancer Inst. 2004;96(2):145.

45. Gajendran VK, Nguyen M, Ellison LM. Testicular cancer patterns in African-American men. Urology. 2005;66(3):602.

46. Zheng T, Holford TR, Ma Z, Ward BA, Flannery J, Boyle P. Continuing increase in incidence of germ-cell testis cancer in young adults: experience from Connecticut, USA, 1935-1992. Int J Cancer. 1996;65(6):723.

47. Rosenberg L, Palmer JR, Zauber AG, Warshauer ME, Strom BL, Harlap S, Shapiro S. The relation of vasectomy to the risk of cancer. Am J Epidemiol. 1994;140(5):431.

48. U.S. Preventive Services Task Force. Screening for testicular cancer: reaffirmation recommendation statement. Ann Intern Med. 2011;154(7):483.

49. Tseng Jr A, Horning SJ, Freiha FS, Resser KJ, Hannigan Jr JF, Torti FM. Gynecomastia in testicular cancer patients. Prognostic and therapeutic implications. Cancer. 1985;56(10):2534.

50. Marth D, Scheidegger J, Studer UE. Ultrasonography of testicular tumors. Urol Int. 1990;45(4):237.

51. Muglia V, Tucci Jr S, Elias Jr J, et al. Magnetic resonance imaging of scrotal diseases: when it makes the difference. Urology. 2002;59:419.

52. Bosl GJ, Motzer RJ. Testicular germ-cell cancer. N Engl J Med. 1997;337(4):242.

53. Shahid SK. Phimosis in children. ISRN Urol. 2012;2012:6.

54. Barone JG, Fleisher MH. Treatment of paraphimosis using the puncture technique. Pediatr Emerg Care. 1993;9(5):298–9.

55. Gausche M. Genitourinary surgical emergencies. Pediatr Ann. 1996;25(8):458–64.

56. Houghton GR. The iced-glove method of treatment of paraphimosis. Br J Surg. 1973;60(11):876–7.

57. Pholman JD, Phillips JM, Wilcox DT. Simple method of paraphimosis reduction revisited: point of technique and review of the literature. J Pediatr Urol. 2013;9:104.

58. Kerwat R, Shandall A, Stephenson B. Reduction of paraphimosis with granulated sugar. Br J Urol. 1998;82:755.

59. Coutts AG. Treatment of paraphimosis. Br J Surg. 1991;78:252.
60. Huang Y-C, Harraz A, Shindel AW, Lue TF. Evaluation and management of priapism: 2009 update. Nat Rev Urol. 2009;5(6):262–71.
61. Levey HR, Segal RL, Bivalacqua TJ. Management of priapism: an update for clinicians. Ther Adv Urol. 2014;6(6):230–44.
62. Cherian J, Rao AR, Thwaini A, Kapasi F, Shergill IS, Samman R. Medical and surgical management of priapism. Postgrad Med J. 2006;82:89–94.
63. Burnett AL, Bivalacqua TJ. Priapism: current principles and practice. Urol Clin N Am. 2007;34:631–42.
64. Jalkut M, Gonzalez-Cadavid N, Rajfer J. Peyronie's disease: a review. Rev Urol. 2003;5(3):142–8.
65. Greenfield JM, Levine LA. Peyronie's disease: etiology, epidemiology, and medical treatment. Urol Clin N Am. 2005;32:469–78.
66. Bella AJ, Perelman MA, Brant WO, Lue TF. Peyronie's disease. J Sex Med. 2007;4:1527–38.
67. Hauck EW, Weidner W. Francois de la Peyronie and the disease named after him. Lancet. 2001;357:2049–51.
68. Hegarty PK, Kayes O, Freeman A, Christopher N, Ralph DJ, Minhas S. A prospective study of 100 cases of penile cancer managed according to European Association of Urology guidelines. BJU Int. 2006;98(3):526.
69. Ornellas AA. Management of penile cancer. J Surg Oncol. 2008;97(3):199.
70. Burgers JK, Badalament RA, Drago JR. Penile cancer. Clinical presentation, diagnosis, and staging. Urol Clin N Am. 1992;19(2):247.
71. Daling JR, Madeleine MM, Johnson LG, Schwartz SM, Shera KA, Wurscher MA, Carter JJ, Porter PL, Galloway DA, McDougall JK, Krieger JN. Penile cancer: importance of circumcision, human papillomavirus and smoking in in situ and invasive disease. Int J Cancer. 2005;116(4):606.
72. Maden C, Sherman KJ, Beckmann AM, Hislop TG, Teh CZ, Ashley RL, Daling JR. History of circumcision, medical conditions, and sexual activity and risk of penile cancer. J Natl Cancer Inst. 1993;85(1):19.
73. Hernandez BY, Barnholtz-Sloan J, German RR, Giuliano A, Goodman MT, King JB, Negoita S, Villalon-Gomez JM. Burden of invasive squamous cell carcinoma of the penis in the United States, 1998-2003. Cancer. 2008;113(10 Suppl):2883–91.
74. Ritchie AW, Foster PW, Fowler S, BAUS Section of Oncology. Penile cancer in the UK: clinical presentation and outcome in 1998/99. BJU Int. 2004;94(9):1248–52.
75. Heyns CF, Mendoza-Valdés A, Pompeo AC. Diagnosis and staging of penile cancer. Urology. 2010;76(2 Suppl 1):S15–23.
76. Delacroix Jr SE, Pettaway CA. Therapeutic strategies for advanced penile carcinoma. Curr Opin Support Palliat Care. 2010;4(4):285–92.

Chapter 13
Hypogonadism: The Relationship to Cardiometabolic Syndrome and the Controversy Behind Testosterone Replacement Therapy

Joel J. Heidelbaugh, Anthony Grech, and Martin M. Miner

Introduction

Testosterone deficiency (TD) in men has commanded substantial attention over the last decade due to the increased longevity of the male population, increased direct-to-consumer advertising in the media, increased awareness of testosterone repletion by medical care providers, and lastly, the approval of more applicable preparations. Testosterone replacement therapy (TRT) has been used successfully in millions of healthy men worldwide to treat diminished libido and erectile dysfunction and to improve physical strength and overall function [1, 2]. Between 2001 and 2011, prescriptions for TRT among men 40 years of age or older in the United States (US) increased more than threefold [3]. Over this period, it has been noted that nearly one-quarter of men who were prescribed with TRT never had their baseline testosterone levels obtained, or monitored throughout treatment, and up to 60 % of levels are drawn by primary care providers [3].

J.J. Heidelbaugh, MD
Departments of Family Medicine and Urology, University of Michigan
Medical School, Ann Arbor, MI, USA
e-mail: jheidel@med.umich.edu

A. Grech, MD
Departments of Family Medicine and Internal Medicine,
University of Michigan Medical School, Ann Arbor, MI, USA
e-mail: agrech@med.umich.edu

M.M. Miner, MD (⊠)
Departments of Family Medicine and Urology, Warren Alpert School of Medicine,
Brown University, 164 Summit Avenue, Providence, RI, USA

Men's Health Center, The Miriam Hospital, 164 Summit Avenue, Providence, RI, USA
e-mail: Martin_Miner@brown.edu

© Springer International Publishing Switzerland 2016
J.J. Heidelbaugh (ed.), *Men's Health in Primary Care*, Current Clinical Practice,
DOI 10.1007/978-3-319-26091-4_13

250 J.J. Heidelbaugh et al.

Epidemiology

The trend of declining serum testosterone, commonly referred to in the literature as testosterone deficiency in aging men, has been well documented. The Massachusetts Male Aging Study, a community-based study of 3339 random men aged 40–79 years, reported an annual decline in total and free T of 0.8–1.6 % and 1.7–2.8 % per year, respectively, in men over 40 years of age [4]. Comparatively, the European Male Aging Study, a population-based prospective cohort study of 3369 men aged 40–79 years from the general population of eight European countries, reported an age-adjusted annual decline in total T of 0.4 % per year [5].

The hypogonadism in men (HIM) study was an observational study of 2162 men in primary care practices 45 years of age or greater that reported an overall prevalence of biochemical hypogonadism of 38.7 % (Fig. 13.1) [6]. This study found a statistically significant relationship between serum testosterone levels less than 300 ng/mL and components of the metabolic syndrome (MetS). This highlights a significant relationship between TD and obesity, with an odds ratio approaching nearly 2.5 (Table 13.1).

The 2010 Endocrine Society Guidelines define hypogonadism as signs and symptoms of low testosterone (e.g., decreased libido, decreased erections, decreased energy, decreased physical strength) in the setting of low first-morning serum T levels defined as less than 300 ng/dL on two separate occasions [7]. TRT has been shown to reliably increase serum testosterone to physiologic levels, improve libido, improve erectile dysfunction, improve overall sexual function, increase energy,

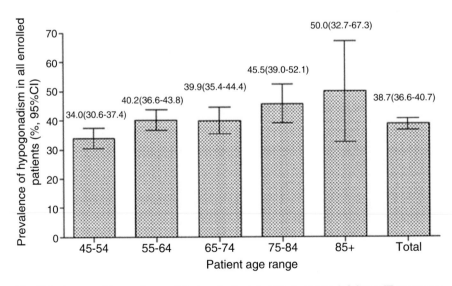

Fig. 13.1 Age-specific prevalence of biochemically defined testosterone deficiency [Testosterone deficiency defined as total testosterone <300 ng/dL or current testosterone therapy. For every 10-year increase in age, risk of TD increased by 17 % (95 % confidence interval [CI], 1.08–1.27)]. Adapted from [6]

Table 13.1 Prevalence of concomitant cardiometabolic conditions in men with total testosterone less than 300 ng/dL

Risk factor	Hypogonadism prevalence (95 % CI)	Odds ratio (95 % CI)
Obesity	52.4 (47.9–56.9)	2.38 (1.93–2.93)
Type 2 diabetes	50.0 (45.5–54.5)	2.09 (1.70–2.58)
Hypertension	42.4 (39.6–45.2)	1.84 (1.53–2.22)
Hyperlipidemia	40.4 (37.6–43.3)	1.47 (1.23–1.76)
Asthma or COPD	43.5 (36.8–50.3)	1.40 (1.04–1.86)
Prostate disease	41.3 (36.4–46.2)	1.29 (1.03–1.62)

Adapted from [6]

improve mood, increase bone mineral density, decrease body fat mass, and increase lean body muscle mass [7, 8]. The Boston Area Community Health (BACH) Survey estimated a crude prevalence of symptomatic androgen deficiency at 5.6 % [9], while it was estimated that only 12 % of symptomatic men were being treated [10]. These trials were the first to describe the magnitude of TD among the aging male population, relative to a decline in various levels of functioning.

Hypogonadism has been identified concomitantly with many comorbid health conditions in men including obesity, cardiovascular disease (CVD), MetS, type 2 diabetes mellitus (T2DM), hypertension (HTN), and dyslipidemia, positing an associative relationship. The exact physiologic mechanisms behind these proposed relationships have still not been inarguably determined. While it has been proposed that hypogonadism may be a direct cause of some or all of these comorbid conditions, a simultaneous condition associated with another underlying process such as senescence, or even a protective evolutionary factor that decreases energy expenditure in men with poor or declining health status, a definitive cause-and-effect answer still remains elusive [8, 11]. Despite such theories, men with hypogonadism have been shown to have less favorable health outcomes compared to the general population and thus may be more susceptible to potential adverse effects associated with TRT, through an associative relationship [7].

Pathophysiology

TD occurs due to a dysregulation in the hypothalamic–pituitary–gonadal axis and is a component of natural senescence in aging men. Decreased levels of gonadotropin-releasing hormone (GnRH) in the pituitary result in decreased levels of serum luteinizing hormone (LH) secreted by the pituitary that in turn directly impact testosterone production at the level of the testes. This is associated with increased serum insulin (insulin resistance) and decreased sex hormone-binding globulin (SHBG). TD results in increased lipoprotein lipase, increased uptake of serum triglycerides, and further increases in visceral adiposity. The final result from this metabolic derangement is an increase in serum aromatase and estrogens that are deposited in visceral fat [14].

Relationship to Metabolic Syndrome

MetS poses a substantial threat to the health of millions of men worldwide, as it has been implicated in adverse morbidity and mortality cardiovascular outcomes. Although no single universally accepted definition exists, the syndrome is ubiquitously characterized by major cardiovascular risk factors including hypertension, hyperlipidemia [specifically elevated triglycerides and reduced high-density lipoprotein cholesterol (HDL-C)], increased fasting glucose, hyperinsulinemia, and increased visceral adiposity [12] (Fig. 13.2). These factors ultimately increase the risk of CVD and T2DM. This syndrome is derived from physical inactivity; obesity; a high-carbohydrate, high-fat diet; and genetic factors. Research over the last decade has examined the role of MetS and testosterone deficiency. MetS has been found to be associated with hypogonadism and erectile dysfunction (ED); thus, MetS is likely a risk factor for the development of ED and underlying endothelial dysfunction [13].

A study by Zitzmann highlights the relationship between hyperinsulinemia and visceral obesity leading to a reduction of endogenous testicular testosterone production [14] (Fig. 13.3). Testosterone has been shown to have negative reciprocal effects on generation of muscle and visceral adipose tissue through influencing the differentiation of pluripotent stem cells and through inhibiting the development of preadipocytes. Testosterone has a protective effect on pancreatic beta cells, exerted by the positive influence of inflammatory cytokines and androgen receptor-mediated pathways. Several epidemiological and interventional studies have posited that TRT may be integral in either preventing or attenuating the MetS in aging men with LOH and in those with concomitant hypogonadism and T2DM [14].

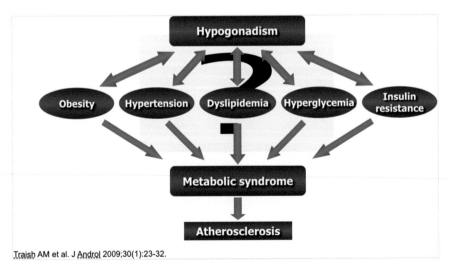

Traish AM et al. J Androl 2009;30(1):23-32.

Fig. 13.2 Relationship between hypogonadism and metabolic syndrome (MetS). Adapted from [12]

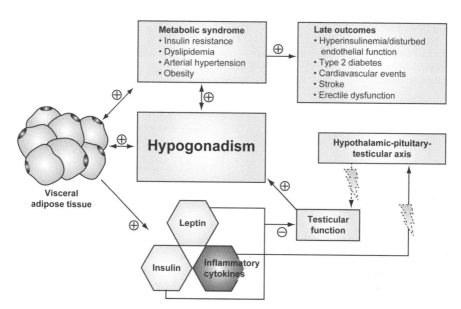

Fig. 13.3 Visceral adiposity is a key component of metabolic syndrome. Lightning signs indicate a disturbance of function. Adapted from [14]

Traish and colleagues have written a series of publications highlighting "the dark side" of the relationship between testosterone deficiency and the metabolic syndrome. This relationship has defined a proven link among reduced plasma testosterone levels, T2DM, and insulin resistance. TRT in the treatment of hypogonadal men has been shown to improve insulin sensitivity, serum fasting glucose levels, and glycosylated hemoglobin levels. Testosterone deficiency has been found to be associated with all of these components, as well as with an increased deposition of visceral fat, which serves as an endocrine organ producing inflammatory cytokines and thus promoting endothelial dysfunction and vascular disease [13, 15].

Measurement of Serum Testosterone

Various assays exist to measure serum testosterone (Fig. 13.4) [16]. Most current literature focuses on measurement of total testosterone, yet bioavailable testosterone assays are becoming more popular as a modality toward more specific identification of the hormone. Most circulating testosterone is bound to sex hormone-binding globulin (SHBG), while approximately 0.5–2 % is unbound to either SHBG or albumin and is considered as free testosterone. All testosterone that is not bound to SHBG is considered to be bioavailable, estimated at approximately 40–50 % of total.

Fig. 13.4 Composition of serum testosterone. *SHBG* sex hormone-binding globulin, *T* testosterone. Adapted from [16]

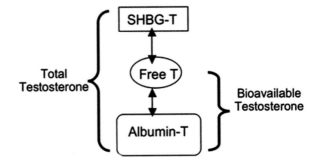

Table 13.2 Should clinicians screen for testosterone deficiency in men?

Yes
Testosterone levels decline as men age
Testosterone deficiency is a real syndrome with real symptoms and improvable metabolic outcomes
Studies suggesting cardiovascular risk associated with TRT have major flaws
TRT has proven benefit in cardiometabolic syndrome
No
Aging adults are a profitable market; TRT has been promoted as a "youth-restoring tonic and disease preventive"
"Pharmaceutical companies use nonspecific symptoms to foster disease states"
No consistent relationship has been proven between testosterone levels and symptoms associated with low testosterone

TRT testosterone replacement therapy
Adapted from [17, 18]

Evaluation and Treatment of the Man with Suspected Testosterone Deficiency

Significant controversy exists over whether or not a man should be screened for potential TD in primary care practices. A recent pro/con debate by Heidelbaugh (pro) and Fugh-Berman (con) published in the *American Family Physician* journal in 2015 highlights the key tenets of this argument (Table 13.2) [17, 18]. A challenge with identifying appropriate symptoms of the man who presents with potential TD lies within the often nonspecific symptoms associated with this disorder (Table 13.3) [7, 19, 20] (Table 13.3) and associated with the comorbid disease states establishing high risk. The Endocrine Society advises against generalized screening. The authors believe that all men who present with largely "organic" ED should be screened with a total testosterone. The Androgen Deficiency in the Aging Male (ADAM) Questionnaire is a validated tool that can help clinicians to screen men appropriately for TD (Table 13.4) [21].

A significant number of comorbid conditions coexist with TD (Table 13.5) [7]. In men with these conditions, a workup for TD should be strongly considered, especially

Table 13.3 Symptoms and signs suggestive of testosterone deficiency in men

More specific signs and symptoms
Reduced libido
Erectile dysfunction (ED)
Reduced intensity of orgasm and genital sensation
Osteoporosis or low bone mineral density
Decreased spontaneous erection
Oligospermia or azoospermia
Very small or shrinking testes
Hot flushes, sweats
Breast discomfort, gynecomastia
Loss of pubic and axillary hair, reduced shaving
Less specific signs and symptoms
Decreased energy or vitality, increased fatigue
Depressed mood
Reduced muscle mass and strength
Poor concentration and memory
Sleep disturbance; increased sleepiness
Mild anemia
Increased body fat, body mass index
Diminished physical or work performance

Adapted from [7, 19, 20]

Table 13.4 ADAM[a] Questionnaire

1. Do you have a decrease in libido?
2. Do you have a lack of energy?
3. Do you have a decrease in strength and/or endurance?
4. Have you lost height?
5. Have you decreased an "enjoyment of life?"
6. Are you sad and/or grumpy?
7. Are your erections less strong?
8. Have you noted a decrease in ability to play sports?
9. Are you falling asleep after dinner?
10. Has there been a recent deterioration in work performance?

Positive screen = YES for no. 1–7 or any three questions

[a] *A*ndrogen *D*eficiency in *A*ging *M*ales

Adapted from [21]

Table 13.5 Risks and comorbid illnesses associated with testosterone deficiency

Metabolic syndrome
Obesity
Hyperlipidemia
Hypertension
Elevated fasting plasma glucose and serum insulin
Diabetes mellitus (type 1 or 2)
Cardiovascular disease (including aortic atherosclerosis)
Elevated C-reactive protein
Chronic obstructive lung disease
Inflammatory arthritis
Low-trauma fracture
End-stage renal disease
HIV-related weight loss
Hemochromatosis
Sellar mass, radiation to the sellar region, or other diseases of the sellar region
Chronic pain syndrome and treatment with opioids
Treatment with glucocorticoids
Radical prostatectomy

Adapted from [7]

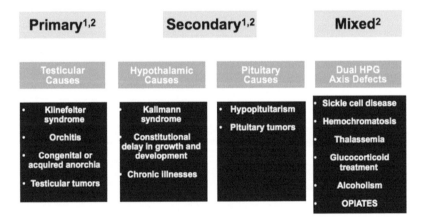

Classification of Hypogonadism

1. AACE Hypogonadism Task Force. *Endor Pract.* 2002;8:439-456;
2. Bhasin S, et al. *J Clin Endocrinol Metab.* 2006;91(6):1995-2010.

Fig. 13.5 Classification of testicular hypogonadism. Adapted from [7]

when concomitant conditions have become difficult to manage (e.g., T2DM, morbid obesity, and other endocrine conditions). Testosterone deficiency is classified as primary, secondary, and mixed disorders (Fig. 13.5) [7]. It is imperative that clinicians appropriately characterize and classify TD in men to propose appropriate treatment.

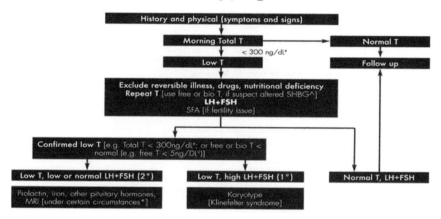

SHBG = sex hormone- binding globulin; LH = luteinizing hormone; FSH = follicle
stimulating   hormone; SFA = sperm functional assessment.
Bhasin S, et al. *J Clin Endocronol Metab.* 2010;95(6):2536-59

Fig. 13.6 Endocrine Society Guidelines for testicular hypogonadism. *SHBG* sex hormone-binding globulin, *LH* luteinizing hormone, *FSH* follicle-stimulating hormone, *SFA* sperm functional assessment. Adapted from [7]

The Endocrine Society Guidelines from 2010 present a schematic to aid clinicians in the evaluation of the man with suspected TD (Fig. 13.6) [7]. By convention, a cutoff of 300 ng/dL has been defined as TD, coupled with the symptoms highlighted in Table 13.3. Currently, there are a variety of widely available testosterone formulations including topical gels and patches, intramuscular injections, subcutaneous pellets, and oral/buccal formulations that provide clinicians and male patients the opportunity to personalize replacement therapy.

Potential Adverse Effects of Testosterone Replacement Therapy

The estimated likelihood of adverse effects of long-term TRT is still essentially unknown, as overall high-quality evidence to recommend its use in most men with TD is lacking. The highlighted studies can be used to guide the clinician in how to best monitor patients on TRT, especially those with the comorbid conditions detailed below.

Risk of Cardiovascular Morbidity and Mortality

Reduced serum testosterone levels have been associated with an increased risk of the development of CVD including ischemic heart disease and stroke, yet whether TD is directly linked to the pathogenesis of CVD, a marker of preexisting CVD, or concomitant manifestation of another underlying disease remains unclear [8, 11]. Low endogenous testosterone levels correlate with an increased risk of adverse CVD events, and endothelial dysfunction and increased atherosclerosis are means by which male hypogonadism may contribute to an increased risk of death [22]. The potential that TD may be involved in the pathogenesis of CVD would create a notion that TRT would result in improved cardiovascular outcomes, yet no current level I evidence exists to support this claim. There are several well-done cross-sectional studies that suggest this association between TRT and improved mortality including CVS mortality.

To date, the literature on the relationship between TRT and CVD has been conflicting, suggesting that TRT has either no beneficial effect on reduction of cardiovascular morbidity or mortality or even a detrimental effect. Two meta-analyses found no differences in cardiovascular events between TRT and placebo groups [23, 24], while a more recent meta-analysis found that TRT increased the risk of cardiovascular events, although the data varied by source of research trial funding. The authors concluded that overall, and particularly in trials not funded by the pharmaceutical industry, exogenous testosterone increased the risk of cardiovascular-related events [25].

A retrospective cohort study of men with serum T levels below 300 ng/dL who underwent coronary angiography in the Veterans Affairs (VA) healthcare system between 2005 and 2011 investigated the association between TRT and all-cause mortality, myocardial infarction (MI), and stroke in 8709 men [26]. Men were excluded if they were started on TRT prior to angiography or prior to obtaining serum T levels. Further exclusion criteria included receiving TRT after suffering an MI. In the study, 1223 men with low serum T levels received TRT while 7486 did not. Their results indicated that TRT was associated with an absolute risk difference of 5.8 % (95 % CI 1.4–13.1 %) increased risk of mortality, MI, or ischemic stroke regardless of the presence of preexisting coronary artery disease.

Several limitations of this trial are noteworthy. First, the raw data in the abstract directly contradicted the authors' conclusions. With regard to the T-treated group, the calculated absolute risk for all CV events was 10 % (123 events in 1223 men) versus the group not treated with T with a calculated risk of 21.2 % (1587 events in 7486 men). This reported outcome was reversed subsequent to possible inappropriate evaluation of the statistical data. In addition, this study excluded 1132 hypogonadal men who had suffered either MI or stroke, prior to initiation of T therapy. Lastly, these findings are in direct contrast to results from a similar VA population that yielded a mortality risk in men treated with T of 10.3 % compared with 20.7 % in untreated men ($P < 0.0001$) and a mortality rate of 3.4 deaths per 100 person-years for T-treated men compared to 5.7 deaths per 100 person-years in men not treated with T [27].

The Testosterone in Older Men (TOM) trial, a double-blinded randomized controlled trial of 209 men of mean age 74 years, was performed to assess effects of TRT in men with low serum T and limited mobility [28]. The primary outcome was to evaluate the change from baseline of maximal voluntary muscle strength in leg press exercise with secondary outcomes measuring chest press, 50-m walking speed, and stair climbing. Although the study demonstrated significant improvements in leg press, chest press, and stair climbing in the TRT group compared to the placebo group, the study was discontinued early due to a higher incidence of adverse cardiovascular effects in the TRT group (hazard ratio = 2.4, $p = 0.05$). Of the 209 men randomized (106 in the TRT arm and 103 in the placebo arm), 23 of the TRT subjects experienced an adverse cardiovascular event compared to only 5 in the placebo arm. The predominant criticism of this study was that there was a high prevalence of hypertension, diabetes, hyperlipidemia, obesity, and metabolic syndrome among the participants, with a substantially advanced age. In addition, subject selection was based solely upon T values, rather than in combination with defined clinical symptoms of TD. Finally, the study was not powered for safety data, and the adverse events were often self-reported with most including what is to be expected at supraphysiologic use of TRT, i.e., edema and dizziness.

Subsequent evaluation of the TOM trial sought to evaluate changes in gonadal hormones and markers of inflammation and coagulation to determine risk factors associated with potential cardiovascular events. In 179 men of mean age 74 years, within the T treatment group, the 6-month increase in serum free T levels was significantly greater in men who experienced cardiovascular events than in those who did not. In multivariable logistic regression analysis, the change in the serum levels of free T was associated with cardiovascular events, again most of which were benign. Older men with limited mobility who experienced cardiovascular events had greater increases in serum free T levels compared to control subjects [28].

A recent cohort study was conducted to assess risk of acute nonfatal MI within 90 days following an initial prescription for TRT in a healthcare database of 55,593 US men [29]. The authors also compared post/pre-rates in 167,279 men prescribed with phosphodiesterase type 5 inhibitors (PDE5I) (sildenafil or tadalafil). In men aged 65 years and older, the relative risks (RR) were 2.19 for those who received TRT and 1.15 for men who received PDE5I. The RR for TRT prescriptions increased with age from 0.95 for men under age 55 years to 3.43 for men aged greater than or equal to 75 years of age.

A limitation of this study centers on utilization of a healthcare database that did not include information on either serologic or diagnostic criteria for men who received TRT, which therefore questions the validity of the appropriateness of therapy in these men. The trial also identified only men with nonfatal MIs, based upon diagnosis of a physician, rather than a structured evaluation and specified criteria standardly set forth in a rigorous randomized controlled trial. In addition, men would have to survive their MIs to be included in the study. Lastly, the authors admit that they were unable to explore whether or not the increase in CVD mortality was related directly to serum T levels or baseline TD.

Elevation of Prostate-Specific Antigen

While TRT for treatment of TD may cause elevations in serum PSA in some men within safe parameters (as outlined in the Endocrine Society Guidelines), it has not been definitively shown to lead to a significantly increased risk of prostate cancer [7]. The saturation model postulates that the androgen receptors on the prostate are saturated at physiologic and even sub-physiologic levels of T such that there is minimal response of the prostatic tissue to TRT. This model also explains how castration results in dramatic regression of prostate cancer, as there is no longer an available substrate for the androgen receptors [30].

A European interventional trial of 200 men investigated changes in serum PSA in hypogonadal men treated with transdermal T over a 6-year period [31]. Only seven men throughout the study were found to have PSA levels above 4.0 ng/mL, six of whom were treated for suspected prostatitis with a resultant interval decrease in PSA. PSA velocity was also reported which ranged from 0.00 to 0.08 ng/ mL. Overall, ten patients at one point in the study had a velocity over greater than 0.4 ng/mL, yet no cases of prostate cancer were observed.

Risk of Prostate Cancer

The theoretical relationship between an increased risk of prostate cancer development and TRT has been a robust debate for decades. It has been demonstrated in several trials that TRT increases serum PSA levels in some men, while androgen deprivation therapy can be used in the successful treatment of advanced or high-risk prostate cancer. The supportive argument posits that by treating men with TRT, thereby increasing PSA levels and administering testosterone to a steroid-responsive cancer, a man's risk of development of prostate cancer is significantly increased. However, prior literature has failed to definitively demonstrate an increased risk in a cause-and-effect relationship. In a meta-analysis, an increased risk for all prostate events was noted while undergoing TRT between treatment and control arms, yet the analysis did not find any significant difference in individual prostate categories including definable prostate cancers, PSA levels above 4 ng/mL, or increases in PSA levels of 1.4 ng/mL [24].

A retrospective study reviewed Surveillance, Epidemiology, and End Results (SEER)–Medicare data on nearly 150,000 men over a 15-year period and compared prostate cancer outcomes in men who had received TRT prior to prostate cancer diagnosis and those who did not [32]. The authors found no statistically significant difference in disease-specific survival, overall survival, or need for salvage androgen deprivation therapy. They also found favorable results with regard to prostate cancer-specific outcomes including tumor grade and clinical staging. Compared to men without prior TRT use, men who used TRT prior to diagnosis were more likely to have moderately differentiated cancer (64.6 % vs. 59.2 %) and less likely to have poorly differentiated cancer (28.3 % vs. 34.2 %). With regard to clinical staging, men with prior TRT use were more likely to be diagnosed with stage T3 disease (4.0 % vs. 3.1 %) and less likely to be diagnosed with stage 4 disease (4.3 % vs. 6.5 %).

A prospective trial followed 81 men (mean age 57 years) for a mean (range) of 33.8 (6–144) months after starting TRT [33]. Only four men were found to develop prostate cancer over 5 years of observation, which is not greater from the incidence in the general population. The baseline PSA of men in this study was 1.32 ng/mL, and among those not diagnosed with prostate cancer, there was no significant difference either at any 12-month interval or at 5 years relative to baseline (1.43 ng/mL). However, among men diagnosed with prostate cancer, there was a significant increase in PSA from baseline by a mean value of 3.2 ng/mL. This finding led the authors to conclude that prostate cancer can be effectively diagnosed and treated while receiving TRT. These findings are consistent with prior data that demonstrated no influence of either T or other androgens on prostate cancer development [34].

The Testim Registry in the United States (TRiUS) and the International, multicenter, Post-Authorization Surveillance Study (IPASS) on long-acting-intramuscular T undecanoate (TU) investigated the safety of these forms of T and reported on both PSA and prostate cancer outcomes [35, 36]. Both studies demonstrated significant elevations in PSA from baseline in their study groups; however, the TRiUS study only demonstrated a nonsignificant increase in men over the age of 65 years. Collectively, in these trials, only one case of prostate cancer was observed during the study periods in over 2000 men. These studies together suggest that while TRT can significantly increase PSA levels, it remains within clinically acceptable ranges and does not increase the risk of prostate cancer.

A recent randomized controlled trial conducted in Malaysia investigated the efficacy and safety of TU in the treatment of aging men with TD [37]. Their study demonstrated a significant elevation in PSA from baseline in the treatment arm compared to the control arm (0.44 vs. 0.15 ng/mL). However, although statistically significant, this elevation was within acceptable limits with an increase in men receiving TU from a mean baseline of 0.80–1.25 ng/mL after 48 weeks.

While TRT is often a lifelong treatment for many men, it is important to note that no randomized controlled trials to date have been large enough and adequately powered to detect differences in prostate cancer risk. One review reported that 6000 men with LOH would need to be randomized both to the TRT and control arms and be treated for an average of 5 years to detect a 30 % difference in prostate cancer incidence [8].

Lower Urinary Tract Symptoms

In similar fashion to the potential increased risk of prostate cancer, it has long been postulated that TRT results in increased prostate volume and worsening due to benign prostatic hyperplasia (BPH). Current literature has thus far been heterogeneous, yet tends to demonstrate that TRT does not worsen LUTS and may actually improve symptoms in some cohorts.

One randomized controlled trial of 46 men evaluated the effects of intramuscular T administration on LUTS in men with known BPH [38]. A significant decrease in International Prostate Symptom Score (IPSS) scores compared to baseline was observed in the group of 23 men who received TRT (baseline mean 15.7 with 12 month mean score of 12.5); however, no difference was observed in the control group (baseline mean 14.0 and 12-month mean score 13.5). Additionally, when compared to baseline, the TRT group was found to have significantly improved maximum urine flow rates (12.9 mL/s improved to 16.7 mL/s) and voided volumes (253–283 mL) whereas no differences were observed in the control group.

A prospective study of 120 men with TD receiving TRT observed that men who experienced improvement in symptoms had significantly higher baseline American Urological Association Symptom Index (AUASI) scores than those who experienced no change or interval worsening in symptoms [39]. Overall, 55 men (45.8 %) reported a less than three-point change in AUASI relative to either worsening or improvement of LUTS; 38 men (31.7 %) had improvement in AUASI of three or more points, while 27 men (22.5 %) had worsening of AUASI three or more points. Nine men (7.5 %) initiated a new medication for treatment of LUTS during the course of the study.

A randomized, double-blind, placebo-controlled trial of 53 men aged 51–82 years with symptomatic BPH, prostate volume 30 cc or greater, and serum total T less than 280 ng/dl were randomized to daily transdermal 1 % T gel plus oral placebo or dutasteride for 6 months [40]. As expected, the TRT+dutasteride (TRT+D) group had significantly smaller prostate volumes compared to the TRT only group (38.6 vs. 58.3 cc, $p<0.05$). While the TRT+D group demonstrated a significant decrease in prostate volume from baseline at 6 months (44.4–38.6 cc), the TRT-only group demonstrated a nonsignificant increase (54.2–58.3 cc). Although significant decreases in IPSS scores were observed in both treatment groups at the end of the study period, there was no significant difference between the two groups (11.1 in TRT only vs. 10.3 in TRT+D). Most significantly, there were no differences in urine flow measures or post-void residual between the two groups. These results further suggest that TRT may offer some minor improvements in LUTS. While this study also demonstrates the desired effect of decreasing prostate volume, it failed to demonstrate any significant improvement in symptom scores or objective measures of urinary function.

At the present time, current evidence does not support an increased risk for worsening LUTS with TRT, and some men may in fact experience mild symptomatic improvement. However, these studies are of small sample size and of short duration of follow-up. More long-term randomized trials are needed before more definitive conclusions can be reached.

Obstructive Sleep Apnea

The potential risk of adverse effects of TRT on sleep, specifically obstructive sleep apnea (OSA), has been a growing area of research and discussion. Our literature search retrieved five studies that evaluated this association [41–45]. However, only one trial addressed TRT in relation to the possible worsening of OSA.

An 18-week randomized, double-blind, placebo-controlled, parallel group trial in 67 men found that TRT in obese men with severe OSA mildly worsened sleep-disordered breathing in a time-limited manner, irrespective of initial T concentrations in the short term (7 weeks), but this worsening resolved after 18 weeks [42]. Testosterone, compared to placebo, worsened the oxygen desaturation index (ODI) by 10.3 events/h and nocturnal hypoxemia (sleep time with oxygen saturation less than 90 %, SpO(2) T90%) by 6.1 % at 7 weeks. TRT did not alter ODI or SpO(2) T90% at 18 weeks compared to placebo. The authors also found that the TRT effects on ODI and SpO(2) T90% were not influenced by baseline T concentrations (T by treatment interactions, all $P>0.35$) [42].

The same authors, using the same cohort, also sought to evaluate body compositional and cardiometabolic effects of TRT with testosterone undecanoate in obese men with severe OSA [43]. This trial concluded that 18 weeks of TRT in obese men with OSA improved several important cardiometabolic parameters including insulin resistance, decreased liver fat, and increased lean muscle mass, but did not differentially reduce overall weight or the metabolic syndrome.

The remaining three trials did not adequately assess the relationship between TRT and OSA but offered some interesting results. One study of 1312 community-dwelling men aged 65 years or older from six clinical centers in the United States determined that low serum total T levels were associated with less healthy sleep in older men, explained by the degree of central adiposity [41]. Another trial evaluated 40 men with severe OSA and 40 control subjects. Serum T in the OSA group was significantly lower compared to controls, and a statistically significant inverse correlation was found between serum T level and depressive symptoms [45]. The third trial yielded positive correlations between changes in serum T and hyperoxic ventilatory recruitment threshold in 21 men with OSA and between changes in hyperoxic ventilatory recruitment threshold and time spent with oxygen saturations during sleep <90 % at 6–7 weeks, but these changes had resolved by 18 weeks [44].

To date, there are no randomized trials focusing on the long-term effects of TRT and OSA. It is recommended that clinicians inquire about symptoms of OSA in men with TD on TRT and to offer a referral for polysomnogram evaluation in men with hallmark symptoms, especially those who are starting testosterone therapy [7].

Erythrocytosis

Erythrocytosis, or polycythemia, is a known side effect of TRT. A meta-analysis of adverse effects of TRT in men with TD found 11 trials that highlighted erythrocytosis as a prominent side effect of a TRT; however, the mechanism behind what causes hemoconcentration and how this may affect men is poorly understood [23]. Only one study has addressed elevated hemoglobin and hematocrit in patients receiving TRT. This study demonstrated that TRT caused statistically significant increased hemoglobin levels. The authors then hypothesized that TRT increased serum erythropoietin, leading to erythrocytosis, yet this was disproven. There were no "serious" patient-centered adverse events (e.g., cerebrovascular accident, vascular occlusive events, venous thromboembolisms) reported during the study period of 36 months [46]. Clinicians are advised to follow the Endocrine Society Guidelines that recommend to check hematocrit at baseline, at 3–6 months, and then annually. If hematocrit is greater than 54 %, then TRT should be stopped until hematocrit decreases to a safe level or the patient on a long-acting T product should undergo phlebotomy; the patient should be evaluated for hypoxia, underlying lung disease, and/or sleep apnea, and then therapy can be reinitiated with a reduced dose [7].

Latest Developments

In August 2015, Basaria and colleagues sought to determine the effect of testosterone on subclinical atherosclerosis progression. @The placebo-controlled, double-blind, parallel group randomized trial involved 308 men 60 years or older with low or low-normal testosterone levels. They determined that over 3 years, testosterone administration versus placebo did not result in a significant difference in the rates of change in either common carotid artery intima–media thickness or coronary artery calcium, nor did it improve overall sexual function or health-related quality of life [47].

Conclusions

The available evidence indicates that TRT is largely considered to be safe in most men, with modest benefit on outcomes in men with MetS, and with a small theoretical risk of adverse events in selected high-risk populations of men with multiple medical comorbidities. TD is associated with an increased risk of development of cardiovascular disease; however, the nature of the relationship remains unclear, and recent evidence suggests that TRT may increase risk of adverse cardiovascular events in men with significant comorbidities. As with any therapeutic intervention, clinicians should discuss the benefits and potential risks of hormone replacement therapy with men prior to initiating treatment, as well as to discuss provisions for ongoing management and surveillance.

As of March 2015, the US Food and Drug Administration (FDA) has required all makers of TRT to include a warning on their information labels stating a possible increased cardiovascular and stroke risk associated with supplemental testosterone use. In contrast, in November 2014, the Coordination Group for Mutual Recognition and Decentralised Procedures–Human (CMDh), a regulatory body representing European Union member states, concluded that there is "no consistent evidence" of an increased risk for heart problems with testosterone products. The story of safety of and efficacy of TRT in older men is yet to be answered.

References

1. Shabsigh R. Hypogonadism and erectile dysfunction: the role for testosterone therapy. Int J Impot Res. 2003;15 Suppl 4:S9–13.
2. Page ST, Amory JK, Bowman FD, et al. Exogenous testosterone (T) alone or with finasteride increases physical performance, grip strength, and lean body mass in men with low serum T. J Clin Endocrinol Metab. 2005;90:1502–10.
3. Baillargeon J, Urban RJ, Ottenbacher KJ, et al. Trends in androgen prescribing in the United States, 2001 to 2011. JAMA Intern Med. 2013;173(15):1465–6.
4. Mohr BA, Guay AT, O'Donnell AB, et al. Normal, bound and nonbound testosterone levels in normally ageing men: results from the Massachusetts Male Ageing Study. Clin Endocrinol. 2005;62:64–73.
5. Wu FCW, Tajar A, Pye SR, et al. Hypothalamic-pituitary-testicular axis disruptions in older men are differentially linked to age and modifiable risk factors: the European Male Aging Study. J Clin Endocrinol Metab. 2008;93(7):2737–45.
6. Mulligan T, Frick MF, Zuraw QC, et al. Prevalence of hypogonadism in males aged at least 45 years: the HIM study. Int J Clin Pract. 2006;60(7):762–9.
7. Bhasin S, Cunningham GR, Hayes FJ, et al. Testosterone therapy in men with androgen deficiency syndromes: an Endocrine Society clinical practice guideline. J Clin Endocrinol Metab. 2010;95(6):2536–59.
8. Corona G, Vignozzi L, Sforza A, Maggi M. Risks and benefits of late onset hypogonadism treatment: an expert opinion. World J Mens Health. 2013;31(2):103–25.
9. Araujo AB, Esche GR, Kupelian V, et al. Prevalence of symptomatic androgen deficiency in men. J Clin Endocrinol Metab. 2007;92(11):4241–7.
10. Hall SA, Araujo AB, Esche GR, et al. Treatment of symptomatic androgen deficiency: results from the Boston Area Community Health Survey. Arch Intern Med. 2008;168(10):1070–6.
11. Corona G, Rastrelli G, Vignozzi L, et al. Testosterone, cardiovascular disease and the metabolic syndrome. Best Pract Res Clin Endocrinol Metab. 2011;25:337–53.
12. Traish AM, Saad F, Guay A. The dark side of testosterone deficiency: II. Type 2 diabetes and insulin resistance. J Androl. 2009;30(1):23–32.
13. Traish AM, Guay A, Feeley R, Saad F. The dark side of testosterone deficiency: I. Metabolic syndrome and erectile dysfunction. J Androl. 2009;30(1):10–22.
14. Zitzmann M. Testosterone deficiency, insulin resistance and the metabolic syndrome. Nat Rev Endocr. 2009;5(12):673–81.
15. Traish AM, Saad F, Feeley RJ, Guay A. The dark side of testosterone deficiency: III. Cardiovascular disease. J Androl. 2009;30(5):477–94.
16. Turek PJ. In: Tanagho EA, McAninch JC, editors. Smith's urology, Chap 46. 17th ed. Stamford: Appleton and Lange; 2003.
17. Heidelbaugh JJ. Yes: screening for testosterone deficiency is worthwhile in most older men. Am Fam Physician. 2015;91(4):220–1.
18. Fugh-Berman A. No: screening may be harmful, and benefits are unproven. Am Fam Physician. 2015;91(4):226–8.
19. Wang C, Nieschlag E, Swerdloff R, et al. ISA, ISSAM, EAU, EAA and ASA recommendations: investigation, treatment, and monitoring of late-onset hypogonadism in males. Aging Male. 2009;12:5–12.
20. Petak SM, Nankin HR, Spark RF, et al. American Association of Clinical Endocrinologists Medical Guidelines for clinical practice for the evaluation and treatment of hypogonadism in adult male patients—2002 update. Endocr Pract. 2002;8:439–56.
21. Mohammed O, Freundlich RE, et al. The quantitative ADAM questionnaire: a new tool in quantifying the severity of hypogonadism. Int J Impot Res. 2010;22(1):20–4.
22. Jackson G, Montorsi P, Adams MA, et al. Cardiovascular aspects of sexual medicine. J Sex Med. 2010;7:1608–26.

23. Fernandez-Balsells MM, Murad MH, Lane M, et al. Adverse effects of testosterone therapy in adult men: a systematic review and meta-analysis. J Clin Endocrinol Metab. 2010;95:2560–75.

24. Calof OM, Singh AB, Lee ML, et al. Adverse events associated with testosterone replacement in middle-aged and older men: a meta-analysis of randomized, placebo-controlled trials. J Gerontol. 2005;60(11):1451–7.

25. Xu L, Freeman G, Cowling BJ, Schooling CM. Testosterone therapy and cardiovascular events among men: a systematic review and meta-analysis of placebo-controlled randomized trials. BMC Med. 2013;11:108.

26. Vigen R, O'Donnell CI, Baron AE, et al. Association of testosterone therapy with mortality, myocardial infarction, and stroke in men with low testosterone levels. JAMA. 2013;310(17):1829–36.

27. Shores MM, Smith NL, Forsberg CW, et al. Testosterone treatment and mortality in men with low testosterone levels. J Clin Endocrinol Metab. 2012;97:2050–8.

28. Basaria S, Coviello AD, Travison TG, et al. Adverse events associated with testosterone administration. N Engl J Med. 2010;363(2):109–22.

29. Finkle WD, Greenland S, Ridgeway GK, et al. Increased risk of non-fatal myocardial infarction following testosterone therapy prescription in men. PLoS One. 2014;9(1):1–7.

30. Morgentaler A, Traish A. Shifting the paradigm of testosterone and prostate cancer: the saturation model and the limits of androgen-dependent growth. Eur Urol. 2008;55(2009):310–21.

31. Raynaud JP, Gardette J, Rollet J, Legros JJ. Prostate-specific antigen (PSA) concentrations in hypogonadal men during 6 years of transdermal testosterone treatment. BJU Int. 2013;111:880–90.

32. Kaplan AL, Hu JC. Use of testosterone replacement therapy in the United States and its effect on subsequent prostate cancer outcomes. Urology. 2013;82:321–6.

33. Coward RM, Simhan J, Carson CC. Prostate-specific antigen changes and prostate cancer in hypogonadal men treated with testosterone replacement therapy. BJU Int. 2008;103:1179–83.

34. Morgentaler A. Testosterone and prostate cancer: what are the risks for middle-aged men? Urol Clin N Am. 2011;38:119–24.

35. Bhattacharya RK, Khera M, Blick G, et al. 2012) Testosterone replacement therapy among elderly males: the Testim Registry in the US (TRiUS. Clin Interv Aging. 2012;7:321–30.

36. Zitzmann M, Mattern A, Hanisch J, et al. IPASS: A study on the tolerability and effectiveness of injectable testosterone undecanoate for the treatment of male hypogonadism in a worldwide sample of 1,438 men. J Sex Med. 2013;10:579–88.

37. Tan WS, Low WY, Ng CJ, et al. Efficacy and safety of long-acting intramuscular testosterone undecanoate in aging men: a randomized controlled study. BJU Int. 2013;111:1130–40.

38. Shigehara K, Sugimoto K, Konaka H, Iijima M, Fukushima M, Maeda Y, et al. Androgen replacement therapy contributes to improving lower urinary tract symptoms in patients with hypogonadism and benign prostate hypertrophy: a randomised controlled study. Aging Male. 2011;14(1):53–8.

39. Pearl JA, Berhanu D, Francois N, Masson P, Zargaroff S, Cashy J, McVary KT. Testosterone supplementation does not worsen lower urinary tract symptoms. J Urol. 2013;190:1828–33.

40. Page ST, Hirano L, Gilchriest J, et al. Dutasteride reduces prostate size and prostate specific antigen in older hypogonadal men with benign prostatic hyperplasia undergoing testosterone replacement therapy. J Urol. 2011;186:191–7.

41. Barrett-Connor E, Dam TT, Stone K, et al. The association of testosterone levels with overall sleep quality, sleep architecture, and sleep-disordered breathing. J Clin Endocrinol Metab. 2008;93(7):2602–9.

42. Hoyos CM, Killick R, Yee BJ, et al. Effects of testosterone therapy on sleep and breathing in obese men with severe obstructive sleep apnoea: a randomized placebo-controlled trial. Clin Endocrinol (Oxf). 2012;77(4):599–607.

43. Hoyos CM, Yee BJ, Phillips CL, et al. Body compositional and cardiometabolic effects of testosterone therapy in obese men with severe obstructive sleep apnoea: a randomised placebo-controlled trial. Eur J Endocrinol. 2012;167(4):531–41.

44. Killick R, Wang D, Hoyos CM, et al. The effects of testosterone on ventilatory responses in men with obstructive sleep apnea: a randomised, placebo-controlled trial. J Sleep Res. 2013;22(3):331–6.

45. Bercea RM, Patacchioli FR, Ghiciuc CM, et al. Serum testosterone and depressive symptoms in severe OSA patients. Andrologia. 2013;45(5):345–50.
46. Maggio M, Snyder PJ, Ceda GP, et al. Is the haematopoietic effect of testosterone mediated by erythropoietin? The results of a clinical trial in older men. Andrology. 2013;1(1):24–8.
47. Basria S, Harman SM, Travison TG, et al. Effects of testosterone administration for 3 years on subclinical atherosclerosis progression in older men with low or low-normal testosterone levels. JAMA. 2015;314(6):570–81.

Chapter 14
Prostate Cancer: A Primary Care Perspective

Robert Langan

Introduction

Prostate cancer is the most common non-skin cancer diagnosed in the United States (US) [1], with an estimated 221,000 cases diagnosed in 2015, and it is the second most common cause of cancer death in men, with a projected 28,000 deaths in 2015 [2]. It is more common in older men, in African Americans, and in men with a first-degree relative with prostate cancer [3]. Since 1999, the incidence of prostate cancer has decreased by approximately 40 cases/100,000 men. Mortality from prostate cancer has also decreased, although the decline has not been as dramatic [4] (Fig. 14.1).

There are a number of proposed reasons why the incidence and mortality have decreased. With the introduction of prostate-specific antigen (PSA) testing in the 1990s, the amount of screening examinations in men increased dramatically. At the same time, there have been improvements in the treatment of prostate cancer and better surveillance tools for men diagnosed with prostate cancer. As the gap between incidence and mortality from prostate cancer widened in the early 2000s, it was proposed that this finding represented an overdiagnosis of prostate cancer without defined clinical significance in many cases that ultimately did not lead to mortality [5].

R. Langan, MD (✉)
Department of Family Medicine, St. Luke's University Hospital, 2830 Easton Avenue, Bethlehem, PA 18017, USA
e-mail: robert.langan@sluhn.org

© Springer International Publishing Switzerland 2016
J.J. Heidelbaugh (ed.), *Men's Health in Primary Care*, Current Clinical Practice,
DOI 10.1007/978-3-319-26091-4_14

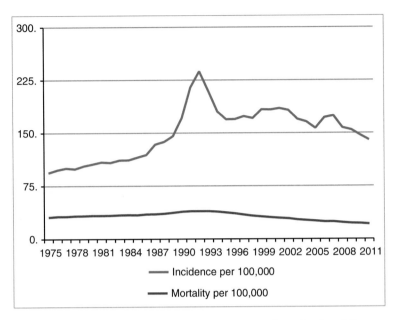

Fig. 14.1 Prostate cancer incidence and mortality 1975–2011. Information from [4]

Prostate-Specific Antigen Testing: History and Early Studies

The PSA is a 240-amino acid serine protease that belongs to the larger family of glandular kallikreins. It was isolated by both Wang and Graves separately in 1979 [6, 7]. It was initially investigated as a marker for detecting semen in cases of rape. In 1987, in an attempt to see if a link existed between elevated PSA levels and adenocarcinoma of the prostate, PSA levels were measured in 2200 samples taken from 699 patients and were found to be elevated in 122 out of 127 patients with newly diagnosed prostate cancer. PSA levels fell following treatment with radical prostatectomy, and rising PSA levels after surgery were associated with recurrence of the disease [8].

Within a few years, the feasibility of using PSA as a screening test for prostate cancer was investigated in 1653 healthy men aged 50 years or greater. Using a cutoff value of greater than or equal to 4.0 micrograms/liter (mcg/l), men with an elevated PSA underwent digital rectal examination (DRE) and transrectal ultrasound (TRUS) of the prostate with biopsies done in men with abnormal DRE or TRUS. In the 107 men with a PSA of 4.0–9.9 mcg/l, 85 required biopsy (85/107, or 79 %) and 19 of those were diagnosed with prostate cancer (19/85, or 22 %). In the 30 men with a PSA above 10, 27 required biopsy (27/30, or 90 %) and 18 had prostate cancer (18/27, or 67 %) (Fig. 14.2). The authors noted that "Our results provide no information about the value of serum PSA measurement with respect to morbidity and mortality" and concluded that the results "suggest that measurement of serum PSA

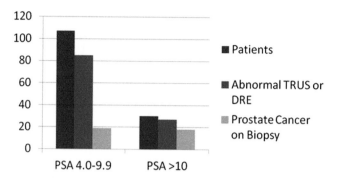

Fig. 14.2 Association between elevated prostate-specific antigen, abnormal biopsy, and prostate cancer diagnosis in initial feasibility study. Information from [9]

and rectal examination combined, with the addition of ultrasonography in patients with abnormal findings, will provide a better method of detecting prostate cancer than rectal examination alone." [9] Despite this, about 95 % of male urologists and 78 % of male primary care physicians older than 50 years report that they have had a PSA test themselves [10].

Other Methods to Screen for Prostate Cancer

In addition to the aforementioned DRE, a number of variations on PSA testing [11–15] have been proposed to attempt to increase the accuracy of prostate cancer screening. The clinical usefulness of these strategies has not been proven, and they are not recommended for use by any major organization. These PSA variations include:

1. Prostate velocity: the rate of change of PSA over a specified period of time
2. Free PSA: the amount of PSA that is not bound to protein
3. PSA density: the amount of PSA per unit volume of the prostate gland (as determined by TRUS)
4. Age-specific PSA levels: using different cutoff values for "normal" PSA based on age
5. Race-specific PSA levels: using different cutoff values for "normal" PSA based on race

An abnormal DRE is in itself considered an indication for referral for prostate biopsy regardless of PSA level [16]. In a cohort of 806 men undergoing prostate biopsy (including 306 men ultimately diagnosed with prostate cancer), 44 % of the men with cancer had an abnormal DRE ($n=136$) and a third of the men with an abnormal DRE had a normal PSA test ($n=43$) [17]. However, a systematic review in 2013 failed to find any major study in which DRE alone was used for screening [18]. No major organization recommends the routine use of DRE in prostate cancer screening; the AUA states that DRE should be considered a "secondary test" with potential utility for determining the need for a prostate biopsy [19].

In addition to PSA-based testing, other markers have been investigated for the early detection of prostate cancer. Prostate cancer antigen 3 (PCA3) is a gene that is overexpressed in specific prostate cancer cell lines but not other prostate conditions, such as prostatitis. It is collected as a urine test after a prostate massage and is currently commercially available. In the Reduction by Dutasteride of prostate Cancer Events (REDUCE) trial, an elevated PCA3 score was correlated with a positive prostate biopsy in men at average risk for prostate cancer with a PSA test between 2.5 and 10 ng/mL [20]. PCA3 was evaluated alone and in combination with the gene fusion TMPRSS2:ERG for the detection of prostate cancer in a trial of 497 men scheduled to undergo prostate biopsy; adding TMPRSS2:ERG to PCA3 significantly improved the sensitivity of PCA3. The authors concluded that adding both tests to clinical practice has the potential to decrease the number of prostate biopsies [21].

A commercially available assay combining PSA, PCA3, and TMPRSS2:ERG is marketed under the name MiPS (http://www.mlabs.umich.edu/files/pdfs/MiPS_FAQ.pdf). The PSA precursor, 2-pro PSA, has also been evaluated as a potential test to improve the ability to detect prostate cancer and avoid unnecessary biopsies [22]. There are currently no cost-effective screening tests that have been studied and shown to reduce morbidity or mortality associated with prostate cancer. A number of other single tests are currently under investigation, yet there is reason to believe that future screening strategies for prostate cancer will involve an assay that combines protein and gene testing [23].

PLCO and ERSPC

In 2012, results of the US-based Prostate, Lung, Colorectal, and Ovarian screening trial (PLCO) were published. Over 76,000 men aged 55–74 years, including 4 % African Americans and 7 % with a family medical history of prostate cancer, were randomized to no screening or screening with annual PSA for 6 years and annual DRE for 4 years and followed for 13 years. Of note, the degree of contamination, defined as the percentage of men in the control group who received screening, reached 50 % by year 6. The incidence of prostate cancer was nonsignificantly higher in the screened group (11 % versus 9.9 %), and mortality was nonsignificantly lower in the screened group (0.38 % versus 0.41 %). The authors concluded that there was no mortality benefit seen from combined screening [24].

In the same year, the results of the European Randomized Study of Screening for Prostate Cancer (ERSPC) were also published. This study, conducted in 7 countries in Europe, included over 180,000 men aged 55–69 years. Men were randomized to either PSA every 4 years or no screening and patients were followed for 11 years. The degree of PSA screening contamination was lower than in PLCO at 20 %.

The incidence of prostate cancer was significantly higher in the screened group (9.6 % versus 6 %) and mortality was significantly lower in the screened group (0.41 % versus 0.52 %). This corresponds to a 20 % relative risk reduction and an absolute risk reduction of seven prostate cancer deaths for 10,000 men screened [25]. It is important to note that both the PLCO and the ERSPC trials included a predominance of white men, which may negatively bias the impact and predictive value of screening African American men, who have the highest statistical risk of developing and dying from prostate cancer.

In 2013, a Cochrane review including five randomized controlled trials and over 340,000 men addressed whether prostate cancer screening reduced prostate-specific mortality or all-cause mortality and whether it had an impact on quality of life or adverse events. The authors concluded that prostate cancer screening did not significantly reduce prostate cancer-specific or overall mortality. Furthermore, harms associated with screening and diagnosis were frequent and moderate in severity and there were also harms associated with treatment. Only screening with PSA was assessed in the review; no evidence of the utility and limitations of DRE or other tests were studied [18].

Taken together, these two large trials and Cochrane review suggest that screening for prostate cancer with serial PSA testing has only a modest reduction in prostate cancer mortality during the first 10 years of initiating such screening. However, both the costs and the risks associated with overdiagnosis of prostate cancer are substantial.

Benefits and Risks of Screening

Characteristics of ideal screening programs include [26]:

1. Evaluation of diseases that have a significant effect on public health and have an asymptomatic period during which detection is possible and disease outcomes are improved by treatment during the asymptomatic phase
2. Tests that are sufficiently sensitive to detect the disease during the asymptomatic phase, are sufficiently specific to minimize false-positive results, and are acceptable to patients
3. Involves populations with sufficiently high prevalence of the disease to justify screening that have access to relevant medical care and are willing to comply with further work-up and treatment

In general, prostate cancer screening programs with PSA testing meets the first and third criteria of an ideal screening program. No studies to date have evaluated the effect of PSA screening on the development of subsequent metastatic disease, so the primary outcome that has been evaluated is reduction in prostate cancer-specific mortality. Based upon the results of the PLCO and ERPSPC trials, there is adequate evidence that the benefits of PSA screening and subsequent early treatment are a reduction of 0–1 deaths for every 1000 men screened and an estimated diagnosis of 1 case of prostate cancer in every 1470 men screened [3].

When a man is told that his PSA test is abnormal, it is often associated with negative psychological effects such as excessive worry about prostate cancer itself, the effects of treatment, and the impact on his life and his family [27], although the magnitude of these effects has not been measured [28]. Transrectal ultrasound (TRUS)-guided biopsy of the prostate, the diagnostic test of choice, is also associated with a number of side effects, such as pain, fever, urethral and rectal bleeding, infection, transient urinary tract symptoms, and, in 1 % of patients, hospitalization due to pain and/or sepsis [29, 30]. The risk of a false-positive PSA test is substantial. In the PLCO trial, there was a 12.9 % cumulative risk of at least one false-positive PSA test after four screening tests [24]. In the Finnish center of the ERPSC trial, 12.5 % of men had at least one false-positive result after three rounds of PSA testing [25]. Conversely, false-negative results also occur, and there is no absolute PSA level below which prostate cancer cannot occur.

In the United States, approximately 9 out of every 10 men diagnosed with localized prostate cancer opted for treatment [31], typically radical prostatectomy and radiation, and these treatments are associated with a number of side effects. In the 2012 United States Preventive Services Task Force (USPSTF) final recommendation statement, it was estimated that there is a 20 % increase in absolute risk of urinary incontinence and a 30 % increase in absolute risk for erectile dysfunction among men who were treated with a radical prostatectomy. The absolute risk of urinary incontinence was estimated to increase by 17 % among men treated with radiation [3]. Thus, the USPSTF recommendation was changed to a D category recommendation, citing that PSA-based prostate cancer screening causes harm. The USPSTF summarized the population-based risks and benefits of prostate cancer screening in the same recommendation statement. They assumed PSA testing every 1–4 years in men at average risk for developing prostate cancer who were aged 55–69 years old and who were followed for 10 years (Table 14.1).

Table 14.1 Effects and harms of prostate cancer screening

Effects of PSA screening on prostate cancer mortality	
Men who will die of prostate cancer without screening	5/1000 men
Men who will die of prostate cancer with screening	4–5/1000 men
Men who will not die of prostate cancer because of screening	0–1/1000 men
Harms of PSA screening and subsequent diagnosis and treatment of prostate cancer	
Men who will have at least one false positive	100–120/1000 men
Men who will have a cardiovascular event due to treatment	2/1000 men
Men who will have a deep vein thrombosis/pulmonary embolism due to treatment	1/1000 men
Men who will have erectile dysfunction due to treatment	29/1000 men
Men who will have urinary incontinence due to treatment	18/1000 men
Men who will die due to treatment	<1/1000 men

Information from [3]

Screening Recommendations

A number of national organizations have published recommendations for prostate cancer screening. This section will discuss recommendations from the United States Preventive Services Task Force (USPSTF), the American Urological Association (AUA), the American Cancer Society (ACS), and the American College of Physicians (ACP).

The 2012 USPSTF recommends against PSA-based screening for prostate cancer (grade D). The authors noted that "all men deserve to know what the science tells us about PSA screening: there is a very small potential benefit and significant potential harms." If patients specifically request PSA screening, the USPSTF recommends that men should be given sufficient information about the relative benefits and harms in order to make an informed choice [3]. The American Academy of Family Physicians (AAFP) endorses the USPSTF statement [32].

The AUA clinical practice guideline for early detection of prostate cancer was updated in 2013. The expert panel recommends against screening any men under the age of 40 years, noting that in this population the incidence of prostate cancer is very low, there is no compelling evidence of the benefit of screening, and the harms of screening are likely high. Similarly, low-risk men (e.g., non-African American and no family history of prostate cancer) between the ages of 41 and 54 years should not be screened, but high-risk men should have individualized discussions about screening. Using the same projected morbidity and mortality data as the USPSTF, the expert panel recommends that men aged 55–69 have a screening strategy that involves "shared decision making" with their physician and incorporates a man's "values and preferences." Finally, the AUA does not recommend prostate cancer screening for men aged 70 years or older or men with a life expectancy of less than 10–15 years. The recommended screening test, if used, is PSA with a 2-year testing interval preferred over an annual test [19].

The ACS clinical practice guideline for prostate cancer screening was last updated in 2010. The ACS recommends that discussions about screening should occur at age 50 years for average-risk men, 45 years for moderate-risk men (African American and/or one first-degree relative diagnosed with prostate cancer prior to age 65 years), and 40 years for high-risk men (two or more first-degree relatives diagnosed with prostate cancer prior to age 65 years). Men with a life expectancy of less than 10 years and men older than 70 years of age and older should not be screened, regardless of risk category. As with the AUA guideline, the ACS recommends that men must be made aware of the risks and benefits of prostate cancer screening and be allowed to make an informed decision. Screening, if performed, should be done with a PSA test. DRE may be considered in conjunction with PSA, but the value is likely low. If the PSA is less than 2.5 ng/mL, it can be repeated in 2 years; if the PSA is 2.5–3.9 ng/mL, it should be repeated in 1 year; and if the PSA is 4 ng/mL or higher, the man should be referred to a urologist for consideration of prostate biopsy [33].

Table 14.2 Current recommended screening of average-risk men for prostate cancer with PSA testing

Organization	Age group of average-risk men (unless otherwise specified)			
	<40 years	40–54 years	55–69 years	>70 years
USPSTF (2013)	No	No	No	No
AUA (2013)	No	No	Shared decision making	No
ACS (2010)	No	Consider screening after risks and benefits are discussed with patient		No
ACP (2013)	No	Discuss limited benefits and substantial risks with patient		No

PSA prostate-specific antigen, *USPSTF* United States Preventive Services Task Force, *AUA* American Urological Association, *ACS* American Cancer Society, *ACP* American College of Physicians

Information from [3, 19, 33, 34]

In 2013, the ACP published its guideline on the early detection of prostate cancer. The guideline recognizes that PSA testing and DRE are the tests generally used for screening, but PSA is more sensitive than DRE. Prostate cancer screening is not recommended for any men under the age of 50 years, over the age of 69 years, or with a life expectancy of less than 10–15 years. For average-risk men between the ages of 50 and 69 years, the ACP recommends that physicians inform men of the limited potential benefits and substantial harms of prostate cancer screening. Furthermore, men who do not express a clear preference for screening should not be offered screening. The ACP concludes that prostate cancer screening is low-value care, "given that the chances of harm with screening outweigh the chances of benefit for most men and that the direct and indirect costs associated with biopsy, repeated testing, aggressive therapy, patient anxiety and missed work are significant [34]." The four current guidelines for prostate cancer screening are summarized in Table 14.2.

Screening Summary

Epidemiologic studies reveal that 9 out of 10 men diagnosed with prostate cancer by screening receive treatment with the goal of complete cure rather than observation [30, 35]. In the 2012 Prostate Cancer Intervention versus Observation Trial (PIVOT), 731 men with localized prostate cancer were randomized to radical prostatectomy or observation. After 12 years, there was no reduction in prostate cancer-specific or overall mortality. In a subset of men with PSA greater than 10 mcg/l, men in the radical prostatectomy group had a 13.2 % reduction in all-cause mortality [36].

What conclusions can be drawn from the available information? First, if the purpose of an effective screening test is to reduce morbidity and mortality from a disease or condition, PSA testing has yet to prove its worth. Secondly, when a test receives widespread adoption and acceptance by patients and the medical community prior to good data proving its effectiveness, it is extremely difficult to dissuade individuals from its use. Thirdly, there is currently no viable alternative to screening with PSA, and many men and physicians feel more comfortable utilizing an imperfect test rather than no test at all. Finally, there is little data to guide the use of PSA screening in high-risk men (African American men and men with a family history of prostate cancer). If patients request PSA screening or physicians choose to discuss PSA screening with their patients, it is crucial that physicians provide adequate counseling to their patients about the limited benefits and substantial harms associated with screening.

Surveillance of Men Diagnosed with Prostate Cancer

Treatment of men with prostate cancer is determined by the tumor size, tumor invasion of lymph nodes, and the presence or absence of metastatic spread—the TMN staging system. In addition, PSA levels and the Gleason score (a pathologic determination of the two most frequent patterns of neoplastic cells seen on a prostate biopsy) [37] are also considered. Finally, patient-specific factors, such as life expectancy, comorbid conditions, the availability of local resources, and the wishes and preferences of the man and his family must be factored into the final treatment decision. Depending upon these components, treatment may include observation, active surveillance, surgery, external beam radiation, brachytherapy, and/or hormonal therapy and involve a coordinated team approach. A detailed discussion of prostate cancer treatment strategies can be found at the National Comprehensive Cancer Network website, available at http://www.nccn.org/professionals/physcian_gls/f_guidelines.asp (registration required).

If treatment of prostate cancer is elected, patients will often return to their primary care physician for "ongoing surveillance" once the course of treatment is completed. The objective of this surveillance is to detect recurrent disease at an early and, presumably, treatable stage. Unfortunately, there are no randomized controlled trials that have evaluated the optimal manner to conduct such posttreatment surveillance [38]. Ongoing surveillance is not recommended if a man has limited life expectancy or is unwilling or unable to undergo further treatment. The National Comprehensive Cancer Network, in their prostate cancer guideline, recommends PSA testing every 6 months for 5 years following the completion of treatment but does not recommend DRE or routine imaging studies [39].

In its 2013 best practice statement [38], the AUA makes several recommendations concerning the posttreatment use of PSA in men with prostate cancer. Periodic PSA testing should be offered to detect disease recurrence after definitive local treatment, although the optimal strategy for initiating adjuvant therapy for recurrence is unknown, as is whether or not PSA testing in such situations improves survival [40, 41]. After radical prostatectomy, PSA should remain undetectable, and a confirmed elevation should prompt reevaluation by the patient's urologist [42]. Unlike surgical follow-up, men who undergo external beam radiation or brachytherapy for treatment will still have a detectable PSA. A 2005 consensus panel concluded that any rise in PSA of 2.0 ng/mL or greater over the posttreatment PSA nadir should be considered a true recurrence that necessitates evaluation [43].

Evaluation of Men with Elevated PSA and Negative Biopsy

TRUS-guided prostate biopsy is the preferred method for evaluating men for prostate cancer, whether due to an abnormal DRE or an elevated PSA test. Extended prostate biopsy schemes (typically 12-core biopsies) have been shown to be superior to 6- and 8-core biopsy protocols [44] without an increase in the rates of major complications [45].

Some findings on prostate biopsy warrant close observation as they may be associated with a higher incidence of subsequently detected prostate cancer. Atypical small acinar proliferation (ASAP) and multifocal high-grade prostatic intraepithelial neoplasia (HGPIN) on prostate biopsy have been associated with a higher risk of prostate cancer on subsequent prostate biopsy. If multifocal HGPIN or ASAP are seen, it is reasonable to have the pathology reviewed since, if prostate cancer is seen, further biopsies are unnecessary [46]. Men with multifocal HGPIN should undergo a repeat biopsy in 3 years [47], while men with ASAP sooner. Repeat "saturation" biopsies of 20 core sites are often done in these situations [48].

Persistently elevated PSA following a negative prostate biopsy has been used as an indication for repeat biopsy, but this strategy has not been well studied. Low levels of percent-free PSA (<12 %) have been shown to be a more sensitive and specific marker than total PSA for the presence of prostate cancer [49]. The role of imaging in determining which men would benefit from repeat prostate biopsy is unclear. In a review of 479 men who had undergone two previous negative prostate biopsies, prostate cancer detection was evaluated using one of two biopsy protocols on subsequent biopsy specimens over a 10-year period. Prostate cancer was uncommonly detected on subsequent biopsies and, when found, was usually clinically insignificant. The authors concluded that there should be a very high threshold to repeat a prostate biopsy after a previous negative biopsy [50].

References

1. US Cancer Statistics Working Group. United States cancer statistics: 1999–2011 incidence and mortality web-based report. Atlanta (GA): Department of Health and Human Services, Centers for Disease Control and Prevention, and National Cancer Institute; 2014.
2. Prostate Cancer Overview. American Cancer Society. January 2015. http://www.cancer.org/cancer/prostatecancer/overviewguide/prostate-cancer-overview-key-statistics
3. Final Recommendation Statement. Prostate cancer: screening. U.S. Preventive Services Task Force. 2014. http://www.uspreventiveservicestaskforce.org/Page/Document/RecommendationStatementFinal/prostate-cancer-screening

4. Howlader N, Noone AM, Krapcho M, Garshell J, Miller D, Altekruse SF, Kosary CL, Yu M, Ruhl J, Tatalovich Z,Mariotto A, Lewis DR, Chen HS, Feuer EJ, Cronin KA (eds) SEER cancer statistics review, 1975-2011. Bethesda, MD: National Cancer Institute. http://seer.cancer.gov/csr/1975_2011/, based on November 2013 SEER data submission, posted to the SEER web site, April 2014.
5. Welch HG, Black WC. Overdiagnosis in cancer. J Natl Cancer Inst. 2010;102(9):605–13.
6. Wang MC, Valenzuela LA, Murphy GP, Chu TM. Purification of a human prostate specific antigen. Invest Urol. 1979;17:159–63.
7. Graves HCB, Sensabaugh GF, Blake ET. Postcoital detection of a male-specific semen protein: application to the investigation of rape. N Engl J Med. 1985;312:338–43.
8. Stamey TA, Yang N, Hay AR, et al. Prostate-specific antigen as a serum marker for adenocarcinoma of the prostate. N Engl J Med. 1987;317:909–16.
9. Catalona WJ, Smith DS, Ratliff TL, et al. Measurement of prostate-specific antigen in serum as a screening test for prostate cancer. N Engl J Med. 1991;324:1156–61.
10. Chan EC, Barry MJ, Vernon SW, Ahn C. Brief report: physicians and their personal prostate cancer-screening practices with prostate-specific antigen: a national survey. J Gen Intern Med. 2006;21:257–9.
11. Carter HB, Pearson JD. PSA velocity for the diagnosis of early prostate cancer. A new concept. Urol Clin N Am. 1993;20(4):665–70.
12. Oesterling JE, Jacobsen SJ, Klee GG, et al. Free, complexed and total serum prostate specific antigen: the establishment of appropriate reference ranges for their concentration and ratios. J Urol. 1995;154(3):1090–5.
13. Benson MC, Whang IS, Pantuck A, et al. Prostate specific antigen density: a means of distinguishing benign prostatic hypertrophy and prostate cancer. J Urol. 1992;147(3 Pt 2):815–6.
14. Oesterling JE, Jacobsen SJ, Chute CG, et al. Serum prostate-specific antigen in a community-based population of healthy men. Establishment of age-specific reference ranges. JAMA. 1993;270(7):860–4.
15. Abdalla I, Ray P, Vaida F, Vijayakumar S. Racial differences in prostate-specific antigen levels and prostate-specific densities in patients with prostate cancer. Am J Clin Oncol. 1999;22(6):537–41.
16. Wolf AM, Wender RC, Etzioni RB, American Cancer Society Prostate Cancer Advisory Committee, et al. American Cancer Society guideline for the early detection of prostate cancer: update 2010. CA Cancer J Clin. 2010;60(2):70–98.
17. Palmerola R, Smith P, Eliot V, et al. The digital rectal examination (DRE) remains important—outcomes from a contemporary cohort of men undergoing an initial 12-18 core prostate needle biopsy. Can J Urol. 2012;19(6):6542–7.
18. Ilic D, Neuberger MM, Djulbegovic M, Dahm P. Screening for prostate cancer. Cochrane Database Syst Rev 2013, Issue 1. Art. No.: CD004720.
19. Carter HB, Albertsen PC, Barry MJ, et al. Early detection of prostate cancer: AUA guideline. J Urol. 2013;190(2):419–26.
20. Aubin SM, Reid J, Sarno MJ, et al. Prostate cancer gene 3 score predicts prostate biopsy outcome in men receiving dutasteride for prevention of prostate cancer: results from the REDUCE trial. Urology. 2011;78(2):380–5.
21. Leyten GH, Hessels D, Jannink SA, et al. Prospective multicentre evaluation of PCA3 and TMPRSS2:ERG gene fusions as diagnostic and prognostic urinary biomarkers for prostate cancer. Eur Urol. 2014;65(3):534–42.
22. Abrate A, Lughezzani G, Gadda G, et al. Clinical use of 2-pro PSA and its derivatives for the detection of prostate cancer: a review of the literature. Kor J Urol. 2014;55(7):436–45.
23. Velonas VM, Woo HH, dos Remedios CG, Assinger SJ. Current status of biomarkers for prostate cancer. Int J Mol Sci. 2013;14(6):11034–60.
24. Andriole GL, PLCO Project Team, et al. Prostate cancer screening in the randomized prostate, lung, colorectal and ovarian cancer screening trial: mortality results after 13 years of follow-up. J Natl Cancer Inst. 2012;104(2):125–32.
25. Schroder FH, ERSPC Investigators, et al. Prostate-cancer mortality at 11 years of follow up. N Engl J Med. 2012;366(11):981–90.

26. Gates TJ. Screening for cancer: evaluating the evidence. Am Fam Physician. 2001;63(3):513–23.
27. Cormier L, et al. Impact of prostate cancer screening on health-related quality of life in at-risk families. Urology. 2002;59(6):901–6.
28. Lin K, Lipsitz R, Miller T, Janakiraman S. Benefits and harms of prostate-specific antigen screening for prostate cancer: an evidence update for the U.S. Preventive Services Task Force. Ann Intern Med. 2008;149(3):192–9.
29. Rosario DJ, Lane JA, Metcalfe C, Donovan JL, Doble A, Goodwin L, et al. Short term outcomes of prostate biopsy in men tested for cancer by prostate specific antigen: prospective evaluation within ProtecT study. BMJ. 2012;344:d7894.
30. Raaijmakers R, Kirkels WJ, Roobol MJ, Wildhagen MF, Schröder FH. Complication rates and risk factors of 5802 transrectal ultrasound-guided sextant biopsies of the prostate within a population-based screening program. Urology. 2002;60:826–30.
31. Welch HG, Albertsen PC. Prostate cancer diagnosis and treatment after the introduction of prostate-specific antigen screening: 1986–2005. J Natl Cancer Inst. 2009;101:1325–9.
32. American Academy of Family Physicians. Clinical Preventive Services recommendation: prostate cancer. http://www.aafp.org/patient-care/clinical-recommendations/all/prostate-cancer.html. Accessed 24 Feb 2015.
33. Wolf AMD, et al. American Cancer Society guideline for early detection of prostate cancer: update 2010. CA Cancer J Clin. 2010;60(2):70–98.
34. Qaseem A, Barry MJ, Denberg TD, Clinical Guidelines Committee of the American College of Physicians, et al. Screening for prostate cancer: a guidance statement from the Clinical Guidelines Committee of the American College of Physicians. Ann Intern Med. 2013;158(10):761–9.
35. Cooperberg MR, Broering JM, Carroll PR. Time trends and local variation in primary treatment of localized prostate cancer. J Clin Oncol. 2010;28:1117–23.
36. Wilt TJ, Prostate Cancer Intervention versus Observation Trial (PIVOT) Study Group, et al. Radical prostatectomy versus observation for localized prostate cancer. N Engl J Med. 2012;367(3):203–13.
37. Epstein JI, Allsbrook Jr WC, Amin MB, Egevad LL, ISUP Grading Committee. The 2005 International Society of Urological Pathology (ISUP) consensus conference on Gleason grading of prostatic carcinoma. Am J Surg Pathol. 2005;29(9):1228–42.
38. American Urological Association. PSA testing for the pretreatment staging and posttreatment management of prostate cancer: 2013 revision of 2009 best practice statement. http://www.auanet.org/education/guidelines/prostate-specific-antigen.cfm. Accessed 24 Feb 2015
39. National Comprehensive Cancer Network. http://www.nccn.org/professionals/physician_gls/f_guidelines.asp (registration required). Accessed 24 Feb 2015
40. Moul JW, Wu H, Sun L, et al. Early versus delayed hormonal therapy for prostate specific antigen only recurrence of prostate cancer after radical prostatectomy. J Urol. 2004;171:1141.
41. Freedland SJ, Moul JW. Prostate specific antigen recurrence after definitive therapy. J Urol. 2007;177:1985.
42. Stephenson AJ, Kattan MW, Eastham JA, et al. Defining biochemical recurrence of prostate cancer after radical prostatectomy: a proposal for a standardized definition. J Clin Oncol. 2006;24:3973.
43. Roach M, Hanks GE, Thames H, et al. Defining biochemical failure following radiotherapy with or without hormonal therapy in men with clinically localized prostate cancer: recommendations of the RTOG-ASTRO Phoenix consensus conference. Int J Radiat Oncol Biol Phys. 2006;65:965.
44. Presti Jr JC, O'Dowd GJ, Miller MC, et al. Extended peripheral zone biopsy schemes increase cancer detection rates and minimize variance in prostate specific antigen and age related cancer rates: results of a community multi-practice study. J Urol. 2003;169:125–9.
45. Berger AP, Gozzi C, Steiner H, et al. Complication rate of transrectal ultrasound guided prostate biopsy: a comparison among 3 protocols with 6, 10 and 15 cores. J Urol. 2004;171:1478–80.
46. Wolters T, van der Kwast TH, Vissers CJ, et al. False-negative prostate needle biopsies: frequency, histopathologic features, and follow-up. Am J Surg Pathol. 2010;34:35–43.

47. Lefkowitz GK, Sidhu GS, Torre P, et al. Is repeat prostate biopsy for high-grade prostatic intraepithelial neoplasia necessary after routine 12-core sampling? Urology. 2001;58:999–1003.
48. Rabets JC, Jones JS, Patel A, Zippe CD. Prostate cancer detection with office based saturation biopsy in a repeat biopsy population. J Urol. 2004;172:94–7.
49. Catalona WJ, Partin AW, Slawin KM, et al. Use of the percentage of free prostate-specific antigen to enhance differentiation of prostate cancer from benign prostatic disease: a prospective multicenter clinical trial. JAMA. 1998;279:1542–7.
50. Zaytoun OM, Stephenson AJ, Fareed K, et al. When serial biopsy is recommended: most cancers detected are clinically insignificant. BJU Int. 2012;110(7):987–92.

Chapter 15
Caring for Men Who Have Sex with Men

Jim Medder

Introduction

While other chapters in this book address issues that apply to men in general, this chapter covers the special and unique aspects of healthcare for men who have sex with men (MSM), whether they self-identify as gay, bisexual, or even heterosexual. *Sexual orientation*, defined as one's physical and/or emotional attraction to the same and/or opposite gender, is a continuum with attraction to women on one end and to men on the other with bisexuality in the middle [1]. In contrast, *gender identity* is one's innate psychological identification as a man, woman, or another gender, e.g., natal males who identify as female are transgender females and natal females who identify as male are transgender males [1].

Prevalence

The prevalence of gay and bisexual men in the USA is difficult to determine with precision and is somewhat controversial. Because of the stigma associated with homosexuality and a reluctance of MSM to self-identify, sexual minority research in general is insufficient and problematic [2]. Currently the best estimate comes from a 2011 analysis of previous surveys, which concluded that 3.6 % of the US adult male population identify as gay or bisexual (2.2 % gay and 1.4 % bisexual) resulting in an estimated total of about four million men. However, 8.2 % (19 million) of the total US population has engaged in same sex behavior at some time, and 11 % report some same sex attraction [3].

J. Medder, MD, MPH (✉)
Department of Family Medicine, University of Nebraska Medical Center,
Omaha, NE 68198-3075, USA
e-mail: jmedder@unmc.edu

© Springer International Publishing Switzerland 2016
J.J. Heidelbaugh (ed.), *Men's Health in Primary Care*, Current Clinical Practice,
DOI 10.1007/978-3-319-26091-4_15

Health Disparities

Compared to heterosexuals, MSM have a higher rate of risky health behaviors and a lower level of accessing healthcare, including preventive services. These health disparities have been attributed to discrimination and bias from all levels of society, including the medical community [4]. Education and training of healthcare providers have been inadequate to address healthcare provider bias and their lack of knowledge of the specific healthcare needs of MSM; the average training on sexual minority or LGBT (lesbian, gay, bisexual, and transgender) topics in US medical schools is 7 h, which is inadequate [5, 6].

Minority Stress Model

The minority stress model helps to explain the negative factors (e.g., stigmatization, discrimination, victimization, and devaluation) that affect sexual minorities. Being a member of a minority group increases stress levels above those that everyone faces from common everyday stressors. Minority stressors are chronic and socially/culturally based and lead to anxiety and depression and secondarily to risky behaviors [2, 4, 7].

Risk Factors/Health Problems

Because of the higher prevalence of risky behaviors and a lower utilization of medical care and preventive services, MSM are believed to be at higher risk for several diseases/conditions: cardiovascular disease (CVD) (e.g., tobacco and alcohol/drug use), mental health issues (e.g., depression, suicide, anxiety), injuries/violence (e.g., intimate partner violence, victimization, and trauma), sexually transmitted infections (STI) and human immunodeficiency virus (HIV) (risky sexual behaviors and alcohol/drug use), and anal cancer (e.g., human papillomavirus (HPV), HIV infection, and receptive anal sex). Other cancers, such as testicular, lung, colorectal, and prostate, may be missed due to avoidance of healthcare services and a lack of timely screening [8–10].

MSM require the same preventive services that all men should receive based on age and risk assessment, but MSM also have specific health issues and preventive services that require special attention. Table 15.1 lists healthcare topics and preventive services specifically recommended for gay and bisexual men.

Welcoming Environment/Cultural Competency

Based on population prevalence, it is estimated that 3–4 % of male patients seen in clinics should be MSM. However, 47 % of MSM in one study never discussed their sexual orientation with their healthcare provider, 28 % felt uncomfortable coming out to their clinician, and 15 % had been treated poorly when they did come out [17].

Table 15.1 Healthcare topics and preventive services specifically recommended for MSM [4, 11–16]

Screening	Recommendation
Tobacco	Screening questions (tobacco use and readiness to quit)
Dietary habits and BMI	Screening questions (eating disorders, body image issues, and weight)
Alcohol/drugs	Screening questions (alcohol and drug misuse/abuse)
Mental health	Screening questions (depression, suicide, and anxiety)
Injuries/violence	Screening questions (intimate partner violence, victimization, and trauma)
Sexual behaviors	Screening questions (5 Ps: partners, practices, protection from STIs, past history of STIs, and prevention of pregnancy)
Gonorrhea/chlamydia	Screening as indicated[a] (test all exposed sites: urethra/urine, rectum, and pharynx)
Syphilis	Screening as indicated[a]
Hepatitis B	Screening as indicated[a]
Hepatitis C	Screening as indicated[a] (one time if born between 1945 and 1965 is recommended for the general population)
HIV	Screening as indicated[a] (one time for age 15–65 years is recommended for the general population)
Anal cancer	Some advocates recommend screening every 3 years with anal Pap and annually/biannually if HIV positive based on CD4 count
Immunizations	Recommendation
Hepatitis A	Vaccinate at any age with 2-dose series if not done previously
Hepatitis B	Vaccinate at any age with 3-dose series if not done previously
Human papillomavirus	Vaccinate at age 13–26 with 3-dose series if not done previously
Preventive medications	Recommendation
Postexposure prophylaxis (PEP)	Start antiretroviral regimen within 72 h of HIV exposure and continue for 28 days; follow-up with periodic HIV testing
Preexposure prophylaxis (PrEP)	Consider once-daily antiretroviral regimen for significant ongoing HIV exposure risk with follow-up HIV/STI testing, side effect monitoring, and safe sex counseling every 90 days
Counseling	Recommendation
Coming-out/support systems, legal concerns, smoking, dietary habits, obesity, alcohol and drug use, depression, violence, safe sex practices, family planning, and HIV prevention	Periodically counsel on topics as indicated based on responses to screening questions and risk factors

[a]Annual screening tests; screen every 3–6 months if high risk

Clinicians who do not know the sexual orientation of MSM provide fewer recommended health services [18–20]. MSM may delay or avoid healthcare because of previous negative experiences with the healthcare system, fear of potential discrimination, and concerns about confidentiality. Clinicians should complete additional training to become culturally and medically competent to identify sexual orientation/gender identity and to address the healthcare issues of MSM [11]. Some of the ways to make the healthcare environment more welcoming to LGBT patients in general include the following [11, 12, 21–23]:

- Advertise in local LGBT-friendly papers and online organizations.
- Sign up as a provider at the Gay Lesbian Medical Association (GLMA) online web site (http://www.glma.org).
- Have LGBT-friendly posters/pictures and literature/handouts in the waiting room.
- Prominently display LGBT signs/logos in office or web site, such as rainbow, safe zone, and Human Rights Campaign equality logo.
- Provide unisex bathroom for transgender patients.
- Train staff and post nondiscrimination policies that include sexual orientation/gender identity.
- Have intake/registration forms that are LGBT inclusive.
- Adapt culturally competent and open communication/history-taking skills.
- Do not assume heterosexuality; use gender-neutral language; don't be afraid to ask.
- Don't assume all MSM are high risk for STI/HIV; ask about behaviors.
- Assure confidentiality; be supportive.
- Have a list of LGBT-friendly resources/referrals available to give to patients.

Taking the History

Sexual Orientation/Gender Identity

Before clinicians can provide culturally appropriate healthcare and preventive services, they need to know the sexual orientation/gender identity of the patient sitting in front of them. Sexual minorities are more likely to self-identify by completing an LGBT-inclusive intake form (paper or computer entry) prior to being seen. Asking open-ended, nonjudgmental, gender-neutral questions about their social situation and history establishes a respectful clinician-patient relationship, which is critical to making patients feel comfortable enough to disclose their sexual orientation/gender identity and to discuss their personal health issues. Clinicians can also identify sexual orientation by asking patients whether they have sex with men, women, or both, but taking this approach may not be directly relevant to patients' reasons for their visits unless they are having sexually related symptoms [24].

Coming-Out/Support Systems

An important component of the gay/bisexual man's history is whether he has accepted his sexual orientation, a process that usually takes several years, and whether he is "out of the closet" and open to families, friends, co-workers, etc. While identifying negative risk factors is important, it is also important to identify positive support systems. MSM who are "out" are usually better prepared to face negative or hostile environments, have fewer risky behaviors, and have more healthy and productive lives overall [12].

Clinicians can help MSM through the process of self-acceptance and coming out to others, but under no circumstances should clinicians "out" anyone without their permission. For gay and bisexual youth who may face the adverse consequences of nonaccepting parents, an assessment of the home environment prior to coming out is especially important. Community support organizations, such as PFLAG (Parents, Families, and Friends of Lesbians and Gays; https://community.pflag.org), can also assist in personal and family acceptance of one's sexual orientation and provide connections to others in the gay/bisexual community for additional social support [25].

Sexual History

See Chap. 9 for information and an algorithm for taking the sexual history; this section will emphasize topics specifically relevant to MSM. The 5 Ps (partners, practices, protection from STIs, past history of STIs, and prevention of pregnancy) is a useful tool/mnemonic for taking the routine sexual history for all patients [8, 26]. After a transition statement that introduces and normalizes the sexual history and assures confidentiality, patients should be asked the following three screening questions:

- Have you been sexually active in the last year?
- Do you have sex with men, women, or both?
- How many people have you had sex within the last year?

Based on the patients' responses, the clinician can stratify patients into low- and high-risk groups for STI/HIV and follow-up with appropriate questions.

Partners Many MSMs consistently use safe sex practices or are in long-term, monogamous relationships. However, MSM with multiple or new partners should be screened with additional questions about sexual behaviors.

A specific point to clarify with MSM who state that they have or live with one partner is whether the relationship is monogamous or not. A *closed relationship* is assumed to be low risk if truly monogamous. *Open relationships* are those in which one or both partners also have sex with other men or, in the case of bisexual men, with women. Because open relationships vary in what activities are allowed or not, ask the partners to describe their activities to assess their risk.

Practices Ask about receptive and insertive penile-oral/anal sex and direct oral-anal exposures to determine appropriate STI exposure/testing sites. Questions about injectable drug use help identify viral hepatitis/HIV risks, and substance use during sex may affect judgment and lead to risky sexual behaviors.

Protection from STIs MSM should be asked about the consistency of condom/barrier use.

Past History of STIs History of previous STIs and the frequency of STI screening tests are important to assess risk status and the patient's need and comfort level for ongoing screening.

Pregnancy Plans Contraception/barrier protection is relevant for the bisexual male.

Finally, clinicians should not forget to ask about sexual function and satisfaction as well as sexual abuse/trauma to complete the sexual history.

Special Health Topics

For the following topics, refer to previous chapters where the topics and their management are discussed in more detail. In this section, issues specifically relevant to MSM are discussed, yet there is overlap with the material provided in the other sections in this textbook that also apply to MSM.

Tobacco Use

Extensive reviews of the literature reveal a strong association of smoking by gay/bisexual men with an odds 2–2.5 times that for heterosexuals [27]. A 2013 national survey found that 26 % of gay men and 29 % of bisexual men smoke compared to 20 % of heterosexual men [28].

Risk factors for smoking by MSM include internalized homophobia, victimization and discrimination, younger age, lower educational level, alcohol use, depression, and stress. Tobacco companies also have specifically targeted the sexual minority population, and the relatively safe haven of bars where MSM congregate and smoking is common has contributed to higher rates of smoking [7].

Dietary Habits

Compared to heterosexual men, eating disorders and body image issues are more common in gay men who are twice as likely to describe themselves as underweight while bisexual men are 2.5 times as likely to think of themselves as overweight. Gay men also have four times the odds of engaging in recent unhealthy weight control behaviors (e.g., fasting, using diet products/laxatives, and purging) [29]. It has been hypothesized that gay men feel greater pressure to be thin than heterosexual males and to achieve the ideal male model look as promoted by the mass media to attract other MSM; the use of performance-enhancing drugs to build muscle ties into the body image problem.

Alcohol/Drug Use

Substance abuse by gay youth is associated with anti-gay school bullying, which leads to associations with other "deviant" peers (defined as those more likely to take risks and not fit in with the norm) [30]. The prevalence in the past year of any substance use disorder was 31.4 % for gay men, 27.6 % for bisexual men, and 15.6 % for heterosexual men [31]. A 2013 national survey found that 39 % of gay men and 52 % of bisexual men drank five or more drinks in one day at least once a year compared to 31 % of heterosexual men [28]. Drugs of abuse are also more commonly used by MSM to manage/reduce stress, and their use may lead to risky sexual behaviors and injuries while under their influence [12].

Mental Health

Substantial mental health disparities exist between gay/bisexual men and heterosexual men including depression, generalized anxiety disorder, panic disorder, eating disorders, and drug and alcohol dependencies; these differences are greater in young gay and bisexual men [32]. Lifetime suicidal ideation and attempts by gay men are 2–4 times greater compared to those of heterosexual men [32, 33], and bisexual men experience more suicide ideation and mental distress than either gay or heterosexual men [34].

Injuries/Violence

Intimate partner violence (IPV) against men partnered with men is up to three times that for men in heterosexual relationships (21.5 % vs. 7.1 %). However, most professionals called upon to assist these men do not receive specific training in sexual minority intimate partner violence management, and few shelters and services are available for this population [35, 36]. Unwanted sex was experienced by 18 % of gay men, 12 % of bisexual men, and 2.2 % of heterosexual men. Childhood violence/maltreatment was recalled by 31.5 % of gay men vs. 19.8 % of heterosexual men [37].

MSM also have more personal violence and knowledge of trauma to close friends/relatives. Types of violence (MSM vs. heterosexuals) include getting beaten (20.7 % vs. 11.7 %), getting mugged (27.5 % vs. 16.2 %), and being stalked (8.1 % vs. 2.6 %) [37]. Gay men have experienced property crime (28.1 %), attempted crime (21.5 %), objects thrown at them (21.1 %), threats of violence (35.4 %), verbal abuse (63.0 %), and employment/housing discrimination (17.7 %); these acts were experienced less often by bisexual men [38].

Crimes against gay men are most often committed by heterosexual men. Gay men are more visible as targets compared to lesbians and bisexuals because gay men are more likely to visit gay-oriented public establishments and to disclose their sexual orientation socially and at work [38].

Sexually Transmitted Infections

STIs, including syphilis, gonorrhea, chlamydia, and HIV, have increased in the past few years for MSM following an increase in unsafe sexual practices. It is believed that some MSM take more risks now because newer HIV medications have changed HIV infection from a death warrant to a chronic, manageable disease. MSM have reported that they also do not like using condoms as they interfere with a feeling of intimacy or they believe that others have the same HIV status as they do and therefore they do not ask about their partner's status [4, 8, 39]. See Chap. 10 for more details and treatment recommendations.

STI Screening Intervals STI screening is recommended annually for all sexually active MSM not in a long-term monogamous relationship if they have had exposures during the past year. Screening is recommended every 3–6 months for those at higher risk who had multiple or anonymous partners or sexual experiences in which either partner used alcohol or illicit drugs [4].

Gonorrhea/Chlamydia While most urethral infections in men are symptomatic, most extragenital gonorrhea/chlamydia infections do not have any symptoms or signs, or they produce mild symptoms that are often ignored [40]. Up to 50 % of chlamydia infections and about 85 % of rectal infections are asymptomatic in men while 53 % of chlamydial and 64 % of gonococcal infections are found in nonurethral sites [40, 41]. In one study of asymptomatic MSM, chlamydia was found in 7.9 % of rectal, 5.2 % of urethral, and 1.4 % of pharyngeal sites while gonorrhea was found in 6.9 % of rectal, 6.0 % of urethral, and 9.2 % of pharyngeal sites [41]. As a result, many infected yet asymptomatic men do not seek treatment and continue to spread the infection.

In screening asymptomatic MSM for gonorrhea and chlamydia, it is important to test not only the urethra/urine (MSM who have insertive penile-oral or penile-anal sex) but also the rectum (MSM who have receptive penile-anal sex) and the pharynx (MSM who have receptive penile-oral sex or direct oral-anal contact). A nucleic acid amplification test (NAAT) is preferred for all testing but especially for extragenital testing because of its greater sensitivity and specificity as compared to culture for those sites [12, 42]. Those with HIV should be tested for gonorrhea/chlamydia quarterly as the incidence is higher in HIV-infected persons (one in seven has asymptomatic infections with 60 % of infections occurring in the pharynx and rectum) [42, 43].

Syphilis With rates of syphilis rising in MSM since 2001, periodic screening for syphilis is also recommended, especially in high-risk populations [13]. MSM account for 75 % of new cases of primary and secondary syphilis; oral sex is considered the primary site of transmission [12].

Hepatitis A Hepatitis A is usually an acute, self-limited infection with fecal-oral transmission. MSM can become infected by sexual activity or direct contact with contaminated fingers or objects. Of new hepatitis A cases, 10 % are estimated to occur in MSM [4]. Testing should only be performed when clinically indicated. Hepatitis A vaccination is recommended as part of the routine childhood immunization schedule and is recommended for MSM at any age if they have not been previously vaccinated [14].

Hepatitis B Hepatitis B is spread by semen or blood and is easily transmitted during sex, being 50–100 times as infectious as HIV. Tattoos and piercings done with infected equipment and injectable drug use are other sources of infection. Hepatitis B can present as an acute infection but also as a chronic asymptomatic infection leading to severe liver damage. Of new hepatitis B cases, 20 % are estimated to occur in MSM. Hepatitis B vaccination is recommended as part of the routine childhood immunization schedule and is recommended for MSM at any age if they have not been previously vaccinated [4, 14].

Hepatitis C Sexual transmission of hepatitis C is not common but does occur, especially among MSM with HIV infection who should be screened periodically. Other risk factors include having another STI, sex with multiple partners, or rough sex. More commonly hepatitis C is spread through contaminated needles used for injectable drugs, piercings, and tattoos [4]. No vaccine for hepatitis C is currently available.

Human Papillomavirus Approximately 75 % of all sexually active adults acquire HPV, often within the first 2 years of starting sexual activity. About 57–61 % of HIV-negative MSM and 72–90 % of HIV-positive MSM will have HPV [44]. Infections are usually asymptomatic, but when symptomatic, HPV expresses itself as genital/anal warts. Because HPV can be spread by direct skin-to-skin contact, condom use is less effective. Multiple partners, alcohol and illicit drug use, and smoking are risk factors [45].

HPV vaccine is recommended for all males and ideally should be given before the onset of sexual activity at age 11–12 years, but it can be given through age 26 years for MSM [14]. Evidence exists that giving HPV vaccine to MSM older than 26 years may be beneficial, but additional studies are needed to confirm this finding [46].

Herpes Simplex Herpes simplex is spread by skin-to-skin or mucous membrane contact, causes painful anogenital ulcers, and may be a risk factor for HIV infection. MSM have high rates of infection, especially young MSM [4, 12]. Testing should only be done when clinically indicated.

Human Immunodeficiency Virus

MSM account for about two-thirds of new HIV cases with 4 % derived from injection drug use. The incidence of HIV has increased 12 % from 2008 to 2010 for MSM, especially in adolescent and young adult MSM (22 % increase). MSM make up over one-half of all persons with HIV in the USA, and about one-third do not know that they are infected [4].

Postexposure Prophylaxis (PEP) An antiretroviral regimen of three drugs (tenofovir, emtricitabine, and raltegravir; alternative regimens are also available) should be started within 72 h after an HIV exposure and continued for 28 days. Periodic HIV testing is recommended at 1, 3, and 6 months following the exposure [15]. Those with recurrent exposures should consider preexposure prophylaxis (see below).

Preexposure Prophylaxis (PrEP) The Centers for Disease Control and Prevention (CDC) [15] and World Health Organization (WHO) [47] recommend that MSM and others whose behaviors place them at a significant risk of getting HIV infection consider the benefits of taking the once-daily antiretroviral combination of tenofovir and emtricitabine. If taken daily, PrEP can reduce the risk of infection up to 92 % without significant complications. A clinical practice guideline [16] and provider's supplement [48] for PrEP were issued in 2014 by the US Public Health Service and include criteria for determining HIV risk and a comprehensive program of every 3-month STI/HIV testing, side effect monitoring, and safe sex counseling [15].

Criteria for taking PrEP for MSM include all of the following [16]:

- Adult man age 18 and older
- Without acute or established HIV infection
- Any male sex partners in the past 6 months
- Not in a monogamous partnership with a recently tested, HIV-negative man

And at least one of the following:

- Any anal sex without condoms (receptive or insertive) in the past 6 months
- Any STI diagnosed or reported in past 6 months
- Is in an ongoing sexual relationship with an HIV-positive male partner

Insurance companies generally are covering the cost of PrEP with the rationale that preventing HIV infections is cheaper than treating HIV/AIDS. The manufacturer (Gilead) also has an online medication assistance program for those without insurance and co-pay assistance for those with insurance.

Anal Cancer

Anal cancer and cervical cancer are caused by the same strains of HPV (see above). Proponents argue for anal Pap screening based on the model for cervical screening and the higher incidence of anal cancer in MSM (20 times) and especially in MSM with HIV (40 times) [45]. However, progression of anal cancer precursors to cancer appears to be much lower than for cervical cancer. No definitive evidence exists that screening reduces the incidence of anal cancer and well-designed prospective trials are needed [49].

While the CDC states that screening can be considered, the US Preventive Services Task Force does not make any recommendations for screening. One common recommendation is for anal Pap screening every 3 years for MSM without HIV; in MSM with HIV, periodicity is based on CD4 counts (biannually if $\geq$500 and annually if <500) [44, 45]. Anal Pap testing is easy to perform by following a few specific guidelines, which are readily available online [50].

Cardiovascular Disease

Studies indicate a higher incidence of CVD in older MSM, assumed to be secondary to the presence of higher rates of smoking and recreational illicit drug use [12]. MSM should receive the same screening tests, preventive medications, and risk factor modification counseling that are recommended for the general population to prevent CVD.

Legal Rights

Legal inequalities are often major stressors that directly impact the health and well-being of MSM. The Supreme Court decision on marriage equality reaffirmed the previously granted rights of sexual minorities to visit their hospitalized same sex partners and to make medical decisions for their partners if they become incapacitated [51]. However, with marriage equality, LGBT couples enjoy additional benefits, including federal legal/tax, social security, spousal/partner health insurance, joint adoption, and family medical leave. While acceptance of LGBT rights are rapidly evolving, others are still denied; discrimination in employment, housing, nursing homes for older adults, and other areas still exists, depending upon the state in which one lives [24, 52].

Special Populations

Youth

Besides the challenges of normal adolescence, sexual minority youth also experience the additional challenges of their sexual orientation, which include higher rates of illicit substance abuse, eating disorders, mental health issues and both attempted and completed suicides, risky sexual behaviors, violence and victimization, and homelessness [23]. About one-quarter of adolescent gay and bisexual males report childhood sexual and physical abuse while about one-half experience peer victimization (bisexuals have slightly higher rates than gay males) [53]. Implementation and support of anti-bullying policies in school may help address some of these issues.

A higher percentage of sexual minority youth (mostly males) are represented among the homeless, comprising 30–40 % of homeless youth. The primary reasons given for being homeless are rejection by family, forced to leave home after coming out voluntarily or involuntarily, or avoiding violence in the foster care system [54]. Homeless adolescents are less likely to stay in shelters and more likely to stay with strangers or in public places, which are associated with more risky sexual behaviors [55].

Families and Children

A 2013 Pew poll found that 40 % of gay men and bisexual men were married, living with a partner, or in a committed relationship with about three quarters of those living together [56]. In addition, a 2012 Gallup poll found that 16 % of MSM were raising children [57]. Many gay men, particularly those in relationships, are choosing to have children through fostering, adoption, or assisted reproductive technology (ART).

Clinicians should ask MSM about their desire to have children and provide counseling as appropriate regarding options for achieving parenthood. Those selecting ART will need to make decisions about which partner will be the sperm donor; selection of an egg/oocyte donor; the relationship, if any, of the gestational carrier and the child after birth; the legal requirements/regulations involved; and options for adoption of the child by the partner who is not the sperm donor [58].

Numerous studies have shown that children raised by same sex parents do just as well as children raised by heterosexual parents as measured by physical, mental, and social health factors, including emotional/behavioral/cognitive functioning, gender role behavior, self-esteem, depression, anxiety, school connectedness, school success, and academic performance with less delinquent/aggressive behavior and substance abuse [59]. The American Academy of Pediatrics (AAP) states that:

> children's well-being is affected much more by their relationships with their parents, their parents' sense of competence and security, and the presence of social and economic support for the family than by the gender or the sexual orientation of their parents. [60]

Older MSM

It is estimated that the US sexual minority population age 65 years and older is 1–3 million people [61]. Compared to heterosexual men, MSM greater than 50 years old are more likely to still smoke and drink excessively, to be disabled, and to have poor mental and physical health. However, MSM have lower rates of obesity and similar rates of physical activity compared to older heterosexual men. Bisexual men are less likely than gay men to be tested for HIV and have higher rates of diabetes mellitus but otherwise have similar risks [62]. Erectile and sexual dysfunction associated with aging is another concern for this population as it is with all men.

About one-half of older MSM live alone compared to 13.4 % of heterosexual men, which is possibly related to having an HIV-positive partner die or growing up at a time when MSM was even less accepted than it is today. With fewer adult children and less family support, caretakers of MSM are less likely to be related and more likely to be from "families of choice." Living alone and lack of support can lead to premature disability/death; however, many elder LGB believe that facing the stigma of being LGB has made them stronger and more capable to face the problems of aging [63]. Assisted living can also be a problem as many gay/bisexual men feel the need to return to the closet upon entering these facilities because of discrimination by staff and other residents. As a result, assisted living facilities specifically oriented toward the sexual minority population and the special services they may need are being built and promoted [61].

Bisexual Men

Bisexual men have greater health risks than gay and heterosexual men in several areas, e.g., lower health access and utilization of screening tests, self-rating of poor/fair health, disability causing limitation in activity, obesity, heart disease, and mental health issues, which are especially high in this group [64]. These differences have been explained by marginalization and lack of support for bisexual men in both the gay/lesbian and heterosexual communities and because bisexual men are less likely to disclose their orientation to healthcare providers [65].

Racial/Ethnic Minorities

African American, Latino, and Asian MSM face the double discrimination of being members of both racial/ethnic and sexual minorities, which results in even higher levels of depression/stress, risky sexual behaviors, and sexual dysfunction. Stigma management strategies adapted by MSM in these groups include concealment of their sexual orientation, avoidance of social situations associated with the stigma, drawing support from external sources to minimize the stigma, and direct confrontation with stigmatizers [66].

According to the CDC, in 2010 the greatest number of new HIV infections among MSM occurred in young black/African American MSM who accounted for 45 % of new HIV infections among all black MSM and 55 % of new HIV infections among all young MSM [67]. Young black men are also disproportionally affected by other STIs [68].

Transgender Men

In the USA, 0.3 % of adults are estimated to be transgender, a number felt to be less reliable than those for the LGB population [3]. Furthermore, the LGB and transgender populations overlap with approximately a quarter of transgender men (female to male or FTM) identifying as having same gender or bisexual orientation [69, 70]. Compared to the LGB population, transgender individuals have higher levels of societal and healthcare discrimination and as a result higher rates of associated risk factors and health issues [12, 69].

Standards of care for transition related to mental health counseling, hormonal therapy, and surgical options for transgender individuals are provided by the World Professional Association for Transgender Health (WPATH) [71] and the Endocrine Society [72]. Providers not comfortable with providing transitional care, especially for those who are starting to transition with hormonal therapy or are ready for surgery, should refer patients to specialists in transgender care. While most (61 %) transgender men are on hormonal therapy (testosterone), fewer (33 %) have undergone any surgical procedures, such as mastectomy, hysterectomy/BSO, and other procedures to create male genitalia [12, 69].

Transgender men may see primary care providers for general healthcare and preventive services, and some who are already on hormonal therapy may only seek medication refills and lab monitoring. However, transgender men specifically present several unique health challenges. Discussion of and attention to female body parts can result in emotional discomfort for transgender men, which should be respected by clinicians. Depending on surgeries undertaken, they may still have breasts, uterus, and ovaries and should receive preventive services and screening tests as indicated for natal females. Some breast tissue may remain after mastectomy and require continued breast/chest exams. Periodic testosterone levels and monitoring for side effects (lipids for dyslipidemia, CBC for polycythemia, and liver function tests) should be performed. Transgender men may still have a pregnancy risk while on testosterone [12].

Conclusion

The establishment of an expectation for periodic health visits with culturally competent providers and staff and the development of innovative, nontraditional school-, work-, and community-based interventions and programs will go a long way toward reducing the health disparities of all MSM [68].

References

1. Sexual orientation and gender identity definitions. Human Rights Campaign. http://www.hrc. org/resources/entry/sexual-orientation-and-gender-identity-terminology-and-definitions. Accessed 11 May 2015.
2. Committee on Lesbian, Gay, Bisexual, and Transgender Health Issues and Research Gaps and Opportunities, Institute of Medicine. The health of lesbian, gay, bisexual, and transgender

people. Building a foundation for better understanding. Washington, DC: The National Academies Press; 2011. http://www.iom.edu/Reports/2011/The-Health-of-Lesbian-Gay--Bisexual-and-Transgender-People.aspx. Accessed 23 April 2015.

3. Gates GJ. How many people are lesbian, gay, bisexual, and transgender? Los Angeles, CA: The Williams Institute, UCLA School of Law; 2011. http://williamsinstitute.law.ucla.edu/research/census-lgbt-demographics-studies/how-many-people-are-lesbian-gay-bisexual-and-transgender/. Accessed 18 April 2015.

4. Gay and bisexual men's health. Centers for Disease Control and Prevention, US Department of Health and Human Services. http://www.cdc.gov/msmhealth/. Accessed 18 April 2015.

5. Obedin-Maliver J, Goldsmith ES, Stewart L, et al. Lesbian, gay, bisexual, and transgender-related content in undergraduate medical education. JAMA. 2011;306(9):971–7. doi:10.1001/jama.2011.1255.

6. Implementing curricular and institutional climate changes to improve health care for individuals who are LGBT, gender nonconforming, or born with DSD. AAMC Advisory Committee on Sexual Orientation, Gender Identity, and Sex Development, Association of American Medical Colleges. 2014.

7. Blosnich J, Lee JG, Horn K. A systematic review of the aetiology of tobacco disparities for sexual minorities. Tob Control. 2013;22:66–73. doi:10.1136/tobaccocontrol-2011-050181.

8. Taking routine histories of sexual health: a system-wide approach for health centers. National LGBT Health Education Center. A Program of the Fenway Institute. 2014. http://www.lgbthealtheducation.org/wp-content/uploads/COM827_SexualHistoryToolkit_August2014_v7.pdf. Accessed 18 April 2015.

9. Top health issues for LGBT populations information and resource kit. Rockville, MD: Department of Health and Human Services, US Substance Abuse and Mental Health Services Administration, Center for Substance Abuse Prevention; 2012. http://store.samhsa.gov/shin/content//SMA12-4684/SMA12-4684.pdf. Accessed 8 May 2015.

10. Ten things gay men should discuss with their healthcare provider. Gay and Lesbian Medical Association. http://glma.org/index.cfm?fuseaction=Page.viewPage&pageID=690. Accessed 8 May 2015.

11. McNair RP, Hegarty K. Guidelines for the primary care of lesbian, gay, and bisexual people: a systematic review. Ann Fam Med. 2010;8(6):533–41. doi:10.1370/afm.1173.

12. Makadon HJ, Mayer KH, Potter J, Goldhammer H, editors. The Fenway guide to lesbian, gay, bisexual, and transgender health. 2nd ed. Philadelphia: American College of Physicians; 2015.

13. Recommendations. US Preventive Services Task Force, Agency for Healthcare Research and Quality, US Department of Health and Human Services. http://www.uspreventiveservicestaskforce.org/. Accessed 28 July 2015.

14. Adult immunization schedules. US Department of Health and Human Services, Centers for Disease Control and Prevention. 2015. http://www.cdc.gov/vaccines/schedules/hcp/adult.html. Accessed 18 April 2015.

15. Preventing new HIV infections. US Department of Health and Human Services, Centers for Disease Control and Prevention. http://www.cdc.gov/hiv/guidelines/preventing.html. Accessed 18 April 2015.

16. Preexposure prophylaxis for the prevention of HIV infection in the United States—2014: a clinical practice guideline. US Department of Health and Human Services, Centers for Disease Control and Prevention. 2014. p. 1–67. http://www.cdc.gov/hiv/pdf/prepguidelines2014.pdf. Accessed 7 May 2015.

17. Hamel L, Firth J, Hoff T, Kates J, Levine S, Dawson L. HIV/AIDS in the lives of gay and bisexual men in the United States. The Henry J Kaiser Family Foundation. 2014. http://kff.org/hivaids/report/hivaids-in-the-lives-of-gay-and-bisexual-men-in-the-united-states/. Accessed 18 April 2015.

18. Petroll AE, Mosack KE. Physician awareness of sexual orientation and preventive health recommendations to men who have sex with men. Sex Transm Dis. 2011;38(1):63–7. doi:10.1097/OLQ.0b013e3181ebd50f.

19. Ng BE, Moore D, Michelow W, et al. Relationship between disclosure of same-sex sexual activity to providers, HIV diagnosis and sexual health services for men who have sex with men in Vancouver, Canada. Can J Public Health. 2014;105(3):e186–91.

20. Bernstein KT, Liu KL, Begier EM, et al. Same-sex attraction disclosure to health care providers among New York City men who have sex with men: implications for HIV testing approaches. Arch Intern Med. 2008;168(13):1458–64. doi:10.1001/archinte.168.13.1458.
21. The Joint Commission. Advancing effective communication, cultural competence, and patient- and family-centered care for the lesbian, gay, bisexual, and transgender (LGBT) community: a field guide, Oak Brook, IL. 2011. http://www.jointcommission.org/assets/1/18/LGBTField Guide_WEB_LINKED_VER.pdf. Accessed 25 July 2015
22. Coren JS, Coren CM, Pagliaro SN, Weiss LB. Assessing your office for care of lesbian, gay, bisexual, and transgender patients. Health Care Manag. 2011;30:66–70. doi:10.1097/HCM. 0b013e3182078bcd.
23. Coker TR, Austin SB, Schuster MA. The health and health care of lesbian, gay, and bisexual adolescents. Annu Rev Public Health. 2010;31:457–77. doi:10.1146/annurev.publhealth. 012809.103636.
24. Ard KL, Makadon HJ. Improving the health care of lesbian, gay, bisexual and transgender people: understanding and eliminating health disparities. Boston: The National LGBT Health Education Center, The Fenway Institute. http://www.lgbthealtheducation.org/wp-content/ uploads/12-054_LGBTHealtharticle_v3_07-09-12.pdf. Accessed 4 May 2015.
25. Parents, Families, and Friends of Lesbians and Gays (PFLAG). https://community.pflag.org. Accessed 10 May 2015.
26. A guide to taking a sexual history. US Department of Health and Human Services, Centers for Disease Control and Prevention. http://www.cdc.gov/std/treatment/sexualhistory.pdf. Accessed 18 April 2015.
27. Lee JG, Griffin GK, Melvin CL. Tobacco use among sexual minorities in the USA, 1987 to May 2007: a systematic review. Tob Control. 2009;18:275–82. doi:10.1136/tc.2008.028241.
28. Ward BW, Dahlhamer JM, Galinksy AM, Joestl SS. Sexual orientation and health among U.S. adults: National Health Interview Survey, 2013. National Health Statistics Reports, Number 77. US Department of Health and Human Services, Centers for Disease Control and Prevention. 2014.
29. Hadland SE, Austin SB, Goodenow CS, Calzo JP. Weight misperception and unhealthy weight control behaviors among sexual minorities in the general adolescent population. J Adolesc Health. 2014;54(3):296–303. doi:10.1016/j.jadohealth.2013.08.021.
30. Huebner DM, Thoma BS, Neilands TB. School victimization and substance use among lesbian, gay, bisexual, and transgender adolescents. Prev Sci. 2015(5);734-43. doi: 10.1007/ s11121-014-0507-x.
31. McCabe SE, Bostwick WB, Hughes TL, West BT, Boyd CJ. The relationship between discrimination and substance use disorders among lesbian, gay, and bisexual adults in the United States. Am J Public Health. 2010;100(10):1946–52. doi:10.2105/AJPH.2009.163147.
32. Lewis NM. Mental health in sexual minorities: recent indicators, trends, and their relationships to place in North America and Europe. Health Place. 2009;15(4):1029–45. doi:10.1016/j. healthplace.2009.05.003.
33. King M, Semlyen J, Tai SS, et al. A systematic review of mental disorder, suicide, and deliberate self harm in lesbian, gay and bisexual people. BMC Psychiatry. 2008;8:70. doi:10.1186/1471-244X-8-70.
34. Pompili M, Lester D, Forte A, et al. Bisexuality and suicide: a systematic review of the current literature. J Sex Med. 2014;11(8):1903–13. doi:10.1111/jsm.12581.
35. Ford CL, Slavin T, Hilton KL, Holt SL. Intimate partner violence prevention services and resources in Los Angeles: issues, needs, and challenges for assisting lesbian, gay, bisexual, and transgender clients. Health Promot Pract. 2013;14:841–9. doi:10.1177/1524839912467645.
36. Roberts AL, Austin SB, Corliss HL, Vandermorris AK, Koenen KC. Pervasive trauma exposure among US sexual orientation minority adults and risk of posttraumatic stress disorder. Am J Public Health. 2010;100(12):2433–41. doi:10.2105/AJPH.2009.168971.
37. Ard KL, Makadon HJ. Addressing intimate partner violence in lesbian, gay, bisexual, and transgender patients. J Gen Intern Med. 2011;26:930–3. doi:10.2105/AJPH.2009.168971.
38. Herek GM. Hate crimes and stigma-related experiences among sexual minority adults in the United States: prevalence estimates from a national probability sample. J Interpers Violence. 2009;24:54–74. doi:10.1177/0886260508316477.

39. Sexually transmitted diseases treatment guidelines, 2010. US Department of Health and Human Services, Centers for Disease Control and Prevention. MMWR. 2010. p. 12–3. http://www.cdc.gov/std/treatment/2010/std-treatment-2010-rr5912.pdf. Accessed 18 April 2015.

40. Healthy People 2010 companion document for lesbian, gay, bisexual, and transgender (LGBT) health. San Francisco, CA: Gay and Lesbian Medical Association; 2001. https://www.nalgap.org/PDF/Resources/HP2010CDLGBTHealth.pdf. Accessed 10 May 2015.

41. Kent CK, Chaw JK, Wong W, et al. Prevalence of rectal, urethral, and pharyngeal chlamydia and gonorrhea detected in 2 clinical settings among men who have sex with men: San Francisco, California, 2003. Clin Infect Dis. 2005;41(1):67–74.

42. Templeton DJ, Read P, Varma R, Bourne C. Australian sexually transmissible infection and HIV testing guidelines for asymptomatic men who have sex with men 2014: a review of the evidence. Sex Health. 2014;11(3):217–29. doi:10.1071/SH14003.

43. Rieg G, Lewis RJ, Miller LG, Witt MD, Mario M, Daar ES. Asymptomatic sexually transmitted infections in HIV-infected men who have sex with men: prevalence, incidence, predictors, and screening strategies. AIDS Patient Care STDS. 2008;22(12):947–54. doi:10.1089/apc.2007.0240.

44. Park IU, Palefsky JM. Evaluation and management of anal intraepithelial neoplasia in HIV-negative and HIV-positive men who have sex with men. Curr Infect Dis Rep. 2010;12(2):126–33. doi:10.1186/1471-2407-12-476.

45. Anal cancer, HIV and gay/bisexual men. New York: National LGBT Cancer Network. http://www.cancer-network.org/cancer_information/gay_men_and_cancer/anal_cancer_hiv_and_gay_men.php. Accessed 20 April 2015.

46. Swedish KA, Goldstone SE. Prevention of anal condyloma with quadrivalent human papillomavirus vaccination of older men who have sex with men. PLoS One. 2014;9(4):e93393. doi:10.1371/journal.pone.0093393.

47. Guidance on oral pre-exposure prophylaxis (PrEP) for serodiscordant couples, men and transgender women who have sex with men at high risk of HIV. Recommendations for use in the context of demonstration projects. World Health Organization. 2012. http://www.who.int/hiv/pub/guidance_prep/en/. Accessed 18 April 2015.

48. Preexposure prophylaxis for the prevention of HIV infection in the United States—2014: clinical providers' supplement. US Department of Health and Human Services, Centers for Disease Control and Prevention. 2014. p. 1–43. http://www.cdc.gov/hiv/pdf/prepprovidersupplement2014.pdf. Accessed 7 May 2015.

49. Machalek DA, Poynten M, Jin F, et al. Anal human papillomavirus infection and associated neoplastic lesions in men who have sex with men: a systematic review and meta-analysis. Lancet Oncol. 2012;13(5):487–500. doi:10.1016/S1470-2045(12)70080-3.

50. Screening: obtaining an anorectal cytology specimen. San Francisco: Department of Medicine, University of California. http://id.medicine.ucsf.edu/analcancerinfo/diagnosis/screening.html. Accessed 9 May 2015.

51. Medicare steps up enforcement of equal visitation and representation rights in hospitals (press release). U.S. Department of Health and Human Services. 8 Sept 2011. http://www.cms.gov/Newsroom/MediaReleaseDatabase/Press-Releases/2011-Press-Releases-Items/2011-09-08.html. Accessed 7 May 2015.

52. Hughes AK, Harold RD, Boyer JM. Awareness of LGBT aging issues among aging services network providers. J Gerontol Soc Work. 2011;54:659–77. doi:10.1080/01634372.2011.

53. Friedman MS, Marshal MP, Guadamuz TE, et al. A meta-analysis of disparities in childhood sexual abuse, parental physical abuse, and peer victimization among sexual minority and sexual nonminority individuals. Am J Public Health. 2011;101(8):1481–94. doi:10.2105/AJPH.2009.190009.

54. Keuroghlian AS, Shtasel D, Bassuk EL. Out on the street: a public health and policy agenda for lesbian, gay, bisexual, and transgender youth who are homeless. Am J Orthopsychiatry. 2014;84:66–72. doi:10.1037/h0098852.

55. Rice E, Barman-Adhikari A, Rhoades H, et al. Homelessness experiences, sexual orientation, and sexual risk taking among high school students in Los Angeles. J Adolesc Health. 2013;52:773–8. doi:10.1016/j.jadohealth.2012.11.011.

56. A survey of LGBT Americans: attitudes, experiences and values in changing times. Pew Research Center. 2013. http://www.pewsocialtrends.org/files/2013/06/SDT_LGBT-Americans_06-2013.pdf. Accessed 8 May 2015.

57. Gates GJ, Newport F. Special report: 3.4% of U.S. adults identify as LGBT. Gallup. October 18, 2012. http://www.gallup.com/poll/158066/special-report-adults-identify-lgbt-aspx?version=print. Accessed 8 May 2015.

58. Greenfeld DA, Seli E. Gay men choosing parenthood through assisted reproduction: medical and psychosocial considerations. Fertil Steril. 2011;95:225–9. doi:10.1016/j.fertnstert.2010.05.053.

59. Perrin EC, Siegel BS, American Academy of Pediatrics Committee on Psychosocial Aspects of Child and Family Health. Technical report: promoting the well-being of children whose parents are gay or lesbian. Pediatrics. 2013;131(4):e1374–83. doi:10.1542/peds.2013-0377.

60. American Academy of Pediatrics Committee on Psychosocial Aspects of Child and Family Health. Policy statement: promoting the well-being of children whose parents are gay or lesbian. Pediatrics. 2013;131(4):827–30. doi:10.1542/peds.2013-0376.

61. Orel NA. Investigating the needs and concerns of lesbian, gay, bisexual, and transgender older adults: the use of qualitative and quantitative methodology. J Homosex. 2014;61(1):53–78. doi:10.1080/00918369.2013.835236.

62. Fredriksen-Goldsen KI, Kim HJ, Barkan SE, Muraco A, Hoy-Ellis CP. Health disparities among lesbian, gay, and bisexual older adults: results from a population-based study. Am J Public Health. 2013;103:1802–9. doi:10.2105/AJPH.2012.301110.

63. Wallace SP, Cochran SD, Durazo EM, Ford CL. The health of aging lesbian, gay and bisexual adults in California. Policy Brief UCLA Cent Health Policy Res. 2011(2);1–8.

64. Conron KJ, Mimiaga MJ, Landers SJ. A population-based study of sexual orientation identity and gender differences in adult health. Am J Public Health. 2010;100(10):1953–60. doi:10.2105/AJPH.2009.174169.

65. Friedman MR, Dodge B, Schick V, et al. From bias to bisexual health disparities: attitudes toward bisexual men and women in the United States. LGBT Health. 2014;1(4):309–18.

66. Choi K-H, Han C, Paul J, Ayala G. Strategies of managing racism and homophobia among U.S. ethnic and racial minority men who have sex with men. AIDS Educ Prev. 2011;23(2):145–58. doi:10.1521/aeap.2011.23.2.145.

67. HIV in the United States: at a glance. US Department of Health and Human Services, Centers for Disease Control and Prevention. http://www.cdc.gov/hiv/statistics/basics/ataglance.html. Accessed 7 May 2015.

68. Lanier Y, Sutton MY. Reframing the context of preventive health care services and prevention of HIV and other sexually transmitted infections for young men: new opportunities to reduce racial/ethnic sexual health disparities. Am J Public Health. 2013;103(2):262–9. doi:10.2105/AJPH.2012.300921.

69. Grant JM, Mottet LA, Tanis J, Harrison J, Herman JL, Keisling M. Injustice at every turn: a report of the national transgender discrimination survey. Washington: National Center for Transgender Equality and National Gay and Lesbian Task Force; 2011. http://endtransdiscrimination.org/PDFs/NTDS_Report.pdf. Accessed 25 July 2015.

70. Auer MK, Fuss J, Höhne N, Stalla GK, Sievers C. Transgender transitioning and change of self-reported sexual orientation. PLoS One. 2014;9(10):e110016. doi:10.1371/journal.pone.0110016.

71. Standards of care for the health of transsexual, transgender, and gender-nonconforming people. World Professional Association of Transgender Health. 2012. http://www.wpath.org/site_page.cfm?pk_association_webpage_menu=1351&pk_association_webpage=4655. Accessed 25 July 2015.

72. Hembree WC, Cohen-Kettenis P, Delemarre-van de Waal HA, Gooren LJ, Meyer 3rd WJ, Spack NP, et al. Endocrine treatment of transsexual persons: an Endocrine Society clinical practice guideline. J Clin Endocrinol Metab. 2009;94:3132–54.

Index

A

Abdominal aortic aneurysm (AAA), 110, 136
Affordable Care Act (ACA), 39
American Cancer Society (ACS), 275
American College of Physicians (ACP), 275, 276
American Urological Association (AUA), 275

B

Benign prostatic hyperplasia (BPH)
    BOO, 200
    histologic diagnosis, 200–201,
        (*see also* Lower urinary tract
        symptoms (LUTS))
    physical examination, 201–204
    prevalence, 200
Bladder outflow obstruction (BOO), 200, 207
Body mass index (BMI)
    anthropometric measures, 71
    evidence-based guidelines, 109
    physical examination, 58
    weight-for-length, 58–59

C

Cardiovascular disease (CVD)
    AAA, 136
    aspirin, 128
    atherosclerosis, 135
    CAD, 137
    CHF, 137, 138
    chronic atrial fibrillation, 133
    diabetes mellitus
        glycosylated hemoglobin, 131

male–female differences, 131
    metformin, 132
    treatment, 131
    dyslipidemia, 134
    epidemiology, 125
    healthy diet, 126, 127
    hypertension, 128, 129
    medication therapy, 132
    obesity, 127
    PAD, 136
    patient-focused management, 132
    physical activity and exercise, 127
    risk factors, 126
    smoking cessation, 128
    stroke, 135, 136
Chlamydia trachomatis, 167, 172
Chronic prostatitis-chronic pelvic pain
    syndrome (CP-CPPS), 217
Congestive heart failure (CHF), 137, 138
Coronary artery disease (CAD), 137

D

Digital rectal examination (DRE),
    201–204

E

Electronic health record (EHR) system
    benefit, 50
    CDSS, 50
    clinical service improvement, 51
    implementation, 51, 52
    interventions, 50, 51
    shared decision making, 50, 51

© Springer International Publishing Switzerland 2016
J.J. Heidelbaugh (ed.), *Men's Health in Primary Care*, Current Clinical Practice,
DOI 10.1007/978-3-319-26091-4

Erectile dysfunction (ED)
  epidemiology, 149
  risk factor, 150
  treatment, 151–153
European Randomized Study of Screening for
      Prostate Cancer (ERSPC), 272–273
Evidence-based guidelines
  adolescent examination
    anthropometric measures, 71
    back and spine, 75
    blood pressure, 71
    breast examination, 75
    components, 70
    dermatologic examination, 74
    healthcare provider, 71
    palpation, 77, 81, 83
    PPEs, 83
    screening test, 83, 85
    visual inspection, 75, 77
    voice and facial hair, 74
  aspirin, 116
  Bright Futures, 57–58
  child examination, 83, 85
    blood pressure, 59, 63
    eyes, 63
    infancy and early childhood, 69
    later childhood, 70
    mouth, 64
    musculoskeletal examination, 68
    neurologic examination, 64
    skin, 68
    spine, 68
    weight/BMI, 58
  chronic disease
    AAA, 110
    diabetes mellitus, 110, 111
    dyslipidemia, 111
    osteoporosis, 111
  colorectal cancer screening, 112
  cost-effectiveness and outcomes, 103
  depression, 108
  executive physicals, 119
  hypothesis, 57
  immunization, 116–117
  insurance coverage, 117
  lung cancer screening, 113
  motivational interviewing, 119
  pancreatic cancer screening, 114
  physical examination
    blood pressure assessment, 108
    BMI, 110
    JNC 8, 109
    obesity, 109
  preventive health examination, 115

prostate cancer screening, 113, 114
recommendations, 106
risk factor assessment, 105
skin cancer screening, 113
STIs
  hepatitis B, 107
  hepatitis C, 107
  HIV, 107
  intensive behavioral counseling, 106
  prevalence rates, 106
  syphilis, 107
testicular cancer screening, 114

G
Guidelines for Adolescent Preventive Services
      (GAPS), 93

H
Health-seeking behavior
  ACA, 39
  African American men's health, 34
  disparities, 35
  health information, 38
  minority men, 33
  navigation, 35, 36
  racial and ethnic minorities, 37
  self-advocacy, 38
  self-confidence, 37
  self-management, 37
  socioeconomic position, 36
  substance abuse, 36
Hepatitis B vaccination, 189
Herpes simplex virus (HSV), 173–174
Herpes simplex virus 2 (HSV2), 170
Human immunodeficiency virus (HIV), 292
Human papillomavirus (HPV)
  epidemiology, 170
  risk factor, 291
  screening, 187
Hypogonadism. *See* Testosterone replacement
      therapy (TRT)
Hypogonadism in men (HIM) study, 250

I
International Prostate Symptom Score
      (IPSS), 201
Intimate partner violence (IPV), 289

J
Joint National Committee (JNC 8), 109

L

Lower urinary tract symptoms (LUTS)
acute bacterial prostatitis, 216
complications, 216
DRE, 215
gram-negative organisms, 215
gram-positive organisms, 216
management, 216
sepsis, 216
acute urinary retention, 212, 213
BOO
AUA symptom, 205, 207
noninvasive uroflowmetry, 207, 208
post-void residual volume, 207
chronic bacterial prostatitis, 217
chronic urinary retention, 213
combination therapy, 210–211
CP-CPPS, 217
definition, 198
etiology, 199
medical therapy
alpha-1 blockers, 208, 209
anticholinergics, 210
5-alpha-reductase inhibitor, 209, 210
phosphodiesterase type 5 inhibitors, 210
neurogenic bladder, 213
pathophysiology, 198
prevalence, 198
prostate gland, 197
serum PSA levels, 206
surgery, 214–215
terminology, 198
TRT, 261–262
urolithiasis, 213
UTI, 205, 212

M

Male infertility
definition, 157
laboratory testing, 158
physical examination, 157
treatment, 158
Masculinity
Asian American men, 23
definition, 22
health behaviors/outcomes, 22, 23
health-related decisions, 26
hegemonic masculinity, 20, 21
machismo, 23
Male Role Norms Inventory, 22
quantitative and qualitative men's
health, 21
social determinants, 25
stress, 23
time, 24
Men who have sex with men (MSM), 193–194
alcohol/drug use, 289
anal cancer, 292
cardiovascular disease, 293
dietary habits, 288
healthcare environment, 284–286
HIV, 292
legal rights, 293
mental health, 289
minority stress model, 284
population
bisexual men, 295
families and children, 294
older MSM, 294–295
racial/ethnic minorities, 295
transgender men, 296
youth, 293
prevalence, 283
risk factors, 284
sexual history, 287–288
sexual orientation/gender identity, 286
STIs
gonorrhea/chlamydia, 290
hepatitis A, 291
hepatitis B, 291
hepatitis C, 291
herpes simplex, 291
HPV, 291
syphilis, 291
tobacco use, 288
violence, 289
Methicillin-resistant *Staphylococcus aureus*
(MRSA), 216
Motivational interviewing (MI), 96, 97, 119

N

Neisseria gonorrhea, 168
Nucleic acid amplification test (NAAT), 83,
184–186

O

Obstructive sleep apnea (OSA), 262–263
Older adolescent and young adult (AYA)
males
in healthcare
clinical resources, 97
infrastructure, lack of, 92, 93
motivational interviewing, 96, 97
physical and mental health behaviors, 96
physician's office staff, 97

Older adolescent and young adult (AYA)
    males (*cont.*)
  masculinity, 93, 94
  morbidity
    chronic diseases, 90
    mental health disorders, 90
    SHR, 91, 92
    substance abuse rates, 91
  mortality rate, 90
  PYD framework, 95
  strength-based communication, 95
  trauma-informed care framework, 94, 95
Over-the-counter (OTC) treatment, 156

P
Patient-delivered partner therapy (PDPT),
    192–193
Patient Protection and Affordable Care Act
    (ACA), 9, 10
Penile disorders
  clinical presentation, 242
  evaluation, 243–244
  Peyronie's disease, 241–242
  phimosis/paraphimosis, 238–239
  physical examination, 243
  priapism, 240–241
  SCC, 242
  treatment, 244
Peripheral artery disease (PAD), 136
Peyronie's disease, 241–242
Positive Youth Development (PYD)
    framework, 95
Postexposure prophylaxis (PEP), 292
Preexposure prophylaxis (PrEP), 292
Premature ejaculation (PE), 154, 155
Pre-participation evaluations (PPEs), 83
Preventive services
  ACA, 9, 10
  behavioral responses, 11, 12
  characteristics, 11
  data extrapolation, 49
  data support, 49
  definition, 2
  EHR, 51, 52
    benefit, 50
    CDSS, 50
    clinical service improvement, 51
    interventions, 50, 51
    shared decision making, 50, 51
  evidence-based information, 11
  features, 11
  health behavior characteristics, 49
  implementation, 46

issues, 48, 49
  life expectancy, 2, 3
  masculinity, 8
  modalities, 46, 47
  patient and physician interactions, 47
  population-based telephone survey, 47
  recommendations, 10, 12
  screening tests, 49
  seasonal influenza vaccine, 47
  social determinants, 7
  stress, 8
  US age-adjusted mortality rates, 4, 5
  USPSTF, 46
Prostate cancer
  evaluation, 278
  PLCO and ERSPC, 272–273
  PSA
    DRE, 271
    PCA3, 272
    testing, 270
    TMPRSS2:ERG, 272
    variations, 271
  screening
    ACP, 276
    ACS, 275
    AUA, 275
    characteristics, 273–275
    PIVOT, 276
    USPSTF, 275
  surveillance, 277–278
  TRT, 260–261
Prostate cancer antigen 3 (PCA3), 272
Prostate Cancer Intervention versus
    Observation Trial (PIVOT), 276
Prostate, Lung, Colorectal, and Ovarian
    screening trial (PLCO), 272–273
Prostate-specific antigen (PSA), 260, 270

S
Scrotal disorder
  appendix testis, 225–226
  epididymitis, 227–228
  Fournier's gangrene, 226
  hydrocele
    causes, 234
    clinical presentation, 234
    communicating/noncommunicating, 234
    complications, 235
    diagnosis, 234
    management/treatment, 235
    physical examination, 234
  orchitis, 227
  testicular torsion

complications, 230
diagnosis, 229
epidemiology, 228
imaging/evaluation, 229
physical examination, 228–229
treatment, 230
varicocele
clinical presentation, 230
dilated and tortuous spermatic veins, 230
evaluation, 232
incidence, 230
physical examination, 230–232
spermatoceles and epididymal cysts,
232–233
treatment, 232
Serum prostate-specific antigen (serum PSA)
levels, 206
Sexual health risks (SHR), 91, 92
Sexually transmitted infections (STIs), 183, 290
chlamydia
epidemiology, 167
screening, 184, 186
clinical care, 165
clinical features, 171–172
epididymitis/orchitis, 173
erectile dysfunction (see Erectile
dysfunction (ED))
genital herpes, 173–174
genital warts, 173
gonorrhea
epidemiology, 168–169
screening, 184, 186
health history
communication methods, 178
information, 176–178
setting, 176
hematospermia, 155
hepatitis B, 107
hepatitis C, 107, 187
history, 146–149
HIV, 107, 188
HPV, 187
epidemiology, 170
treatment, 191–192
HSV
epidemiology, 170
treatment, 191
infertility (see Male infertility)
intensive behavioral counseling, 106
male circumcision, 175
MSM (see Men who have sex with men
(MSM))
NAATs, 184–186
OTC treatment, 156

painful ejaculation, 155, 156
partner management, 192–193
physical examination, 178–179
premature ejaculation (see Premature
ejaculation (PE))
prevalence rates, 106
prevention, 189–190
public health, 165
risk assessment, 174–175
risk-reduction counseling
adolescents, 181
behavioral changes, 180
cultural and belief issues, 181–183
USPSTF, 179
syphilis, 107
epidemiology, 169
screening, 188
test of cure, 193
urethritis
clinical syndromes, 172
treatment, 190–191
Squamous cell carcinoma (SCC), 242

T
Testicular cancer
clinical presentation, 236
diagnosis, 237
germ cell tumors, 236
incidence, 235
physical examination, 236
risk factors, 236
treatment, 238
Testosterone replacement therapy (TRT), 250
cardiovascular morbidity
cohort study, 258, 259
endothelial dysfunction, 258
meta-analyses, 258
TOM trial, 259
developments, 264
erythrocytosis, 263
LUTS, 261–262
OSA, 262–263
prostate cancer, 260–261
PSA, 260

U
United States Preventive Services Task Force
(USPSTF), 46, 275
Urethritis, 172, 190–191
Urinary tract infection (UTI), 205, 212
US Centers for Disease Control and
Prevention (CDC), 166

V
Varicocele
    clinical presentation, 230
    dilated and tortuous spermatic veins, 230
    evaluation, 232

incidence, 230
physical examination, 230–232
spermatoceles and epididymal cysts,
    232–233
treatment, 232